Assisting in Long-Term Care

Barbara Hegner, MSN, RN

Professor
Nursing and Life Science Department
Long Beach City College (CA)

Esther Caldwell, MA, PhD

Consultant in Vocational Education (CA)

Delmar Publishers Inc®

WITH THE LATEST INFECTION CONTROL TECHNIQUES

W9-CGU-122

NOTICE TO THE READER

Delmar Staff
Administrative Editor: Leslie Boyer
Developmental Editor: Marjorie A. Bruce
Production Editor: Carol Micheli
Publications Coordinator: Karen Seebald
Cover Design Coordinator: Susan Mathews
Text Design Coordinator: Linda Johnson

For information, address Delmar Publishers Inc.
Two Computer Drive West, Box 15-015
Albany, New York 12212

COPYRIGHT © 1988
BY DELMAR PUBLISHERS INC.

10 9 8 7 6 5

Printed in the United States of America
Published simultaneously in Canada
by Nelson Canada,
A division of The Thomson Corporation

Library of Congress Cataloging in Publication Data

Hegner, Barbara R.
  Assisting in long term care.

  Includes index.
  1. Nurses' aides. 2. Long-term care of the sick.
I. Caldwell, Esther. II. Title [DNLM: 1. Homes for
the Aged. 2. Long Term Care — methods. 3. Nurses'
Aides. 4. Nursing Homes. WT 30 H464a]
RT84.H44   1988   362.6′1   87-20084
ISBN 0-8273-2959-8 (soft)

CONTENTS

SECTION II The Nursing Assistant 42

SECTION III

The Resident 124

SECTION IV Basic Science Concepts 190

SECTION VI   Seeking Employment 488

PROCEDURE COMPETENCY EVALUATIONS

PREFACE

Thousands of long term care facilities provide nursing care and support for people to care for themselves. The inability of these people to provide self care stems from both physical impairments and the aging process.

In the years to come, the population of long term residents will swell, requiring an expanded and better prepared stable working force. The workers must be able to meet the physical and psychological needs of those in their care. Several factors will make this a growing need.

First: The numbers of elderly are steadily increasing and although most of these older people will remain independent but supported in the community, that small percentage who are institutionalized will translate into growing numbers of actual people needing care. This trend will continue well into the twenty-first century.

Second: Changes in funding of medical care through government programs, a major source of care funding, have already forced a reevaluation of how long acute care will be provided. The reevaluation process is prompting more early discharges from acute care facilities than ever before. Additional care must then be provided in less acute and less costly settings. The need for home care providers, skilled nursing homes, intermediate care facilities and board and care facilities will continue to grow. Each setting will require prepared people to do the work.

Third: There is now a tremendously high turnover rate among workers in nursing homes. Nurse's aides or orderlies account for almost one half of all nursing home employees. This group of people provides the major physical care and emotional support for the burgeoning population of the elderly and physically impaired nursing home residents.

The high (75%) yearly turnover rate for these nursing assistants point to the poor level of preparation, the degree of difficulty of the work, and the unmet expectations of the workers. Unless these factors are addressed, the instability and dissatisfaction of the working force will not be corrected.

Over the last decade, the quality of care provided in nursing homes has become a public issue. As a result, studies have been conducted and regulations tightened. More states are spelling out the level of skill and training required of workers in long term care settings but there is as yet no consistent national standard and requirements are minimal at best. Teachers of these workers will play a vital role in determining which standards will ultimately prevail.

Assisting in Long-Term Care has been developed to help entry level nursing assistants to achieve a level of skill and background information that will enable them to become certified and successful in the field of long term care. Additional suggestions for using the text with experienced workers desiring certification are included in the teacher's guide.

The material in this text is written in simple language with new vocabulary emphasized and fully illustrated. The objectives included at the beginning of each lesson of study let students know the specific expectations to be achieved and give directions to the course of study. Simple questions at the end of each lesson help the learner put the material into perspective and provide both the learner and teacher with a method of checking to see how well the objectives have been met.

The comprehensive achievement reviews for each section and procedure competency evaluations give the teacher and student a tool to assess how well the subject matter has been mastered.

Some materials, such as diagrams, may be used as references, but in the short period available to most teachers the emphasis should be placed on the skill and safety of hands-on procedures and the student's behavioral response to the basic human needs of those in their care.

SECTION I   THE PLACE OF EMPLOYMENT

LESSON 1   Care Facilities

OBJECTIVES

After studying this lesson, you should be able to:

- List the types of people requiring long term care.
- List six names applied to long term care facilities.
- Describe the main areas in a long term care facility: the typical resident unit and its equipment, the dining room, day room, and nurses' station.
- Define and spell all vocabulary words and terms.

Different types of long term care facilities are designed to provide the specific care needed by residents with different needs. There are also specific types of people needing long term care. They include those who:

Facilities offer differing levels of care.

- need help in regaining the ability to care for themselves (rehabilitation).
- cannot, because of illness or disability, care for themselves, figure 1–1.
- are terminally ill and need care until they die. Such care is known as *hospice care*.
- are old and infirmed and need continuous care (geriatric care).

Geriatrics is that branch of medicine that is concerned with the medical problems and care of the elderly. Nursing assistants who are especially trained to care for this group of people are called *geriatric nursing assistants*.

Geriatric nursing assistants are men and women who work in a variety of facilities designed to provide long term care and treatment for the elderly. The names of the facilities differ and to some degree indicate the extent of service offered.

The majority of your residents will probably fall into the geriatric care category. They come because they need assistance and security and there is no one in the community able to provide for them.

1

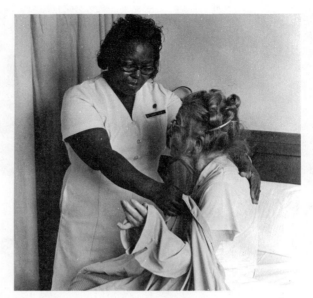

FIGURE 1–1. People need long term care when they can no longer care for themselves. (From Brooks, *The Nurse Assistant,* copyright 1978 by Delmar Publishers Inc.)

TYPES OF FACILITIES

Names that apply to long term care facilities include the skilled nursing facility, intermediate care facility, convalescent home, rest home (nursing home), and board and care facility. All provide housing, protection and assistance as needed to meet individual needs. Most also provide some health care. Placement in a **long term care facility** (*LTC* or *LTCF*) is determined by the level of care and type of services needed. Much of the service is supported by governmental agencies.

The *skilled nursing facility* (SNF) offers professional nursing care to chronically ill or disabled persons and those who are recuperating but do not require the high-cost services of an acute hospital setting. Many of these people are elderly; some are in **terminal** (last) stages of life. Their needs are multiple and require the services of many skilled professionals. Highly trained team members provide this specialized care. The care is aimed at assisting those people to achieve and maintain as high a level of wellness and independence as possible. Physicians, professional nurses, and pharmacy services are readily available. Other support personnel and specialists are available as required, figure 1–2. Skilled nursing facilities are able to provide many, but not all, of the services that are offered in the acute hospital setting. Their emphasis is on rehabilitation (whenever possible), rather than acute care.

Rehabilitation (as applied to elderly persons), is the process of assisting residents to do as much as they can, as well as they can, and for as long as they can. Residents of any age who are admitted primarily for rehabilitation usually stay about three months before they are discharged. The cost of care in such an SNF is high and, as soon as appropriate, residents are transferred, usually to a less expensive care setting such as an *intermediate care facility* (ICF), or nursing home, figure 1–3.

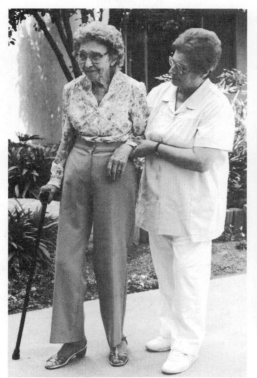

FIGURE 1–2. *The staff of a skilled nursing facility offers professional and supportive care.*

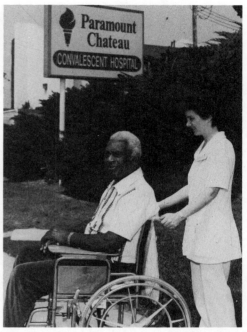

FIGURE 1–3. *Residents are transferred to a usually less expensive care setting as soon as their condition permits.*

In the *intermediate care facility*, the rehabilitation effort is continued, but at a less intensive level and requiring fewer highly trained specialists. Supervision and care is still provided, however, on a twenty-four hour basis. When a person in an ICF has made as much progress toward self care as seems possible, that person is again transferred. It might be to his/her own home or, if further help is necessary, to a still less intensive care facility such as a board and care home.

People who are no longer able to care for themselves in their own homes because of disability or disease, or physical or mental handicap, may also become residents of a nursing home through direct admission from the community. Many people who have disabilities can continue to remain in their own homes because of the assistance of community support groups such as homemaker/home health aides.

Convalescent homes, *rest homes,* or *nursing homes* are names applied to those facilities which provide room and board and assist residents in carrying out their activities of daily living. Some nursing care is available, but these facilities offer a more home-like atmosphere. Rehabilitation efforts are continued as part of an ongoing program.

Nursing assistants are employed in each of these facilities to assist in the physical and psychological care of the residents under the supervision of licensed or registered nurses. They contribute enormously to the success of the nursing staff in meeting resident needs. Much of their work is devoted to offering emotional support and encouragement, figure 1–4.

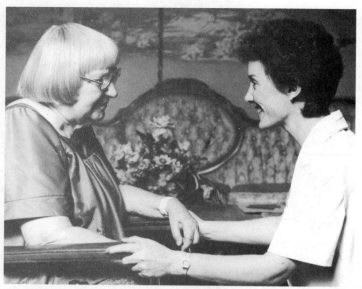

FIGURE 1–4. *Nursing assistants provide a valuable service when they give emotional support.*

Before we go any further, please note that you have seen the term **resident** used several times in the previous paragraphs. We now need a definition of the term before we proceed any deeper into this lesson. Briefly, then, the term *resident* is used by LTC employees to describe any person who lives in an LTC facility and makes it his or her main home, figure 1–5.

STANDARDS

All facilities must adhere to standards which are set by official public agencies. These standards govern the:

- care which is given,
- safety of the facility, and
- sanitary conditions.

Representatives of the various agencies visit each facility and check to be sure that the facility is maintaining the standards. The standards help assure both the quality of care and the safety of the residents.

MAIN AREAS IN A LONG TERM CARE FACILITY

Each facility varies to some degree in physical layout but essential elements are common to all.

The Room

The resident's room is called the **resident unit** or *patient unit*. In each unit an adjustable bed, bedside stand, overbed table, chair, and some storage area is provided for each person, figure 1–6.

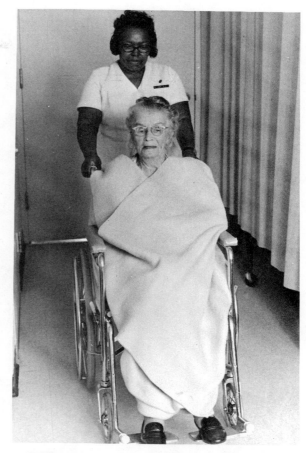

FIGURE 1–5. People who make their homes in long term care facilities are called residents. (From Brooks, *The Nurse Assistant*, copyright 1978 by Delmar Publishers Inc.)

Resident rooms may be designed for occupancy by a single individual, but usually accommodate two or more persons. In some instances, as many as six resident units are in a single room.

When several residents share a single room, conflicts can sometimes develop. You must be tactful as you try to balance the rights of each of the individuals.

The Bed

The bed is usually adjustable for height; it can be raised during care (eliminating bending for the care giver), and lowered so that residents can get into or out of bed safely. The head and bottom of the bed can also be positioned for resident comfort.

Each bed is equipped with side rails for safety. Residents who remain in bed should have the side rails up and securely in place at all times unless a signed side rail release has been obtained.

Side rails should also be securely in place when residents are prepared for sleeping and at any other times that the security of the resident is at risk, figure 1–7. For example, side rails should always be up when the resident is confused. When giving personal care, only the side rail nearest the care giver should be lowered.

Secure side rails are an important safety measure.

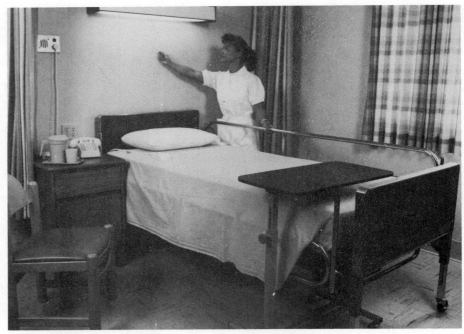

FIGURE 1–6. Standard furniture included in each resident unit.

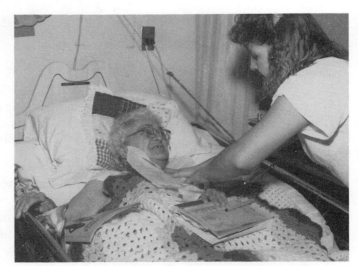

FIGURE 1–7. Side rails must be up and securely in place for the safety of the resident.

Since beds may differ in the way they are controlled, the assistant should be thoroughly familiar with the mechanisms before attempting to operate the bed. Some of the beds are electric, others are adjusted by hand with a crank.

Personal Equipment

The bedside stand in each unit is equipped with articles for that resident's personal care and use and should not be shared.

The equipment included in each unit is kept in two areas of the bedside stand. The top shelf, figure 1–8, is a "clean area" and holds a:

- wash basin
- kidney-shasped emesis (vomit) basin
- soap brush

The **emesis basin** is usually used when carrying out personal care procedures such as brushing the teeth.

The bottom shelf is a "dirty area" and holds the:

- bed pan and/or urinal
- toilet tissue

The drawer holds personal toilet articles such as:

- toothbrush
- toothpaste
- denture cup
- comb

Each unit will be equipped with a chair and some form of signaling device, such as a *call bell*. Call bells may be attached to the wall or may be part of a more complex panel attached to the side rail, figure 1–9. The panel may also control a radio, television, or telephone. Call lights are also located in the bathroom and shower area. When a resident needs assistance and uses the call bell, a light at the nursing station is activated, showing the room number of that resident who called, figure 1–10.

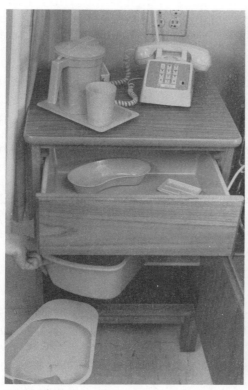

FIGURE 1–8. The drawer and top shelf contain clean equipment.

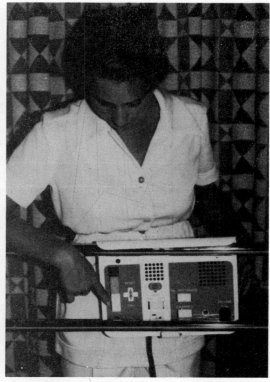

FIGURE 1–9. Each unit is provided with means of signalling for assistance.

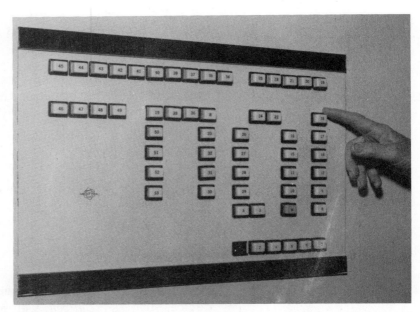

FIGURE 1–10. When the resident rings, a signal is activated and a light shows at the nursing station indicating the room.

An overbed table, which is adjustable in height, may be placed over the bed, providing a place to serve meals or to hold equipment during care.

In some facilities, residents are also permitted to bring some personal belongings from their home. This is especially true if this is apt to be the final residence for a particular person. Because of limited space, however, residents are requested to bring only those personal articles they care most for.

Dining/Day Room

Residents who are able are encouraged to eat in a **communal** (group) setting, so each facility has a common dining room. Long tables that can accommodate many residents, as well as smaller tables where intimate groups can eat, are provided.

Dining rooms often function as *day rooms* where residents can meet for activities and socialization at times other than meal times, figure 1–11. Larger facilities may have separate day rooms and dining rooms.

Since talking, watching television, and card playing are enjoyable activities for those whose physical abilities are limited, often a television set, playing cards, and other quiet games are available. Group exercises, singing, and parties that celebrate a special occasion such as a resident's birthday or a holiday are also usually held in the day room or dining room.

Nurses' Station

Official records are kept in the nursing station.

Every facility will have an area where records of care are kept, figure 1–12. This area is called the **nurses' station**. Part of the nurses' station will be set aside for the control and dispensing of medications; no one but authorized persons are permitted in this area. Authorized persons include the physician, the pharmacist, the registered nurse and the licensed vocational/practical nurse (LVN or LPN). This part of the nurses' station is kept locked when unattended.

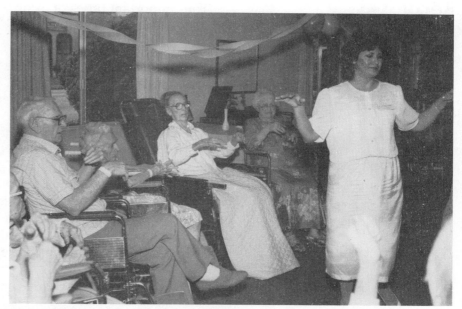

FIGURE 1–11. Group activities take place in the day room.

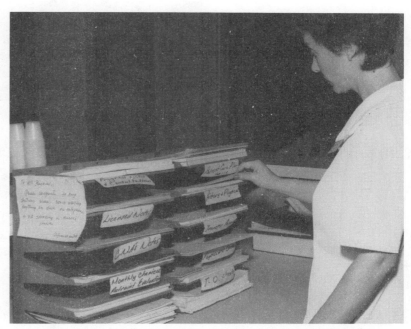

FIGURE 1–12. Official records are kept in the nurses' station.

Reports of resident needs and care are usually given within the nurses' station. This is **confidential** (private, personal) information and should not be shared within hearing of the residents. Nursing assistants will use this area to record their observations and the care given. It is in the nurses' station that directions and assignments are received.

Records

Four important types of records are found in the nurses' station. They are the:

1. procedure book
2. policy book
3. resident's chart
4. Kardex or assignment sheet

The **procedure book** explains how care is to be given. The **policy book** outlines the rules that govern the facility and explains what will be done for the residents, figure 1–13. The resident's chart contains a record of the care given and the progress reported, as well as information about the resident. The assignment sheet or **Kardex** contains information about the specific care to be given to a particular resident. The information on the Kardex reflects a plan called the *care plan* that has been developed for each individual resident.

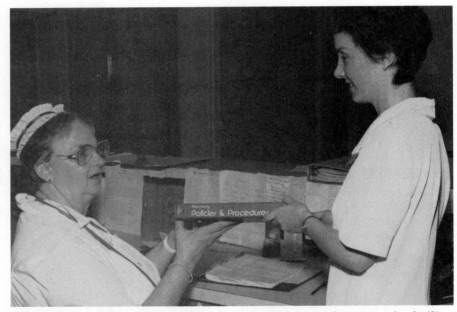

FIGURE 1–13. The policy book outlines the rules which govern the facility.

SUMMARY

Nursing assistants play a vital role in the care of the residents in long term care facilities. Although different types of facilities provide differing *levels* (nursing needs of the resident) of care, all strive to help each resident become and remain as independent as possible. One thing that they all have in common is illustrated in figure 1–14. Special names applied to each facility suggest the type and level of care provided and, although the physical setup of each type of facility may differ in some respects, each shares certain areas in common—such as the resident unit, day room, and nurses' station.

All Care Facilities Provide
- Physical Care
- Emotional Care
- Help with Activities of Daily Living (ADL)
- Rehabilitation
- Safety and Security
- Opportunities for Social Interaction

FIGURE 1–14. Care facility functions.

VOCABULARY

communal
confidential
convalescent home
emesis basin
geriatrics

Kardex
long term care facility
policy book
procedure book

rehabilitation
resident
resident unit
terminal

SUGGESTED ACTIVITIES

1. With other members of your class, visit different types of long term care facilities in your area.

2. Tour your facility, noting the locations of the nurses' station, day room, dining room, and resident units.

3. Examine an unoccupied resident unit to become familiar with the equipment.

REVIEW

A. Brief Answer/Fill in the Blanks

1. Name three types of long term care facilities (LTCF).

   a. _____

   b. _____

   c. _____

2. Name three areas that are common to all long term care facilities.

   a. _____

   b. _____

   c. _____

3. List five pieces of equipment that you would expect to find in the bedside table in a resident unit and indicate on which shelf you would store each item.

   a. _____

   b. _____

   c. _____

   d. _____

   e. _____

4. The process of assisting residents to do as much as they can, as well as they can, and for as long as they can is called _____.

5. A kidney shaped basin found in the bedside table used when brushing the teeth is called an _____.

6. List five things provided for residents in all facilities.

   a. _____

   b. _____

   c. _____

   d. _____

   e. _____

B. Matching. Tell where the following items or areas would be found.

1. _____ bedside stand   a. nurses' station

2. _____ medication storage   b. dining room

3. _____ meal service area   c. resident unit

4. _____ emesis basin   d. day room

5. _____ bed

6. _____ group activities area

7. _____ television

8. _____ reports

9. _____ resident's health record

10. _____ Kardex

CLINICAL SITUATION

Amelia Brown is in the process of recovering from a stroke. She is 79 years old and, although she has progressed to the point where she no longer needs the services of an acute care hospital, she will still require weeks of rehabilitation before she can return to her home. To which facility would she most likely be transferred from the acute care setting?

Answer: _____.

LESSON 2 The Care Givers

OBJECTIVES

After studying the lesson, you should be able to:

- List three care givers who visit the resident to meet special needs.
- Name the care giver who most often helps the resident carry out the activities of daily living (ADL).
- Define and spell all the vocabulary words and terms.

The care givers in a long term care facility include all the people who are responsible for the well being of the residents, whether continuously or as the need is realized. Both professional staff and nursing assistants participate in this care by giving direct and continuous service, figure 2–1. Other care givers such as the physical therapist or dentist provide specific, but occasional, services when needed by an individual resident. Another care giver who may only occasionally see the resident is the professional **speech therapist** who might visit a resident recovering from a stroke only once each week until the resident is able to communicate more effectively.

SPECIFIC CARE GIVERS

Each care giver has a specific function. Some care givers plan and direct the care that will be given—doctors and nurses are among this group. Each care giver on the team—the nursing assistant in particular—contributes to the overall care given. The resident, who receives the care, benefits from the skill of each member, and depends on this care, so it is important for all team members to understand the role each member fulfills, figure 2–2.

Depending on the type of long term care facility, residents may receive more direct physical care or supportive care and, in some cases, more direct acute care. Most of this direct care is given by the nursing staff.

THE NURSING STAFF

The nursing staff in a long term care facility is composed of a director of nursing, a charge nurse (who is a licensed or registered nurse)—either an RN or an LPN—and nursing assistants.

The *director of nursing* must be a registered nurse. This person has had, besides nurse's training, some additional training in adminis-

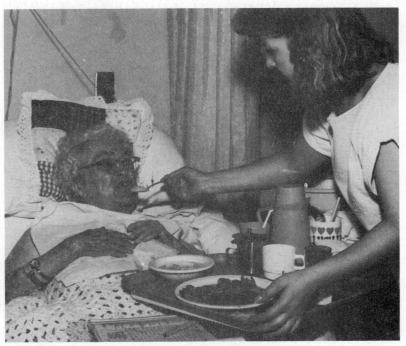

FIGURE 2–1. Nursing assistants give direct continuous care to residents.

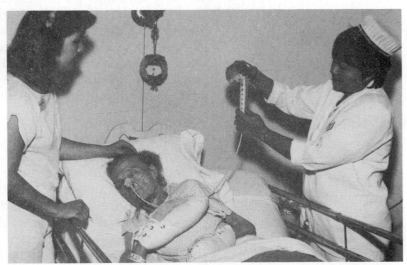

FIGURE 2–2. Nursing assistants work with other staff members to provide care.

The Nursing Staff
  Director
  Charge Nurses
  Staff Nurses
  Assistants

tration. The director of nurses is at the head of the nursing staff and is responsible for all nurses and residents in the facility. To assist the director of nursing, *charge nurses* are assigned to be responsible for specific groups (numbers) of residents. The charge nurse may be either a registered nurse or a licensed practical or vocational nurse. All these nurses have completed specific nursing education and testing. The charge nurses, in turn, have several nurses under their direct supervision. The charge nurse and her *assisting nurses* supervise the **nursing assistants** who work on a day to day basis directly with the residents.

THE PHYSICIAN

At least once a month a **physician** and health care team visits each resident. The health and well being (**status**) of the resident is evaluated. The doctor writes orders for care, figure 2–3. The doctor may also take part in care conferences. This is where many different care givers help in the evaluation and develop a plan of care specific to the individual resident's needs.

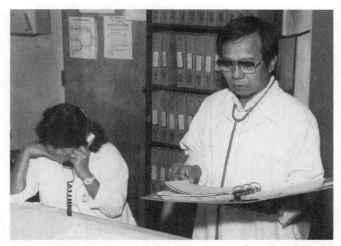

FIGURE 2–3. *The physician writes orders for the care to be given.*

THE DIETITIAN

Each team member contributes to the well being of the resident

A **dietitian** plans and supervises the preparation of resident meals, figure 2–4. In some facilities, the staff eat with the residents in a family atmosphere. Special meals and supplements are provided for those residents requiring **therapeutic diets** (special diets designed to meet a specific resident's needs). For example, a person who suffers from congestive heart failure might be put on a sodium restricted diet. Therapeutic diets are ordered by the physician.

SPECIAL THERAPISTS

The *physical therapist* (**physiotherapist**) works to improve the resident's ability to get around (**mobility**), figure 2–5. After an initial evaluation, a plan is developed to help restore and maintain optimum body functioning. Many times the nursing assistant helps to carry out the program prescribed by the therapist; for example, the range of motion exercises which are part of daily care.

The **occupational therapist** assists residents to find more satisfying ways to fill the time in the long term facility. The occupational therapist can also teach the resident new skills and new ways of doing basic self care to overcome specific handicaps or disabilities. Not only can crafts and handiwork help fill long hours, but they may also provide financial assistance to the resident; for example, the facility might sponsor a craft fair where such items can be sold to visitors, the staff, or other residents. Creative work can give new purpose to living.

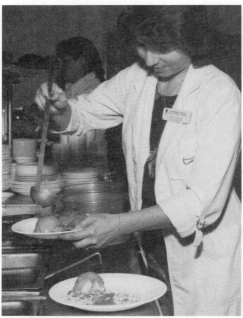

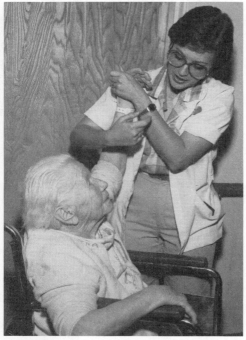

FIGURE 2-4. *The dietitian plans the resident meals and supervises their preparation.*

FIGURE 2-5. *The physiotherapist works with the resident to improve mobility.*

The **social worker** helps the resident make adjustments to changes in his/her life. Sometimes this means working out financial arrangements (figure 2-6), or working through family relationships to improve support and communications.

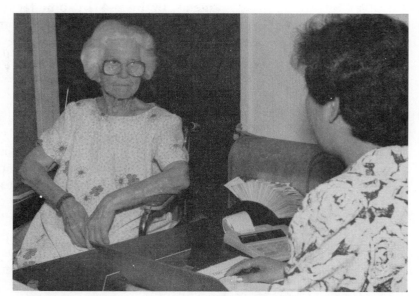

FIGURE 2-6. *The social worker helps residents work out financial problems.*

The **audiologist** also visits the residents. Hearing may diminish with age, and people who do not hear well feel isolated and alone.

The audiologist evaluates their hearing ability and helps adjust hearing devices.

The **dental hygienist** examines, cleans, and evaluates the teeth and dental needs of the residents. If help is needed, or poorly fitted dentures need to be repaired, visits to the **dentist's** office are arranged. Not only is the maintenance of good nutrition very difficult when teeth are in poor condition or dentures fit improperly, but choking is also a major concern with improperly fitting dentures.

The **podiatrist** is another special care giver who comes to visit the resident periodically. Many older persons have foot and toenail problems that make **ambulation** (walking) very difficult. The podiatrist examines and may treat foot problems, which increases the resident's comfort and mobility.

As you can see, many people are special care givers. Some directly and continually, others when specifically needed. In some way each contributes to the total care given each resident.

Total care takes into account the emotional, spiritual, and social needs, as well as the physical needs of each person. Care givers keep this fact in mind as they carry out their assignments.

SUPPORT SERVICES

Many other workers provide **support services**. These include those who:

- maintain the building
- perform housekeeping duties (figure 2-7)
- work in the kitchen
- do the laundry
- care for the grounds
- handle administrative duties
- provide special outside services such as X ray (figure 2–8)

It can be seen that many people work together, each contributing his or her skills so that every resident receives the very best care, figure 2–9.

VOCABULARY

ambulation (AMB)	nurses' station	social worker
audiologist	nursing assistant	speech therapist
dental hygienist	occupational therapist	status
dentist	physician	support services
dietitian	physiotherapist	total care
mobility	podiatrist	therapeutic diet

SUGGESTED ACTIVITIES

1. Visit a facility to see how the care givers work together to provide resident care.

2. Invite a nursing assistant to visit your class and describe the work of different care givers.

3. Invite several of the professionals listed to visit the class and explain their roles and responsibilities.

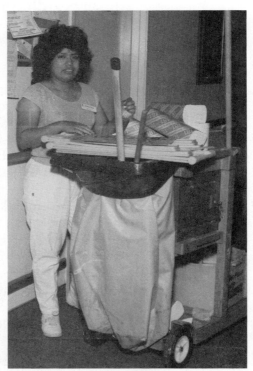

FIGURE 2–7. *Housekeepers keep the facility clean.*

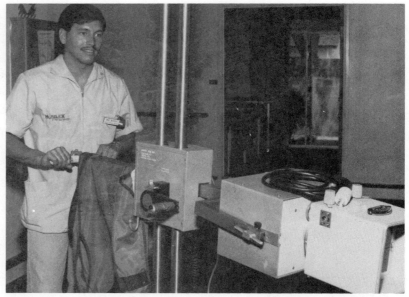

FIGURE 2–8. *The X-ray technician visits when a resident has been injured and a fracture is suspected.*

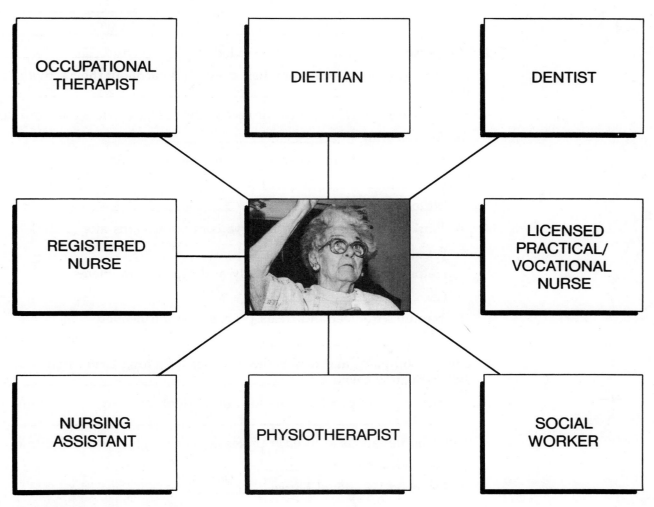

FIGURE 2–9. The care givers.

REVIEW

A. Brief Answer/Fill in the Blanks

1. Name three members of the nursing staff who are care givers in a long term care facility.

   a. _____

   b. _____

   c. _____

2. The person who receives care is called a _____.

3. The care giver who most often helps residents carry out their activities of daily living is the _____.

4. Name the care givers who provide each of the special services listed in *a* to *f*.

   a. Tests hearing (_____)

   b. Examines teeth and checks dentures for proper fit

      (_____)

   c. Writes orders for resident care (_____)

   d. Works with residents to imporve communications after a stroke

      (_____)

   e. Helps residents work out family and financial problems

      (_____)

   f. Examines the feet and treats problems when needed

      (_____)

5. One person plans and directs meal service for a long term care resident. This person is called a _____.

6. The nursing staff provides care for the resident. In charge of the nursing staff is the _____.

7. Write the initials used in each professional care giver listed in *a* to *c*.

   a. Registered Nurse _____

   b. Licensed Vocational Nurse _____

   c. Licensed Practical Nurse _____

B. Matching. Match the words on the right with the statements on the left.

1. _____ Refers to health and well being of resident

2. _____ Helps resident improve mobility

3. _____ Person who plans diet

4. _____ Helps resident make adjustments to changes in their lives

5. _____ Takes care of resident's teeth

6. _____ Ambulate (walk)

7. _____ The ability to get around

8. _____ Activities of daily living

a. status
b. AMB
c. Dentist
d. Dietitian
e. ADL
f. mobility
g. Social Worker
h. Physiotherapist

**CLINICAL
SITUATION**

Ms. Patterson is 79 years old and you are asked to help the podiatrist who is visiting her. You would expect the podiatrist to do what?

Answer: _____

LESSON 3 Functioning as a Team

OBJECTIVES

After studying this lesson, you should be able to:

- State at least five residents' rights.
- Name the person under whose authority care is given.
- Describe the proper lines of communication in a long term care facility.
- Correctly report and record information about the residents.
- Define and spell all the vocabulary words and terms.

The residents in your care are complex human beings. Each has special needs to be met and rights to be protected. When a resident is admitted to a non-skilled or skilled care facility, they must be secure in the knowledge that each member of the staff will know and respect these rights and needs.

RESIDENTS' RIGHTS

Residents have rights which must be protected.

Residents have the right to be treated as individuals with dignity, support, and encouragement. All staff members must be aware of these rights as they carry out their care.

In general, residents have the following rights (figure 3–1):

To be respected and protected from harm both physically and verbally. Speaking to a resident as a child or by pet names is not respectful. Last names, with Mr. or Mrs., should be used unless the resident specifically asks you to do otherwise.

To be informed about the cost and availability of services. The business personnel usually will communicate this information upon admission and whenever it is necessary. You should be familiar with the special services offered and the times they are available.

To refuse treatment. You may not force a resident to undergo any treatment as long as he or she is aware of the need. Make a report and record the refusal.

To be free of physical and mental abuse. You must never say unkind things or be rude to residents. You may not threaten them in anyway. You must perform procedures in a gentle way and never intentionally hurt anyone in your care. Residents may not even be restrained without specific written orders, and then only under special circumstances.

87144. Personal Rights

(a) Each resident shall have personal rights which include, but are not limited to the following:

(1) To be accorded dignity in his/her personal relationships with staff, residents, and other persons.

(2) To be accorded safe, healthful and comfortable accommodations, furnishings and equipment.

(3) To be free from corporal or unusual punishment, humiliation, intimidation, mental abuse, or other actions of a punitive nature, such as withholding of monetary allowances or interfering with daily living functions such as eating or sleeping patterns or elimination.

(4) To be informed by the licensee of the provisions of law regarding complaints and of procedures to confidentially register complaints, including, but not limited to, the address and telephone number of the complaint receiving unit of the licensing agency.

(5) To have the freedom of attending religious services or activities of his/her choice and to have visits from the spiritual advisor of his/her choice. Attendance at religious services, either in or outside the facility, shall be on a completely voluntary basis.

(6) To leave or depart the facility at any time and to not be locked into any room, building, or on facility premises by day or night. This does not prohibit the establishment of house rules, such as the locking of doors at night, for the protection of residents; not does it prohibit, with permission of the licensing agency, the barring of windows against intruders.

(7) To visit the facility prior to residence along with his/her family and responsible persons.

(8) To have his/her family or responsible persons regularly informed by the facility of activities related to his care or services including ongoing evaluations, as appropriate to the resident's needs.

(9) To have communications to the facility from his/her family and responsible persons answered promptly and appropriately.

(10) To have his/her visitors, including ombudspersons and advocacy representatives, visit privately during reasonable hours but without prior notice, provided that the rights of other residents are not infringed upon.

(11) To wear his/her own clothes; to keep and use his/her own personal possessions, including his/her toilet articles; and to keep and be allowed to spend his/her own money.

(12) To have access to individual storage space for private use.

(13) To have reasonable access to telephones, to both make and receive confidential calls. The licensee may require reimbursement for long distance calls.

(14) To mail and receive unopened correspondence.

(15) To receive or reject medical care, or other services.

(16) To receive assistance in exercising the right to vote.

(17) To move from the facility.

(b) All persons accepted to facilities, or their responsible persons, shall be personally advised and given a copy of these rights at admission. The licensee shall have all residents or their responsible persons sign a copy of these rights and the signed copy shall be included in the resident's record.

(c) Facilities licensed for seven (7) or more shall prominently post, in areas accessible to the residents and their relatives, the following:

(1) Procedures for filing confidential complaints.

(2) A copy of these rights or, in lieu of a posted copy, instructions on how to obtain additional copies of these rights.

(d) The information in (c) above shall be posted in English, and in facilities where a significant portion of the residents cannot read English, in the language they can read.

NOTE: Authority cited: Section 1530, Health and Safety Code. Reference: Sections 1501, 1530, and 1531, Health and Safety Code.

FIGURE 3–1. Patients' rights.

To have information about them kept confidential. The ethical code prevents you from sharing any information about residents of a personal nature with others outside the facility.

To expect that an effort will be made by the staff to **help them meet their spiritual, emotional, and social needs** (figure 3–2). Planned group activities, communal eating rooms and special religious services help promote a sense of social, emotional, and spiritual well-being.

You help to ensure and protect residents' rights each time you give care in the proper manner.

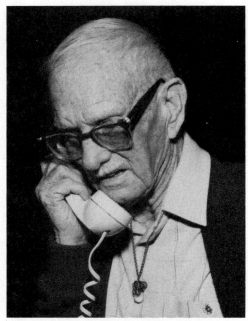

FIGURE 3–2. Residents have the right to make private calls.

DIRECTIONS FOR CARE

Authority and direction in care

The physician admits the resident and writes orders for the care to be given. A medical **diagnosis** (statement of the medical problems) is included in the orders. Medications, diet, and other special procedures are prescribed as needed. The doctor's orders become part of the legal health record (**chart**) of the resident. Because residents of LTC facilities are not acutely ill, the physician visits less often but at least once each month. If changes in the resident's condition make it necessary for orders to be more frequently changed, the physician may be contacted by the charge nurse at any time.

ADMINISTRATIVE ORGANIZATION

Although the physician is the authority for care, the facility is mananged and directed by a Board of Directors which delegates certain authority to others. This organizational pattern represents the lines of authority. You should become familiar with the lines of authority in your own facility.

An example of a line of authority is that from the Board of Directors to an administrator. The administrator is assisted in the work by heads of various departments. For example, the Housekeeping and Maintenance Departments are responsible for the cleanliness of the facility and the supervision of the housekeeping personnel. Another department under the administrator is the Nursing Care Department. Nursing assistants work within this group.

The head of the Nursing Department is the nursing supervisor (Director of Nurses) who is a registered nurse. Working under the nursing supervisor are charge nurses who may be registered nurses or licensed vocational nurses. The charge nurse is responsible for a special group of residents and makes specific assignments for, and supervises the nursing assistants. Study figure 3–3 to see where the nursing assistant fits in. The line of authority or command is also used as a guide for communication.

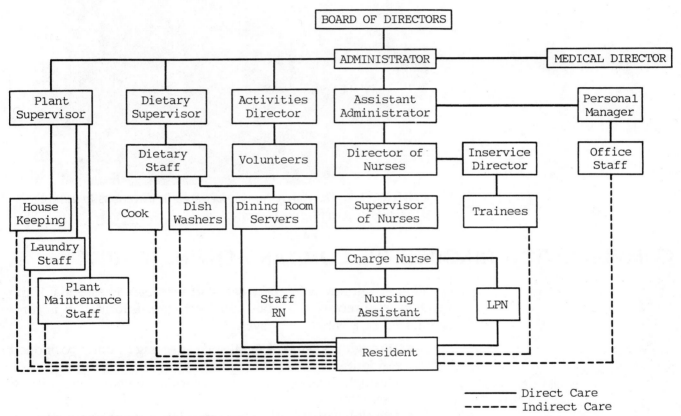

FIGURE 3–3. The nursing assistant reports directly to the charge nurse.

As you can see, the authority for care is passed from the physician to the nursing supervisor, to the charge nurse, and on to the nursing assistant. Your immediate supervisor is the instructor or charge nurse, or someone designated as your supervisor, figure 3–4. Your supervising nurse will give you your assignment and you will report your observations and the completion of the assignment to this same person. She or he becomes your primary line of communication. It is important that you know and follow the proper chain of command.

All assignments must be completely understood before doing them, since each person is responsible for the care they give. Any questions about your assignment should be directed to this same person for clarification. Never attempt to carry out an assignment for which you have not been trained. Inform the supervisor and ask for help. Never feel embarrassed. It is better to ask for help than to injure a resident.

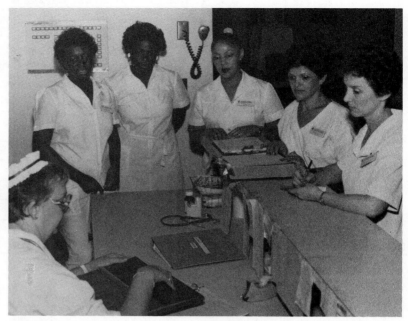

FIGURE 3–4. The charge nurse gives specific directions to nursing assistants who will give the care.

COMMUNICATION THROUGH THE COMMAND CHAIN

Good communication between staff members is essential if the resident is to receive the safest and best care. Information is communicated in a variety of ways:

- Through the sense of sight, such as seeing a poorly positioned resident.
- Through hearing, such as hearing someone cry out in discomfort.
- Through verbal (oral) communication, such as words describing how much a resident has eaten.
- Through **body language,** which sometimes sends a message different from the words being said.

Body language can sometimes be more effective than verbal communication in getting a message across (figure 3–5).

As a nursing assistant it is important that you communicate with other members of the nursing team and with the residents in a clear, correct manner. Three things are needed for successful communication:

- a message
- a sender
- a receiver

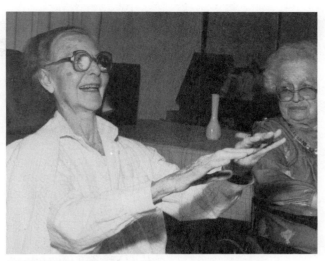

FIGURE 3–5. This resident's body language expresses her joy.

The same message must be sent and received if communication between two people is to be successful.

Some messages are sent with words. This is called **verbal (oral) communication**. Other messages are **nonverbal communications**. These messages are sent without words. They are sent by:

- facial expression
- tone of voice
- body posture

ORAL COMMUNICATIONS

Communications must be accurate and clear. Messages may by mixed.

Listen carefully to directions and assignments that are given to you. It is your responsibility to ask for further clarification if something is unclear. Listen not only to the words but be aware of the body language of the speaker. Does the resident say she feels well while at the same time she is rubbing her abdomen? Listen for the *choice* of words and *tone* of the speaker. Has the charge nurse emphasized that the resident should be given an enema *before* the bath rather than *after*? Be sure your own language is accurate so that you will not confuse the listener by the message you send.

Barriers to Effective Communications____

Special communication skills may be needed in some circumstances. The resident who cannot speak may still be able to hear; the deaf person may still be able to read lips; and a blind person may have no difficulty speaking or hearing. A resident who is confused or speaks a different language may have great difficulty understanding anything but the simplest words or directions. Attitudes can also influence the effectiveness of communications. For example, if you are open and receptive to what someone is saying, you hear more, but if you are angry or anxious you are apt to miss some of the key words. Even when it is difficult, you must attempt to develop some communication with all residents.

Telephone Etiquette

At some time while you are on duty it may be necessary to answer the telephone, figure 3–6. This should be done by identifying yourself, your title, and your location. For example, if you are on the second floor in the south wing you might answer in this way: "Two, south, Miss Johnson, Nursing Assistant, speaking."

- Identify the facility
- Identify yourself
- Identify your location
- Be courteous
- Find out who is calling
- Find out who is wanted
- Take a message if needed
- Thank the caller for calling

FIGURE 3–6. Telephone etiquette.

Facility phones are for facility business and should never be used for personal calls. There are pay phones for such calls, figure 3-7.

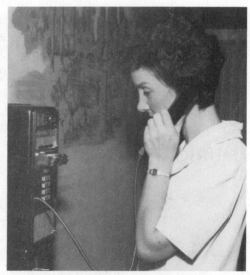

FIGURE 3–7. Pay phones should be used for personal calls.

Oral Report

Report
off- going staff—on-coming staff

The oral report is another instance when effective oral communication is vital, particularly during the shift report. Before beginning their assignment, the on-coming staff receives a report from those who have cared for the residents during the previous shift. The oral shift report is a method used to make sure that all members of the nursing staff fully understand the care to be given each resident. From the report, you should learn about changes in, or special needs of, each resident. Staff members should take notes during report time and ask questions freely.

Usually you will make an oral report to your charge nurse just before you finish your shift. Be sure to include the names and conditions of each resident assigned to your care and any observations you have made. Be accurate and complete but brief.

During your shift, never leave your assigned area without letting your supervisor know of your whereabouts and briefly reporting on your residents.

WRITTEN COMMUNICATIONS

The Care Plan

Many team members give some care to a single resident. To make sure each contributes in a positive way to the overall goals of care, the needs of each resident are outlined and documented in the nursing *care plan*, figure 3–8.

NURSING CARE PLAN SUMMARY		NAME WALLACE, ELEANOR Room 16 B Date 9/8/

Person To Be Contacted If Emergency:
TURNER, AUDRY 762-5005
Name   Phone
684 PARK ST. DALLAS, TEXAS
Address

Name   Phone
Address

Pastor, Rabbi, Priest:
REV. BRUCE WILLIAMS 762-5872
Name   Phone
419 BRIGHT ST. (PROT.)
Address
Social Security No. 024-14-4282
Medicaid No. M-682-6881
Medicare No. 024-14-4282
Former Occupation, Hobbies or Interests:
OFFICE MANAGER - READING, KNITTING, BOWLING
Funeral Home/Donor Institution:

Name   Phone
Address
BH 24
Rev. 10-81

INTAKE
Feeds Self B ✓ (Chair) ____ (Bed) ____ (Out of Room) ✓
✓ Feed - Help D ____ ____ ____
Feed Patient S ____ ____ ____
Nourishment

OUTPUT
Urinary
✓ Continent ____ Incont. ____ Catheter
Bowel
✓ Continent ____ Incont. ____ Colostomy

ACTIVITY
ASST. Up - Ad Lib ____ Chair ____ Stretcher
____ Stand ____ Lift ____ Am't Help
Walk - Self ✓ Walk - Help MOD Am't Help
Passive Exercises LEFT ARM LEFT LEG
Restraint (Type)
____ Always ____ As Needed In Bed
____ Always ____ As Needed In Chair

HYGIENE
Century Tub Bath M - F days/time
Bed Bath days/time
Teeth Natural ✓ Artificial
Shampoo - Beauty Shop THURS. 10 AM
- Century Tub ____ Regular Shampoo ____ Special Shampoo

THERAPY
Physical Therapy WED. - SAT. 9:30/A.M. days/time
Speech Therapy MONDAY 3:00/P.M. days/time
Activities - Group TUES. - THURS. 1:00/P.M. days/time
- Individual days/time

OTHER
____ Hearing Problem SHORT TERM GOAL - IMPROVE MOBILITY AND SPEECH SKILLS.
____ Sight Problem
✓ Speech Problem LONG TERM GOAL - DISCHARGE TO HOME CARE.
____ Behavior Problem
____ Other

FIGURE 3–8. *Nursing care plans are prepared for each resident.*

The nursing care plan is developed during a care conference attended by members of the nursing and medical staffs and other consultants as needed. Sometimes the resident and family also participate. The specific needs of the resident are discussed, and suggestions made by the team members for meeting these needs are noted. The charge nurse then lists the long and short term goals for the resident, including appropriate measures to attain them. This information is transferred to a simple nursing care form which is available to the entire staff and usually is kept in a Kardex at the nursing station. The plan is always shared with the resident, since it is his or her plan. The nursing care plan is a required part of the resident's health record.

The goals of the plan center are designed to help the resident fulfill the basic human needs and his or her own special needs, and to successfully carry out the **activities of daily living (ADL)**, figure 3–9.

NEED	FACTORS AFFECTING NEED NOT BEING MET
Nutrition	Poorly fitting dentures, digestive disorders, lack of appetite
Elimination	Constipation, urinary catheters, colostomy
Oxygen intake	Respiratory disease, poor ventilation
Activity	Requires walker or cane for support; confined to wheelchair; foot problems
Communication	Stroke, hearing loss, vision loss, memory loss, confusion; speaks a different language
Spiritual/emotional support	Anxious, depression, feelings of dependency; unable to attend usual religious service
Rest	Restless, up to bathroom frequently; frequent short rest periods required; poor sleeping patterns
Hygiene	Unable to reach entire body; confused; poor transfer and ambulation ability

FIGURE 3–9. Activities of Daily Living (ADL): Special situations requiring special help.

Basic human needs include the ability to:

- maintain nutrition
- eliminate wastes
- be active (mobile)
- have rest
- communicate with others
- breathe efficiently
- carry out proper hygiene (figure 3–10)
- satisfy spiritual needs
- receive emotional support

The ADL are the activities that every person performs each day in caring for themselves. The basic human needs are met through the ADL, and when the resident is unable to carry out these activities for himself or herself, the staff must provide care.

All staff members use the care plan as a guide and as a tool for assessing or evaluating the effectiveness of the care they give.

The nursing assistant plays three important roles in relation to the care plan:

1. To contribute to and be aware of the care plan for each assigned resident and to know of any changes.
2. To follow the plan when giving care, carefully observing and assessing the resident's response.
3. To report and, when assigned, document observations through charting.

Documentation

A document is an official record. The resident's care, response, and progress is documented in the resident's chart. Nursing **documen-**

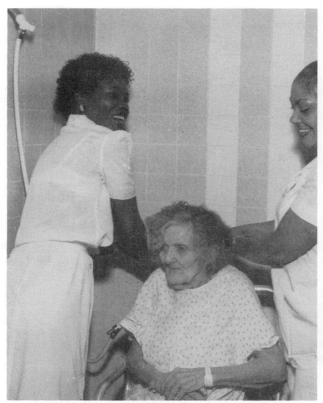

FIGURE 3–10. This resident needs help meeting her need to carry out proper hygiene.

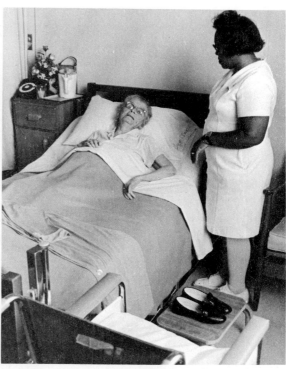

FIGURE 3–11. The assistant is carrying out the resident's need for activity as she prepares her to get out of bed. (From Brooks, The Nurse Assistant, copyright 1978 by Delmar Publishers Inc.)

tation must be made in the resident's health record at least once each week in the unskilled care facility and at the close of each shift in the skilled care facility since the condition of these residents is more subject to rapid change.

Written documentation describes the results of the original goals that the team developed in the care plan. The charge nurse may be responsible for all written documentation (charting) or part of the documentation may be a nursing assistant's responsibility.

A resident's health care record (**chart**) is a legal document and in legal situations may be called to court. It is important that everything be correct and easy to read. All charting and records must be in clear, simple, and accurate language and printed or written carefully so that there is no misunderstanding of the meaning. If you follow the established rules of charting, there will be no problem.

Each chart relates to only one resident, so it is unnecessary to use the term resident or to use the resident's name. Phrases rather than sentences should be used and there should never be erasures or empty spaces on the record. Each entry must be in ink so that it becomes a permanent record; no erasable ink or correction liquid is allowed.

If you use medical terms in your charting, make sure they are correct. A medical dictionary can be found in most units as well as an approved list of the terminology used in your facility.

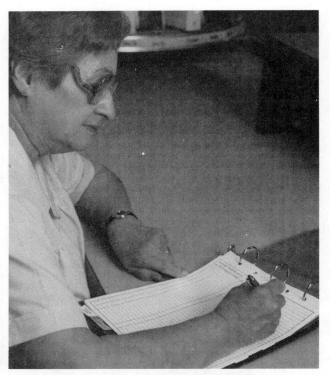

FIGURE 3–12. *The resident's health record is a legal document and must be carefully and correctly written.*

To help you broaden your medical vocabulary, some examples of combining forms and frequently used symbols and abbreviations are listed in figure 3–13. Combining forms allow *beginnings* of some words (**prefixes**) to be combined with the *endings* of other words (**suffixes**) to form acceptable words. For example, dys– is a prefix meaning painful; –uria is a suffix meaning urine. A resident might tell you that it hurts when she goes to the bathroom "to pass water." You would report this fact to the charge nurse as *dysuria* and chart it in the same way. Many of the symbols, abbreviations, and combining forms will be found on assignment sheets and resident health care records. You must chart only for yourself and only when the task or assignment has been completed, figures 3–14 and 3–15.

The *time* of an entry must be noted when the entry is made. Usually the color of the ink and letters A.M. or P.M. indicate whether the entry was made between 12 midnight and 12 noon or between 12 noon and midnight. Increasingly, however, times are being recorded in international or military time, figure 3–16. With this system time is not indicated by A.M. or P.M., but the 24 hours of each day are identified by the numbers 0100 (1 A.M.) through 2400 (12 A.M., midnight). The last two digits indicate the minutes of each hour (from 01 to 59). Thus, 0101 would be one minute after 1 A.M.; 1210 would be ten minutes after 12 P.M. (noon); 1658 would be 4:58 P.M., or two minutes before 5 o'clock; and so on. Make sure you know how time is recorded in your facility and use the proper system.

Time

a.c.—before meals
p.c.—after meals
A.M.—morning
P.M.—evening or afternoon
h.s.—hour of sleep (bedtime)
hr.—hour
b.i.d.—twice a day
t.i.d.—three times a day
q.i.d.—four times a day
q.2h.—every 2 hours
p.r.n.—whenever necessary
stat.—at once
ad. lib.—as desired

Miscellaneous

ADL—activities of daily living
dc.—discontinue
spec.—specimen
noct.—at night
O$_2$—oxygen
n.p.o.—nothing by mouth
p.o.—by mouth
per—by
tinct.—tincture
q.s.—sufficient quantity
ung. or oint.—ointment
c̄—with
s̄—without
lb.—pound
wt.—weight
ht.—height
b.m.—bowel movement
p.o.—postoperative
Rx—treatment (take)
Dr.—doctor
Dx—diagnosis

Diagnosis

A.D.—Alzheimer's Disease
C.H.F.—congestive heart failure
A.S.H.D.—arteriosclerotic heart disease
M.I.—myocardial infarction (refers to death of tissues due to loss of blood supply)
C.V.A.—cerebral vascular accident, also known as stroke
U.R.I.—upper respiratory disease or infection
M.S.—multiple sclerosis
C.O.P.D.—chronic obstructive pulmonary disease
T.I.A.—transient ischemic attack (ministroke)

Measurements and Volume

oz.—ounce
cc.—centimeter
ml.—millimeter
L.—liter
qt.—quart
pt.—pint

Prefixes

a—from, without. Example: *a*nemia—without adequate blood
ante—before. Example: *ante*mortem—before death
cardi—pertaining to the heart. Example: *cardi*algia—pain in the heart

contra—against, opposed. Example: *contra*indicated—against the usual treatment
dys—pain or difficulty. Example: *dys*uria—painful urination
hyper—above, in excess of. Example: *hyper*tension—high blood pressure
hypo—under, a deficiency of. Example: *hypo*tension—low blood pressure
path—disease. Example: cardio*pathy*—disease of the heart
pneum—lung. Example: *pneum*onia—a condition involving the lungs

Suffixes

algia—pain. Example: neur*algia*—pain in nerve
asis or osis—state, condition, or process. Example: arterioscler*osis*—a condition of hardening of the arteries
ectomy—removal of. Example: laryng*ectomy*—removal of the larynx, (voice box)
emia—blood. Example: glyc*emia*—sugar in the blood
itis—inflammation. Example: gastr*itis*—inflammation of the stomach
oma—tumor. Example: lip*oma*—fatty tumor
ostomy—creation of an opening. Example: col*ostomy*—surgical opening into the large bowel (colon)

FIGURE 3–13. Commonly used charting abbreviations and combining forms (prefixes and suffixes).

Use all senses to make accurate observations.

Observation

Making careful, accurate **observations** of the residents in your care is one of your major responsibilities. Your observations must be *objective*. That is, you must report only facts, not opinions. For example, if you take a tray from a resident and find only half the food eaten, an objective observation would include the amount of food consumed. A *subjective* opinion might be that the resident isn't hungry.

You must observe the resident's environment for anything that might be a safety factor and report it at once. Your observations should include:

- the general condition of the resident
- the resident's response to the care plan goals
- anything unusual about the resident

• Check for: Right resident Right chart Right room
• Fill out new headings completely
• Use correct color of ink
• Date and time each entry
• Make entries in proper time sequence
• Make entries brief, objective, accurate
• Spell each word correctly
• Print or write clearly
• Leave no blank spaces or lines between entries
• Do not use the term *resident*
• Do not use ditto marks
• Sign each entry with first initial, last name, and job title
• Make corrections by drawing one line through entry; then print the word "error" and your initials above

FIGURE 3–14. *Charting guide: how to chart.*

WHAT TO CHART	SAMPLE
Amount of assistance needed in ADL	Needs help dressing
Safety measures taken	Side rails up
Amount of food eaten	20% food eaten
Intake and output of fluids	1500 ml dark yellow urine
Procedures carried out	B.P. 148/98
Resident's physical and emotional responses	Face flushed, resists fluids, threw cup against wall
Complaints of discomfort	Difficulty breathing when lying down
Difficulties in communication	Does not respond to questions, repeats word "mama" over and over
Unusual odors	Greenish, foul drainage from area on left hip
Anything else unusual	Unable to move left arm, skin cyanotic

FIGURE 3–15. *What to chart.*

	INTERNATIONAL		INTERNATIONAL
AM	**TIME**	**PM**	**TIME**
12 midnight	2400	12 noon	1200
1	0100	1	1300
2	0200	2	1400
3	0300	3	1500
4	0400	4	1600
5	0500	5	1700
6	0600	6	1800
7	0700	7	1900
8	0800	8	2000
9	0900	9	2100
10	1000	10	2200
11	1100	11	2300

FIGURE 3–16. International time.

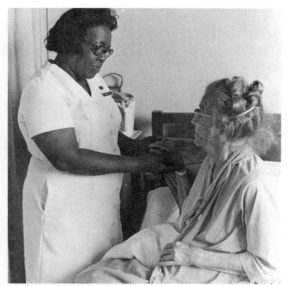

FIGURE 3–17. Carefully observe the resident whenever you give care. (From Brooks, *The Nurse Assistant,* copyright 1978 by Delmar Publishers Inc.)

For example, the skin color of all residents is important, but it is particularly important in the resident with a breathing problem.

As you become more experienced you will make many observations almost automatically. For example, you will quickly note if the urinary drainage bag is above the floor, if the handle on a bed is protruding so that someone might be hurt, or if the rubber tip of a cane is worn. You will also note the resident's body position and mentally record any changes since your last encounter. Often you may sense a problem or change even before you discover its nature. Remember, your observations and **assessments** must be promptly and accurately communicated to your charge nurse.

Use all your senses when making observations. Obviously, *seeing* is one of the most useful ways of making observations, but your sense of smell may let you know that infection is present, your sense of touch make you aware of a resident's rising temperature. The coldness or bluish color of the resident's skin may indicate poor circulation, or the dryness of the skin may tell you the person isn't taking in enough water. Your sense of hearing allows you to receive all kinds of communications about how residents feel. Be an active listener and remember to listen not only to the words but also to the tone of voice. Both reveal much about the true meaning of the message. You must also use your sense of hearing to determine heart rate and blood pressure.

Keep a paper pad and pencil or pen in your uniform pocket and jot down your observations so that you will not forget to report and record them. After you have recorded your observations and assessments and what you have done, be sure to destroy completely any notations you have jotted down before leaving the facility at the end of your shift.

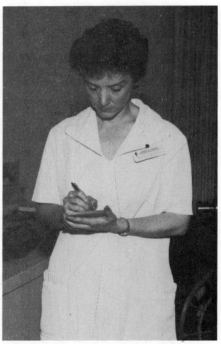

FIGURE 3–18. Keep a small note pad to make notes of your observations.

PROCEDURE: Charting

1. Check to be sure you have the correct chart.
2. Fill out new chart headings completely.
3. Use the correct color of ink.
4. Print or write clearly, spelling each word correctly.
5. Give date and time of each entry.
6. Leave no blank lines or spaces between entries.
7. Correct any errors in the entry by drawing a line through the errors and printing the word "error" and your initials above.
8. Use phrases instead of complete sentences.
9. Do not use the term resident or the resident's name.
10. Make each entry brief but accurate and complete.
11. Sign each entry properly, designating your job classification.

VOCABULARY

activities of daily living
  (ADL)
assessment
body language
care plan

chart
diagnosis
documentation
nonverbal
  communication

observation
prefix
suffix
verbal (oral)
  communication

SUGGESTED ACTIVITIES

1. Invite the charge nurse to explain how residents are informed of their rights.
2. Review several care plans. Look for common elements in each.
3. Draw a chart showing the lines of authority for the residents' care.
4. Practice charting.

REVIEW

A. Brief Answer/Fill in the Blanks

1. The authority for resident care is the _____.

2. The nursing assistant's first line of communication and authority is the _____.

3. The form that lists short and long term goals is known as the _____.

4. People involved in development of the care plan goals include the _____, _____, _____, and sometimes the resident and his family.

5. Name five activities of daily living (ADL).

    a. _____

    b. _____

    c. _____

    d. _____

    e. _____

B. True or False. Answer the following true (T) or false (F).

1. _____ Entries on the nursing care plan can be made in pencil, since it is only a temporary record.
2. _____ All entries on the resident's chart must be signed, with no spaces between entries.
3. _____ The term *resident* or the resident's name must be used with each entry on the resident's chart.
4. _____ Using international time, 1 P.M. is properly written as 1300.
5. _____ The resident is to ambulate q.i.d. This means you will assist him or her to walk three times a day.
6. _____ The resident has the right to be fully informed about, and to participate in, the planning of his or her own care.
7. _____ Residents have the right to be treated with respect.

C. Matching. Match the correct definition with each abbreviation.

1. _____ TIA
2. _____ q.s.
3. _____ p.o.
4. _____ c̄
5. _____ stat.
6. _____ s̄
7. _____ ad lib.
8. _____ p.r.n.

a. sufficient quantity
b. by mouth
c. without
d. at once
e. mini-stroke
f. with
g. whenever necessary
h. as desired
i. without

CLINICAL SITUATION

Mr. Ramirez, an 83-year-old Spanish-speaking man, has just been admitted to your facility. The doctor states that he has difficulty breathing because of emphysema and that he had a stroke 6 months ago. He cannot move his left arm or leg but his speech is unaffected. His dentures do not fit well and he seems rather emotional.

In reviewing his care plan, which ADL do you think might require the most support?

Answer: _____

_____

_____

SECTION 1 Achievement Review

A. **Multiple Choice.** Select the one best answer and circle the correct letter.

1. An intermediate care facility provides
   a. acute care
   b. room and board only
   c. continual rehabilitative care
   d. home atmosphere

2. The resident unit
   a. is the resident's personal space
   b. is always shared with several others
   c. is usually a private room
   d. contains equipment shared with others

3. Each resident unit has
   a. side rails on the bed for safety
   b. a call bell mechanism
   c. equipment for personal hygiene
   d. all of the above

4. The area of the facility where official records are kept is called the
   a. day room
   b. dining room
   c. nurses' station
   d. resident unit

5. The rules governing the facility and the care to be given are found in the
   a. resident's health record
   b. Kardex
   c. dietary list
   d. policy and procedure books

6. The authority for resident care comes from the
   a. charge nurse
   b. physician
   c. social worker
   d. dietitian

7. The physician who provides care of the resident's feet is the
   a. podiatrist
   b. audiologist
   c. speech therapist
   d. physical therapist

8. The person providing the most direct care and assistance to the resident is the
   a. director of nursing
   b. physician
   c. nursing assistant
   d. charge nurse

9. The people who provide the care of the resident are called the
   a. team
   b. nursing pool
   c. contributors
   d. supporters

10. The resident's record states that the resident has had a T.I.A. You recognize this to mean a/an
    a. heart attack
    b. gall bladder problem
    c. inability to urinate
    d. small stroke

11. A resident's record
    a. is a legal record or document
    b. must be made in pencil
    c. can have erasures
    d. need not be signed

12. The care plan reads F.F. p.o. You understand this to mean
    a. increase fluids with meals only
    b. give intravenous fluids
    c. encourage fluids by mouth
    d. limit fluid intake

13. The care plan states physiotherapy at 1530. You will plan to assist the resident to the physiotherapy area at
    a. one o'clock
    b. two o'clock
    c. half past four o'clock
    d. half past three o'clock

14. The resident complains of pain on urination. You would correctly chart this as
    a. dysphagia
    b. dysuria
    c. dysmenorrhea
    d. anuria

15. You must always remember that all residents have
    a. hearing problems
    b. rights
    c. confused periods
    d. severe handicaps

B. **Matching.** Match the correct word or abbreviation at right that stands for each phrase in the left hand column.

16. _____ resident's current condition

17. _____ specific directions for the care to be given and goals to be sought

18. _____ making an official record of care given

19. _____ assisting residents to become as independent as possible in caring for themselves

20. _____ three times a day

21. _____ activities of daily living

22. _____ at once

23. _____ specialist who tests hearing

24. _____ nursing assistant's first line of communication

25. _____ 2 P.M. in international time notation

Choices
a. rehabilitation
b. ADL
c. charge nurse
d. audiologist
e. 1400
f. care plan
g. 1700
h. t.i.d.
i. charting
j. status
k. stat.
l. director of nursing
m. podiatrist
n. b.i.d.

C. Circle six activities of daily living.

C	O	M	M	U	N	I	C	A	T	I	O	N	S	E
D	Y	O	A	Z	C	K	Q	R	L	E	T	B	P	I
F	X	B	R	E	A	T	H	I	N	G	Y	B	I	E
P	B	I	N	L	B	A	M	H	O	D	K	T	R	D
A	C	L	P	I	J	R	G	B	Q	C	P	A	I	X
N	R	I	O	M	C	P	B	N	A	R	E	S	T	C
N	U	T	R	I	T	I	O	N	M	N	E	D	U	A
E	T	Y	C	N	O	N	E	Z	Y	R	I	D	A	O
C	O	N	O	A	A	N	B	T	E	N	Y	O	L	L
H	E	M	O	T	I	O	N	A	L	N	E	E	D	S
O	H	Y	G	I	E	N	E	F	W	X	U	V	I	G
S	T	B	L	O	N	E	W	S	C	O	U	G	H	S
P	V	T	E	N	B	S	T	E	M	P	A	O	T	C

D. Write a brief statement about the type of care provided by each care giver pictured.

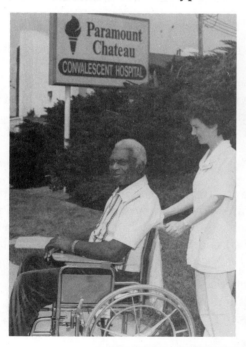

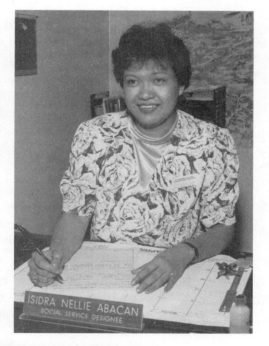

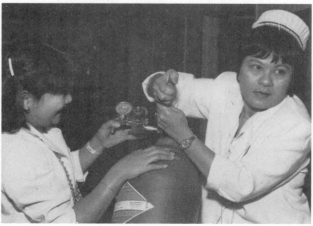

SECTION II

THE NURSING ASSISTANT

LESSON 4 Personal Characteristics

OBJECTIVES

After studying this lesson, you should be able to:

- List six characteristics needed to be a successful nursing assistant.
- Describe how to dress properly for work.
- Explain the responsibilities the nursing assistant has for personal and professional growth.
- Define and spell all the vocabulary words and terms.

SPECIAL CHARACTERISTICS

Nursing assistants are selected, educated, and trained to assist in giving nursing care. These assistants are very special people who feel pride in themselves when they fulfill their role with enthusiasm and dedication in their chosen field, figure 4–1. They will be successful if they:

Nursing Assistants are specially trained care givers.

- possess maturity and sensitivity
- can be satisfied with small gains
- bring a positive attitude to their job (figure 4–2)

Not everyone can be a successful, satisfied nursing assistant. Nursing assistants care for many older people who can no longer independently care for themselves. These are people who need to feel confident and secure with those entrusted with their welfare. Some of them may be confused, while others need a great deal of patience and assistance in carrying out even the most intimate parts of their own personal hygiene.

Sensitivity and Maturity

Because the residents have so many needs, the nursing assistant must have great **sensitivity** in order to recognize both those needs that are expressed and those that are not expressed. The need for dry, clean linen is obvious if the bed is wet, but the need for a close human relationship may be less obvious. It is just as important to

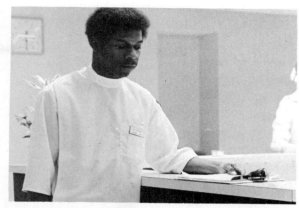

FIGURE 4-1. This nursing assistant was hired because of his maturity and sensitivity. (From Brooks, The Nurse Assistant, copyright 1978 by Delmar Publishers Inc.)

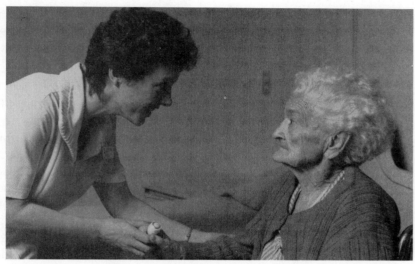

FIGURE 4-2. This nursing assistant brings a positive attitude to her job.

be aware of and to meet the residents' emotional needs as well as the physical needs, figure 4-3.

The sensitive, mature worker quickly recognizes both the physical and emotional needs and willingly reaches out. **Maturity** means that you will be able to control your emotions. Angry responses have no place in the facility. Courtesy and respect must characterize the way you relate to residents and co-workers alike. The mature individual can accept and profit by constructive evaluation and criticism, turning each into a learning experience. It also requires maturity and sensitivity to make the judgments and **assessments** (observations) that are part of a nursing assistant's job. Maturity is not a matter of age; it is a question of attitude.

In the acute hospital, patients who have been very ill or who have had extensive surgery can make rapid, dramatic gains as their health improves. They usually go home to an anxious family waiting to

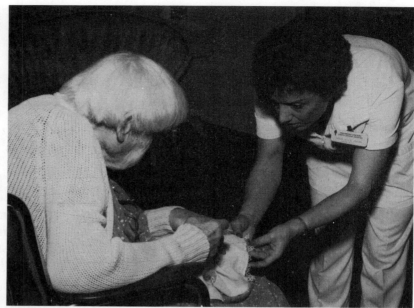

FIGURE 4–3. *The nursing assistant expresses her appreciation of the tatting that the resident is doing.*

Maturity
Dependability
Accuracy
Patience
Skill
Empathy
Sensitivity

receive them. The resident in a long term care facility makes small strides at best—for example, re-learning to hold a spoon or walking a corridor with the help of a cane. They *are* home, and all too often the staff becomes their only family and friends. The enthusiasm and patience that the nursing assistant brings to his or her work can spread like sunshine throughout the unit. A smile or the recognition of a resident's successful efforts can brighten the day for those in your care.

Older people move slowly, often think slowly and in general have more difficulty in doing the things that younger people do with ease. That is why it sometimes takes great patience to encourage residents to feed themselves. The task could be accomplished in a much shorter time if the nursing assistant did the feeding. Although much more quickly accomplished, it would be far less satisfying to the residents. By doing the feeding for the resident you tend to make him/her feel less and less independent.

Dependability and Accuracy

Dependability and **accuracy** are also essential qualities of the nursing assistant. You demonstrate these qualities when you:

- arrive on duty at the proper time (figure 4–4)
- come prepared to do your job
- carry out your assignment in the correct way you have been taught

Empathy

The ability to put yourself in another person's position is called *empathy.* Being able to see a situation from another person's point of view helps you become more sensitive to that point of view.

Just for a moment, pretend you are one of the residents. What kind of a nursing assistant would you want to help you? Imagine what it must be like to:

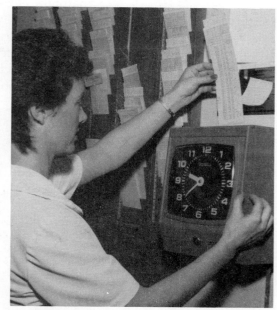

FIGURE 4–4. You demonstrate your depend-ability when you arrive for duty on time.

- have to sit for hours in a geri chair
- have thoughts you cannot express in words
- need to go to the toilet and have to wait for help
- take a bath but need help
- not be able to feed yourself
- have a tube in your bladder to drain urine
- be away from family and friends

As you do this, you will soon begin to develop a feeling for the situation of the resident, and your empathy for the residents in your care will begin to grow.

COMMUNICATION SKILLS

The ability to communicate with the residents is a skill that will develop with experience, but it is founded on an attitude of concern and caring. It is not always the words we choose that are helpful but the way in which they are said. Tone of voice, facial expression, and even the tender way you touch all communicate a sense of honest caring to the resident. Looking directly at the resident as you speak and addressing him or her respectfully by name are also indications of caring.

Listening actively is a special skill and is more than just being physically present. When you listen actively, your attention is on the speaker. You maintain eye contact and do not interrupt while the other person is speaking. You ask questions that encourage the speaker to continue and respond to specific questions being asked, figure 4–5. To communicate effectively:

- face the resident
- speak slowly

- maintain eye contact
- listen carefully
- do not be in a hurry
- use touch occasionally
- be careful of body language
- do not sit too closely

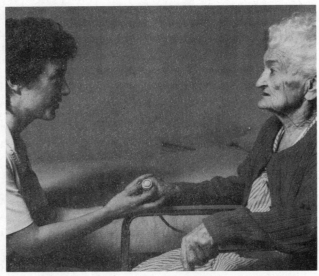

FIGURE 4–5. Communicating effectively takes time, patience, and skill.

ATTITUDE

Perhaps the most important single characteristic that you bring to your job is your **attitude**. All the other characteristics described are an outer reflection of your inner feelings, of your attitude toward your self and others.

Residents have the right and need to be cared for in a calm, unhurried atmosphere, and your attitude and behavior are critical in providing such an environment.

REDUCING STRESS

Your work as a nursing assistant is physically and emotionally demanding because you must give so much of yourself to those in your care. You will need:

- sufficient rest
- good nutrition
- satisfying recreation to do your best and to stay healthy

Burnout (total mental and emotional—and sometimes physical—fatigue) among those working with either the sick or infirmed is very high. You can reduce the stress that leads to burnout by balancing your work with rest and recreation, figure 4–6. You can also learn stress reducing techniques to help you. Food and cigarettes are used by some people to reduce stress but this can cause serious health problems. To reduce stress:

- try sitting for a few moments with your feet up
- shut your eyes and take some deep breaths
- with your eyes shut, picture a special place you like and in your mind take yourself there
- take a warm relaxing bath
- listen to some quiet music
- carry out a specific relaxation exercise
- make yourself a cup of herbal tea and drink it slowly

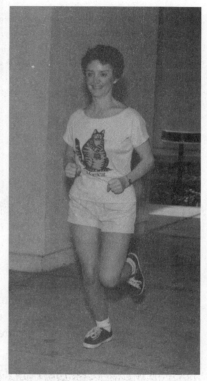

FIGURE 4-6. Work should be balanced with recreational exercise.

PERSONAL HYGIENE

Good personal hygiene is essential.

You will be in close physical contact with the residents, so it is essential that your personal hygiene and grooming is the very best, figure 4-7. Good grooming starts with a daily bath and the use of a deodorant to control body odors. Careful attention to the cleanliness of teeth and nails is also important; teeth should be cleaned at least twice each day and fingernails kept trimmed and smooth. Hair should be neatly arranged and controlled. Beards and mustaches should be neatly trimmed and makeup should be moderate.

Do not smoke while in uniform, since clothing picks up the odor of tobacco, which is offensive to many people. Strongly scented after-shave lotions and perfumes can also be offensive, so use them sparingly.

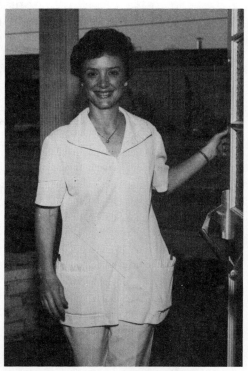

FIGURE 4-7. *Your grooming declares the pride you have in yourself.*

UNIFORMS ▪▪

The uniform of nursing assistants in long term care facilities is often a matter of preference, but a specific color or type may be required. Whatever the dress code for your facility is, it must be followed.

The uniform includes shoes and stockings. Shoes are usually white and should be cleaned daily, and white shoelaces should be laundered frequently. Since nursing assistants spend many hours on their feet, good, comfortable, well-fitting shoes are a worthwhile investment.

Bracelets, rings, earrings, and necklaces are not to be worn (although most facilities do permit the wearing of a wedding ring). The reason for this is that jewelry tends to harbor germs and may scratch or otherwise injure a resident.

A watch with a second hand and an identification badge are part of your official uniform. You will need the watch to carry out certain procedures and the identification badge lets other staff members know who you are and helps residents to remember your name. As previously mentioned, you should keep a pen and pencil and a small note pad in your uniform pocket to jot down your observations of the residents and their responses to care.

Always remember that your appearance declares your pride in yourself and your work and that you are a representative of your facility to residents and visitors. You are ready to work if you:

- demonstrate personal cleanliness
- use an antiperspirant or deodorant
- wear an appropriate, clean uniform
- wear clean shoes and stockings, including clean shoelaces
- have arranged your hair so that it is restrained and neat
- have (if you are a man) your beard and mustache trimmed
- have your fingernails trimmed smoothly
- do not use strong perfumes or after-shave lotion
- wear a watch with a second hand
- carry a pen, pencil, and note pad in your uniform pocket
- have identification badge properly pinned on your uniform
- do not smoke while in uniform

CONTINUE TO GROW

Your training program prepares you to perform as a beginning level nursing assistant. You have both the opportunity and responsibility to continue your education and personal growth, figure 4–8. If you are willing to do so, you may learn much from team leaders, charge nurses, and other nursing assistants.

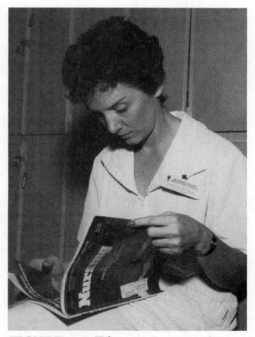

FIGURE 4–8. Take every opportunity you can to increase your knowledge.

Seek out opportunities to grow.

The procedure and policy books that are kept at the nursing station are ready references when you have questions about a new procedure or how to handle a new situation. Become familiar with each of these sources and with the medical dictionary on your unit. Use the dictionary to look up and learn the correct spelling of medical words and terms. In fact, set a goal for yourself to increase your vocabulary by at least two new words each week. Practice using them. Remember your immediate line of communication and always ask for help when in doubt. Always be ready to learn.

Many facilities subscribe to professional magazines that are available for staff use. If this is true of your facility, take advantage of this opportunity to increase your knowledge and grow.

Care planning conferences can be an excellent way to expand your knowledge base. Listen carefully. Remember, learning is a lifetime challenge.

VOCABULARY

accuracy   empathy
attitude   maturity
burnout   sensitivity
dependability

SUGGESTED ACTIVITIES

1. Invite a nursing assistant to discuss ways he or she has found to increase nursing skills and knowledge.

2. Discuss ways that burnout can be avoided.

3. Carefully observe the nursing staff on your unit and note the kinds of uniforms being worn.

4. Locate the medical dictionary and the procedure and policy books on your unit.

5. In a room where you will not be disturbed by the telephone or by others, try this relaxation exercise (approximately 5 minutes):

   - sit in a comfortable chair
   - shut your eyes
   - rest your hands comfortably in your lap
   - concentrate your thoughts on visualizing a seashore
     - hear the waves
     - see the sun
     - hear the sea gulls
     - feel the warmth of the sand
     - feel the coolness of the water
   - stay in this place for a short time, and then gradually let your consciousness return to the room

   You should feel refreshed and relaxed.

REVIEW

A. Brief Answers/Fill in the Blanks

1. List six characteristics of a successful nursing assistant.

   a. _____

   b. _____

   c. _____

   d. _____

   e. _____

   f. _____

2. Sensitivity helps the nursing assistant be aware of obvious and less obvious resident _____.

3. Three ways the nursing assistant demonstrates dependability are

   a. _____

   b. _____

   c. _____

4. When the nursing assistant has empathy he or she can more easily understand what the resident is _____.

5. Two book sources for help in promoting your professional growth include the _____ and _____.

6. Describe briefly the proper dress for work.

   _____

   _____

   _____

   _____

7. The nursing assistant should not smoke while in uniform because

   _____

   _____ .

8. The basis for successful practice as a nursing assistant is largely due to

   _____ .

9. Body odors can be controlled by

   a. _____

   b. _____

   c. _____

10. Most facilities permit some jewelery to be worn, which usually includes _____ and _____.

CLINICAL SITUATION

Pat Doyer has had a very difficult and trying day. He is a nursing assistant at the Branchwater Home. One of the residents in his care was very confused and kept asking the same question over and over again, expecting an answer each time. Pat had been very patient, but now that his shift was over, he was tired, felt uptight, and wondered if he had made a mistake in choosing to become a nursing assistant. How would you describe what is happening to Pat? What would you suggest he do about it?

Answer: _____

_____

_____

LESSON 5 The Successful Worker

After studying this lesson, you should be able to:

- Explain how medical ethics guide the nursing assistant's conduct.
- Identify three legal problems and explain how to avoid them.
- List five ways to efficiently use on-duty time.
- Demonstrate proper body mechanics.
- Define and spell all the vocabulary words and terms.

THE ETHICAL CODE

The **ethical code** is a set of moral rules that guide the behavior of nursing assistants and all other care providers. Care givers voluntarily agree to abide by the rules when they accept their positions. Carefully following the rules protects the residents and the nursing assistant.

Ethics — a moral guide for behavior

One of the most fundamental parts of the code is the concept that life is precious. The saving of life and the promoting of health are primary goals for all health workers. This basic rule must be kept in mind even though the residents in your care may have a limited life span and have health problems that may never be fully cured. Following the ethical code, you must do everything you can to support each resident, to improve the quality of life, and to make him or her as comfortable as possible. Even after death, the code requires respectful care of the body.

CONFIDENTIAL INFORMATION

Your work brings you awareness of information of a personal nature about the residents and their families, figure 5–1. Many times you will become a substitute family and friend of those in your care and this will lead to sharing of many intimacies. The ethical rule says that although the residents share their personal business with you, you must not burden the resident with your problems and information about your personal life. Furthermore, you may not repeat information of a personal nature about any resident to your family or colleagues; this information is confidential. Neither may you use any information gained in this way to your advantage. If, for example, the son of a resident is in real estate and tells his mother that his

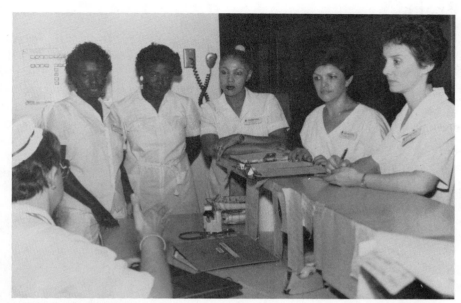

FIGURE 5–1. Personal information about residents must be kept in confidence.

company is planning to buy property to put up a new office building, you cannot pass this information on to any relative or friend in the real estate business, since they could buy this property first and then sell it for a profit.

You must keep all personal information to yourself, unless it affects the health and well being of the resident. For example, one of the married residents tells you that things are not going well between her husband and herself, and she seems very depressed after he leaves. You could share this information with the charge nurse, who might decide to counsel the resident or alert a social worker to the need for counseling. This information, however, should *not* be shared with a co-worker: to do so in a casual conversation is **gossip**, figure 5–2. Gossiping is unacceptable behavior in one who follows the ethical code. Privacy is a fundamental resident right and it is guaranteed through adherence to the code. Remember, this is a code that you promised to follow when you accepted your privileged position as a nursing assistant.

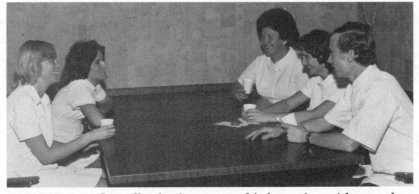

FIGURE 5–2. Casually sharing personal information with coworkers is gossip.

RESPECT

Residents and their families are to be treated with respect at all times. Respect is demonstrated in the way in which we relate to those in our care, figure 5–3. We show respect when we use the name the resident prefers, when we support their chosen spiritual expression, even though it differs from our own, and when we talk with them in a mature manner. Don't speak to residents as if they are children, and do not call them by nicknames unless specifically requested to do so. Neither ignore nor humor a resident—both behaviors are disrespectful. Each resident is a unique person who deserves to be treated with dignity and respect.

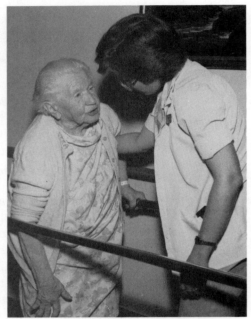

FIGURE 5–3. Respect is demonstrated in the words we choose and they way we say them.

TIPPING

All residents are charged for the care which they receive. You receive a salary for those services which you agreed to perform when you were employed. At no time should a resident's financial resources determine the extent and type of care and services provided; these should be based solely on need. There is no place for **tipping** in the field of health care. Tactfully refuse a tip that is offered and tell the resident of your continued desire to be helpful.

LEGAL RELATIONSHIPS

The moral responsibilities of the ethical code are related to our legal responsibilities. Legal laws are a set of rules which also must be followed. Not to do so is wrong and is punishable. Following these rules protects both you and the resident.

Illegal Acts
— Verbal
— Physical
— Written

Repeating inaccurate, harmful information about a resident is **slander**; putting this same information into writing is **libel.** As well as being illegal, slander and libel are violations of the ethical code which emphasizes loyalty, honesty, and truthfulness. Each person is responsible for his or her own moral behavior, but in a team situation this concept extends beyond the individual.

Loss of facility equipment and personal belongings of residents increases the expense of care and causes the affected resident and family members great anguish. Taking that which does not belong to you is **stealing** and it is a crime; if you witness stealing by someone else and do not report it, then you are **aiding and abetting** the crime. Aiding and abetting is just as wrong and illegal as if you yourself are stealing. If you witness any crime being committed, you are to report it immediately to your charge nurse.

PHYSICAL ABUSE

The ethical code protects the physical welfare of the residents as well as of the care givers. We promise to do no harm as we carry out our responsibilities. Residents must never be roughly handled or abused physically or verbally. They may not be physically restrained unless they are a danger to themselves or to others, and then only with a specific physician's order, for a limited time, in an approved manner. Determining that restraints are necessary is not a nursing assistant's decision.

NEGLIGENCE

As a trained nursing assistant, you are expected to carry out your work in a proper manner, following the procedures as you have been taught. If you fail to perform your duties safely and competently, you will be guilty of **negligence**. Trying to perform tasks for which you have not been prepared and which are not within the usual scope of a nursing assistant's duties is known as **malpractice**. For example, failing to clean up a spill that causes a resident to slip and fall would be considered *negligence*; inserting a nasogastric tube, which is a professional's responsibility, would be *malpractice*. Both actions are illegal.

WILLS

Providing for those left behind when one dies becomes even more pressing as the individual grows older. It is natural for elderly residents to consider writing a will for that purpose. Writing or witnessing such a document is a legal matter for which nursing assistants are not prepared. Refer all matters of this nature to the charge nurse so that she can make proper arrangements.

ORGANIZATION OF TIME

Nursing assistants have busy assignments to carry out during their on-duty time. The better organized you are, the more easily you will accomplish your tasks. There are several ways in which you can help yourself become more organized.

Organization leads to
efficient completion of
tasks

Report on duty at the correct time. Your job is your first responsibility and there are people depending on you. If you are ill, you must call the facility as soon as you know that you will be unable to work so that someone can cover your responsibilities. If you have personal responsibilities that might affect your availability, you should discuss these with your employer at the time you are hired. Be sure that you and your employer are in agreement as to how these responsibilities are to relate to your on-duty time.

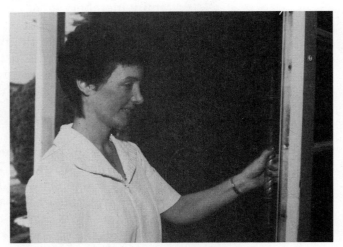

FIGURE 5–4. This nursing assistant arrives to work on time ready to do her best.

Listen to the report and review your assignment. Note any changes in the care plans and any special orders that are to be followed. Make special note of orders that must be carried out at a specific time. Don't assume that because a resident has been at the facility for a long time, orders remain the same.

Think through your assignment and plan your work to save steps and energy. Take a few moments to rearrange your plans if something unexpected develops during your shift.

Remember that you are employed and paid to work for a whole shift. Don't waste time chatting with co-workers. Be on time returning from breaks and lunch and do not leave early without permission.

PROPER BODY MECHANICS ▪▪▪▪▪▪▪▪▪▪▪▪▪▪▪▪▪▪▪▪▪▪▪▪▪▪▪▪▪▪▪▪

Proper body mechanics, which will help protect both you and residents from injury, begins with good posture in all positions. Keeping your back straight but not stiff, you should use your strong arm and leg muscles to push, pull, or lift. Keep your feet separated since a widened base of support makes you steadier.

Always size up the job to be done before attempting to do it. Ask for help or use mechanical assistance such as the **Hoyer lift sheet**, or turning sheet when the resident is very heavy or unable to help. Be willing to work as a team when necessaary to help other co-workers.

The six rules listed below will help your muscles work better for you, figure 5–5.

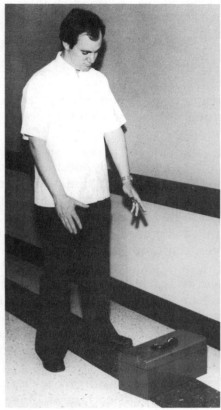

FIGURE 5–5A. *Keep the feet well separated and keep your back straight.*

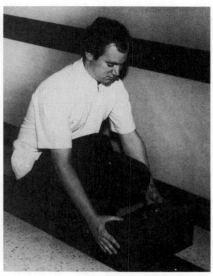

FIGURE 5–5B. *When picking up an object, bend from the hips and knees.*

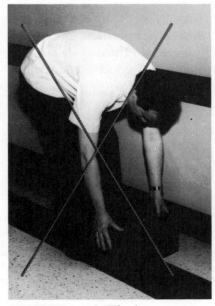

FIGURE 5–5C. *The incorrect way to pick up an object.*

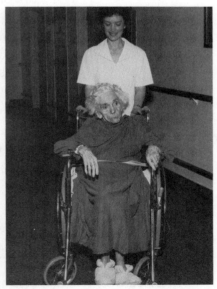

FIGURE 5–5D. *Note the proper posture of both the assistant and the resident.*

FIGURE 5–5. *Proper body mechanics.*

Proper body mechanics save energy and prevent injury.

1. Keep your back steady. Your spinal muscles are small and not designed for heavy lifting.
2. Bend from the hips and knees to get closer to the object to be lifted. Do not bend from the waist.
3. Keep feet separated, about 12 to 15 inches, as a good base for support.
4. Use the weight of your body to help push or pull.
5. Use the strongest muscles to do the job.
6. Avoid twisting your body as you work.

The same principles of good body mechanics can be applied to positioning the resident. **Alignment** (good positioning) is important in keeping the body functioning at its best. The position of the resident who is confined to bed should be changed at least every one or two hours. Pillows can be used for support. The resident who is in a wheelchair or geri chair must have his or her position changed just as often.

Frequent position changes help prevent skin breakdown and improve circulation. Lying or sitting in one position for an extended period results in discomfort and stiffening of joints, which is painful and **debilitating** (weakening); furthermore, it may cause permanent muscle shortening, called **contracture**, and bedsores (**decubitus ulcers**).

It can be very helpful if residents in wheelchairs are able to lift themselves even for a few seconds each hour. Often, you may need to remind the resident to do this.

SUMMARY

The work of a nursing assistant is demanding, but you can meet the challenge if you:

- follow what you have been taught
- are guided by medical ethics
- apply the principles of good management
- use good body mechanics

VOCABULARY

aiding and abetting	decubitus ulcer	malpractice
alignment	ethical code	negligence
body mechanics	gossip	slander
confidential	libel	stealing
contracture	Hoyer lift sheet	tipping
debilitating		

SUGGESTED ACTIVITIES

1. Discuss with classmates and your instructor examples of information that must be kept confidential.

2. Explore with classmates the ways in which the ethical code will influence your work as a nursing assistant.

3. Using proper body mechanics, practice lifting, moving, and carrying objects.

REVIEW

A. Brief Answer/Fill in the Blanks

1. Nursing assistants _____ agree to live up to the ethical code when they accept employment.

2. Information of a personal nature about a resident must be kept _____.

3. Casually sharing personal information about a resident with other staff members is _____.

4. Using information learned while you are working for your own personal gain is _____ the ethical code.

5. If an assistant repeats harmful, _____ information about a resident or anyone, it is considered to be _____.

6. Taking facility property or things which belong to a resident or co-worker is _____.

7. Residents must never be handled roughly or _____ physically or verbally.

8. Nursing assistants are paid for the work they do and the service they give; therefore _____ is not permitted.

9. One way to show respect for a resident is to call him/her by _____.

10. A nursing assistant who performs a task which he or she has not been taught to do is guilty of _____.

B. Identification. Which of the following pictures demonstrates the use of proper body mechanics. (Circle the correct letter.)

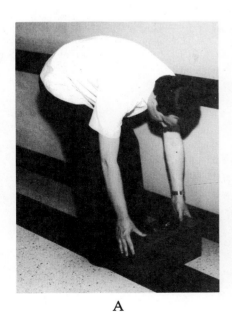

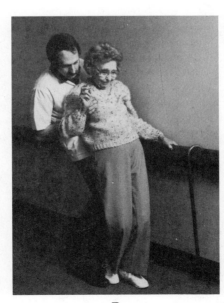

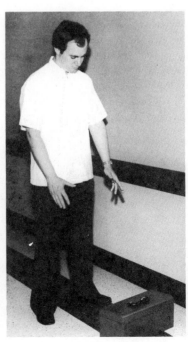

A   B   C

C. Multiple Answer. List five ways of efficiently using on-duty time.

1.

2.

3.

4.

5.

CLINICAL SITUATION

As you are getting linen from the linen cart, you glance into a room where another assistant is dusting the bedside stand and see her slipping the resident's bracelet into her pocket. What must you do?

Answer: _____

_____

_____

LESSON 6 Specific Duties and Responsibilities

OBJECTIVES

After studying this lesson, you should be able to:

- Discuss your job description.
- Explain how interpersonal relations influence the effectiveness of care.
- Identify the forms that outline assignments.
- List ten duties that the nursing assistant performs.
- Define and spell all the vocabulary words and terms.

THE JOB DESCRIPTION

The job description explains what and how you will perform.

Nursing assistants working in long term care facilities carry out many of the same tasks as those working in the acute setting. The activities and responsibilities of the nursing assistants are stated in the policy book as a **job description**. Before accepting employment, you should review the job description to be sure you can perform the work required. Each facility has a policy book that describes the role and responsibilities of each staff member. The way in which each task should be performed in a particular facility is found in the procedure book, figure 6–1. Find each of these books in your unit and become familiar with them. Both books are usually found in the nurses' station.

Each facility varies basic **procedures** in some ways in order to meet individual circumstances. You will learn how to carry out all the tasks of a nursing assistant but it is your responsibility to know any differences preferred in your facility. Differences in procedure may be explained during the orientation period after employment. Another way to be sure of how procedures should be performed is to check the procedure book for exact details.

Co-workers may make helpful suggestions but their information may not always be reliable. Be open to their suggestions, but if they are not in accord with the basic procedures you have learned, check the procedure book or consult with the charge nurse. Be willing to learn new techniques and different ways to do something, but take the instruction from your charge nurse or in-service educator. If you are asked to perform a procedure that you have not learned but it is within the scope of an assistant's tasks, ask for a demonstration and for supervision until both you and your supervisor are confident in your ability to carry out the procedure correctly and safely.

The job description also explains how your employer expects you to perform. Your specific **assignments** will be based on the job description.

STAFF RELATIONS

It is part of the general staff's responsibility to be friendly and cooperative with all members of the team. This kind of relationship promotes a sense of **harmony** which is very important in maintaining a calm atmosphere, figure 6–2. Older residents are very adversely affected by any disharmony between staff members. Naturally, there will be some staff members with whom you will be more friendly, but while you are in the facility, you must be supportive of and pleasant to everyone. If a staff member or resident complains to you about another nursing assistant, tactfully refuse to comment. If you believe that the criticism is justified and that a danger to the resident exists, suggest that the matter be referred to the charge nurse to handle.

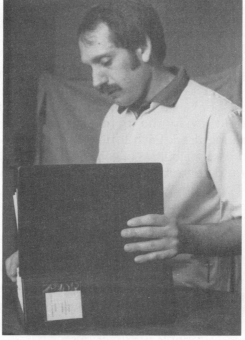

FIGURE 6–1. The procedure book describes how procedures are to be performed.

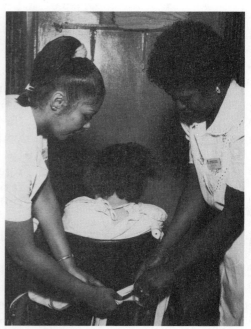

FIGURE 6–2. Harmony is promoted when staff members work in a cooperative manner.

Never criticize your co-workers to the residents. Listen to residents and offer to help with legitimate problems, but real problems are best worked out quietly between the parties involved. Always remember, that the effectiveness of care is greatly affected by interpersonal relationships. Good relationships enhance the care while poor ones can destroy the best of good intentions.

ASSIGNMENTS

The charge nurse makes out assignments based on the needs of the residents and availability of staff, figure 6–3. At times your care load will be lighter than usual and at times much heavier. Remember that the staff works as a team, and be cooperative and ready to help when someone needs it. Although you will be responsible for the care of specific residents, do not ignore a resident who is not part of your assignment and who needs help.

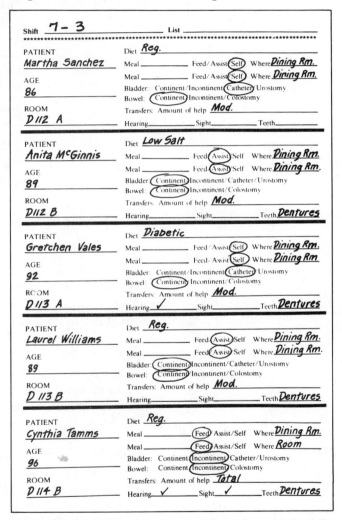

FIGURE 6–3. *The assignment card can be carried while on duty as a reminder of the care to be given.*

Assignments are based on resident needs.

Never allow any resident to be uncomfortable or in danger. For example, a resident who needs assistance to walk becomes impatient waiting in the day room for her assistant to help her return to her room. She stands up and starts unsteadily down the hall. As a nursing assistant, you see potential danger, and so you would assist her to her room even though she is not part of your specific assignment, figure 6–4. Protecting the resident and keeping the environment safe, clean, and uplifting are included in the responsibilities of every staff member.

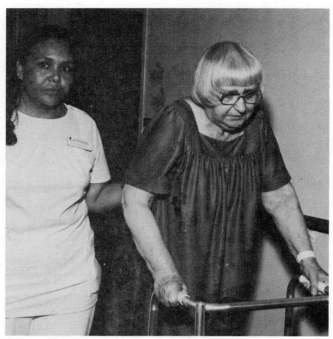

FIGURE 6–4. The nursing assistant saw a need for support by a resident and quickly moved to assist.

Forms

Care facilities use various forms in making out specific assignments. Some of these records remain in the nurses' station and are checked off upon completion so that all staff members know by looking at the form that a particular task has been performed. When a procedure such as position change is frequently done, a reminder checklist may be kept at the bedside, figure 6–5. However, in some facilities, no records are kept at the bedside.

Other forms may be carried by the nursing assistant as a reminder of the specific care to be given. None of these forms may leave the facility.

Unfinished Assignments

Be sure to report any difficulty you have in performing a procedure or carrying out an assignment. Inform the charge nurse of any tasks that are not completed at the time indicated. This can be very important. For example, you are assigned to test the urine of a resident for sugar and acetone before each meal so the nurse can give needed insulin. You have been busy and have not carried out this procedure before the food tray arrives. Inform the charge nurse right away. Do not serve the tray to the resident. Food intake is balanced by insulin administration. The amount of insulin to be given depends on the results of the urine testing. If the resident eats the meal without the intended insulin, the effects could be very serious.

SPECIFIC DUTIES

The duties of a nursing assistant can be divided into four groups of activities:

FRAMINGHAM HOME
POSITION–CHANGE BEDSIDE RECORD

NAME _Smith, Emily_   ROOM NUMBER _118 B_

DATE	TIME	POSIT.	SIGNA.	DATE	TIME	POSIT.	SIGNA.	DATE	TIME	POSIT.	SIGNA.
4/17	7 AM	Dorsal Recombent	JH.								
	9 AM	Left Sims	JH.								
	11 AM	Prone	JH.								

FIGURE 6–5. Some records are kept at the bedside for convenience, such as the position change record.

Nursing assistants assist in ADL, special procedures, support services, documentation.

1. Assisting in the activities of daily living (ADL).
2. Carrying out special procedures.
3. Performing support services.
4. Documentation (keeping records).

Activities of Daily Living (ADL)_____

Much of the nursing assistant's duties involves an important area—that of helping residents carry out the ADL that meet their physical, emotional, spiritual and social needs. As discussed in Lesson 3, the major physical needs of the resident include:

- being clean
- receiving proper exercise and positioning
- receiving proper nourishment
- being able to eliminate wastes

The nursing assistant can also help residents to find the spiritual, social, and emotional support they need, by a caring, respectful, and cheerful attitude and by making the environment as pleasant as possible.

Special Procedures___

Special procedures are needed to care for residents with individual needs that can be met only by special nursing techniques. For example, a resident who has high blood pressure must have his or her blood pressure taken and the temperature, pulse, and respiration of a resident with a fever must be monitored. Special procedures include:

1. Taking the blood pressure.
2. Taking the temperature.
3. Monitoring the pulse rate.
4. Counting the respiration rate.
5. Measuring urine and testing it for sugar and acetone.
6. Giving enemas.
7. Inserting suppositories.

Support Services_____

The third group of tasks relates to services that support the nursing care and includes (figure 6–6):

1. Supplying drinking water.
2. Placing and removing serving trays.
3. Making beds.
4. Caring for equipment.
5. Carrying messages.

Each activity makes the nursing care better and more effective. For example, elderly persons often do not drink enough fluids, and part of your assignment is to encourage them to drink more liquids. Keeping drinking water fresh encourages residents to consume more. Other residents may be on restricted or measured fluids. In this case, part of your job will be to limit intake and to keep a record of the intake.

Documentation_____

The fourth group of nursing assistant activities involves **documentation** of observations and assessments, figure 6-7. This group of tasks includes:

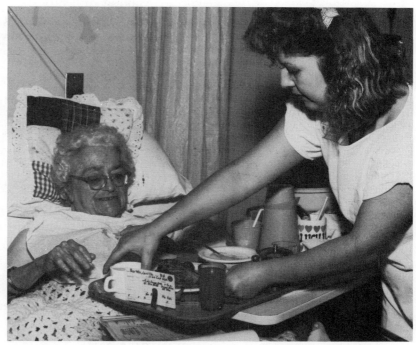

FIGURE 6–6. Serving trays is a nursing assistant function.

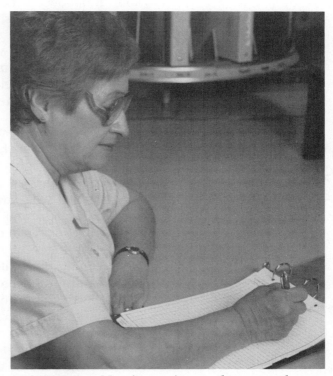

FIGURE 6–7. Nursing assistants document the care they give.

1. Making oral reports.
2. Preparing written reports.
3. Contributing to the development and evaluation of the care plan (figure 6–8).

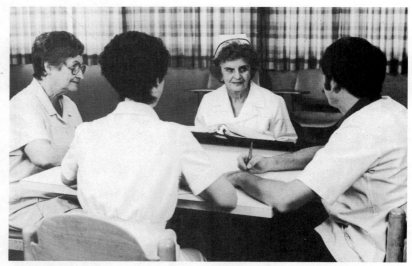

FIGURE 6–8. Nursing assistants make valuable contributions to the care plan.

Your initial observations of the resident are important in formulating both the long and short term goals of the care plan and to serve as a base of comparison for future changes in the resident's condition. Since you spend so much time in direct contact with the residents, your observations can provide much information of value. Again, because of your closeness to the residents, your assessment or evaluation of the resident's response to the care plan goals can be very significant.

Some Common Nursing Assistant Duties_____
(figures 6–9 to 6–12)

- Admitting, transferring and discharging the resident
- Answering lights
- Applying an ace bandage
- Assisting with the physical examinations
- Bathing residents
- Caring for residents' dentures
- Caring for residents' hair
- Cleaning the unit
- Cleaning utility rooms
- Collecting specimens
- Giving a back rub
- Giving foot and nail care
- Irrigating a colostomy
- Preparing an isolation unit
- Providing post-mortem care
- Shaving residents
- Using special equipment, such as the Hoyer lift
- Weighing and measuring residents
- Documenting care given

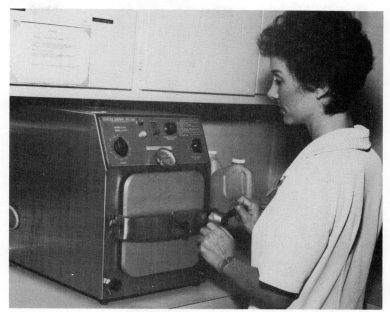

FIGURE 6–9. *Cleaning equipment and sterilizing in the autoclave are common nursing assistant assignments.*

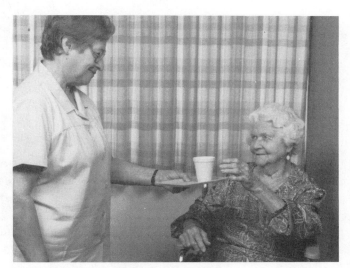

FIGURE 6—10. *Nursing assistants serve nourishment to the residents.*

Nursing assistants are important members of the nursing staff. The tasks that they perform are essential to the well-being of the resident and the smooth operation of the facility, figure 6–13.

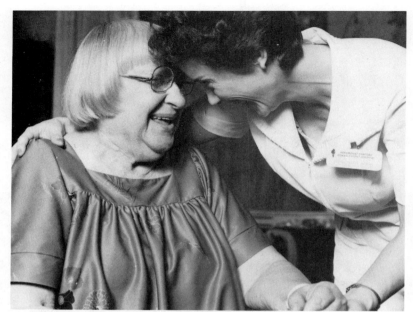

FIGURE 6–11. *Nursing assistants offer emotional support.*

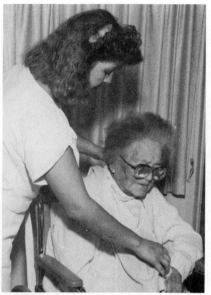

FIGURE 6–12. *Nursing assistants keep residents safe. This nursing assistant is applying a postural support.*

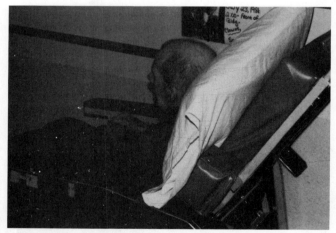

FIGURE 6–13. *Notice that this resident, who is not assigned to your care, has slipped down in the geri-chair.*

VOCABULARY

assignments	job description
harmony	procedure

SUGGESTED ACTIVITIES

1. Talk with nursing assistants in your facility about the tasks they perform.

2. Locate the procedure book and policy book on your unit and become familiar with them.

3. Write a sample job description for a nursing assistant based on what you have learned in the lesson.

REVIEW

A. Brief Answer/Fill in the Blanks

1. If you were unsure of how to perform a specific procedure that you have been taught, you might review the procedure in the _____.

2. A statement of the role and performance expectations of the nursing assistant is called the _____.

3. Such a statement as in #2 is found in the _____.

4. List two sources, other than the procedure manual, that will help you to increase your knowledge and skills.

   a. _____

   b. _____

5. The _____ must be informed if an assignment is not completed on time.

6. List three tasks a nursing assistant performs to aid the resident to carry out activities of daily living.

   a. _____

   b. _____

   c. _____

7. List two tasks related to documentation.

   a. _____

   b. _____

8. List two tasks related to support services.

   a. _____

   b. _____

9. List two tasks that require specific nursing skills.

   a. _____

   b. _____

10. Disharmony between staff members has a _____ effect on the residents.

B. True or False. Answer the following true (T) or false (F).

1. _____ All facilities carry procedures out exactly the same way.

2. _____ You are responsible only for the safety of residents assigned to you.

3. _____ Forms used for assignments containing resident information must never be taken out of the facility.

4. _____ It is permissible to criticize a supervisor in front of the resident as long as the supervisor does not hear you.

5. _____ The harmony of the facility requires cooperation on the part of all staff members.

CLINICAL SITUATION

As you walk down the corridor, you notice that Mr. Whitely, who is in a geri chair, has slipped down toward the foot of the chair and that one foot is on the floor in an awkward position. The nursing assistant that Mr. Whitely is assigned to for care is at lunch. What should you do?

Answer: _____

_____

LESSON 7 Safety Concepts

OBJECTIVES

After studying this lesson, you should be able to:

- Identify the persons responsible for resident safety.
- Identify situations that might lead to accidents, and take proper action.
- Explain ways of controlling the spread of infection.
- Demonstrate proper handwashing and isolation techniques.
- Demonstrate the correct procedure for opening a sterile package.
- Define and spell all vocabulary words and terms.

Safety is everyone's responsibility.

There are many reasons why residents are potential accident victims. It is these very reasons that make accident prevention a prime concern and responsibility of the entire staff. If one reviews the reasons why residents are in a care setting, it is easy to see the need for extreme caution.

FACTORS AFFECTING RESIDENTS' SAFETY

Confusion and vision and hearing loss make residents very vulnerable to injury, figure 7–1. In addition, older people suffer from many weaknesses. Heart, lung, and kidney malfunction is very common and may require the administration of medicines. Older residents are more apt to react unfavorably to the drugs they take, and the number of drugs needed can lead to the possibility of serious drug interactions. Some drugs have side effects that cause confusion and diminished memory.

Most residents are elderly and frail; their sense of balance is diminished, their reaction time is lengthened, and their reflexes are slowed. A fall, once started, is difficult to stop. Distances are misjudged, and confusion and lightheadedness can hinder the ability of the resident to protect himself or herself from injury.

Falls are the most common accidents among older people, but accidental ingestion of toxic products and burns are other common mishaps.

Confusion

It is obvious that a generally confused resident needs constant supervision, but often residents experience temporary confusion, perhaps because the light is dim or because they awaken suddenly

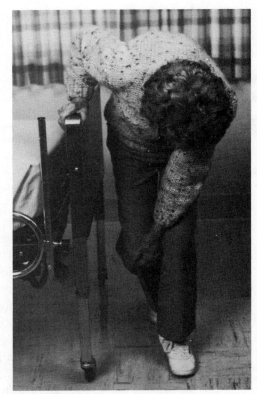

FIGURE 7-1. This resident was injured as she reacted to what she mistakenly believed was happening.

at night. Some residents in their confusion misinterpret circumstances and become injured, reacting to what they believe is happening. For example, Mrs. Bowman thinks she hears Miss Gibson in the next room calling out for help. She gets up suddenly, loses her balance, stumbles, and skins her knee on the bed frame. Despite her injury, she manages to get into the next room, only to find her friend sleeping peacefully. Mrs. Bowman was mistaken.

Toxic Products

Watch for potential hazards such as falls and burns.

A confused resident may mistakenly drink cleaning solution picked up from an unattended cleaning cart or nail polish from another resident's dresser. Serious injury can result from such actions. Therefore, all potentially harmful agents such as cleaning fluids are stored in a locked cabinet away from the resident areas.

Burns

As people age, they are more easily burned because of lowered sensitivity to temperature. This may occur even when water is heated to a temperature that younger individuals can tolerate. Extreme caution must be taken with bath water, foot soaks, and hot packs. Hot water bags and heating pads are to be avoided unless specifically ordered by the physician. Never leave an older person alone while he or she is in the tub. A resident may not only be burned, but there is also the possibility of drowning.

Hot liquids such as coffee and tea are easily spilled when held by trembling hands. Always make certain that residents who feed themselves know the placement of hot liquids and that you have arranged the food tray in such a way that there is clear access to cups or glasses. Check the temperature of soups and other liquids before serving them to the resident.

SAFETY MEASURES

There are many things that you can do to help safeguard your residents. In general, you should:

- always be on the lookout for situations that might contribute to an accident.
- correct and/or report any of these situations before a fall does occur and injuries take place.
- carry out assignments properly.
- use and store equipment correctly.

Situations Contributing to Accidents

Hazards that may cause accidents may be directly related to the residents. For example:

1. Be sure that residents' shoes and slippers fit properly and that laces are securely tied, figure 7–2; poorly fitting slippers offer inadequate support and contribute to instability.
2. Garments (e.g., nightgowns, robes) of residents should be shortened to ankle length.
3. Encourage residents to use rails along hallways and grab-bars in tubs and toilets. They are there to aid residents as they ambulate or rise and sit.

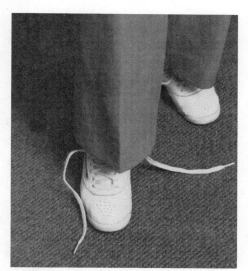

FIGURE 7–2. Untied shoes present a real danger to the resident.

Correct or Report Situations

The following precautions will help to keep the environment of the residents safe:

1. Articles must be kept off the floor to avoid the possibility of tripping.
2. All carpeting should be secured so that a toe will not be caught and a fall occur.

3. Adequate light should be maintained. Adequate light and bright no-glare colors increase visibility. Poor lighting casts misleading shadows. A night light left on in residents' rooms and in the bathrooms or hallways usually doesn't interfere with sleeping and increases the safety of these areas greatly.
4. Spills of any kind should be cleaned up immediately; even small spills can be dangerous.

Carry Out Assignments Properly

Resident safety is promoted when procedures are carried out carefully as taught and orders are correctly followed. Review a resident's care plan daily to be sure orders have not been changed. Changes can occur overnight. For example, when you left the day before, a resident was up and about with minimal supervision; today she is anxious and confused because of a slight stroke during the night. If you fail to provide adequate supervision, the resident may wander into an unsafe area such as the utility room and may be injured.

Use and Store Equipment Properly

Injury can sometimes occur when equipment is improperly used or stored or when it is left unattended. Postural supports and soft restraints, properly applied, can be protective, figure 7–3. Improperly applied, they can fail and a resident may fall from a chair or dislodge a **gavage** (feeding tube). They must be checked frequently to be sure they are not too restrictive.

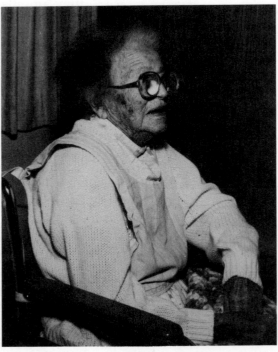

FIGURE 7–3. Properly applied postural restraints help protect residents from falling.

Nursing assistants must know how to safely operate equipment such as lifts, **gurneys** (stretchers), geri chairs, and wheelchairs before attempting to use them. Care should be taken to return all equipment to its proper location when not in use. Be alert to possible malfunctioning equipment such as slipping brakes, split straps (figure 7–4), or faulty plugs. Frayed wires can cause serious electrical fires. Report any potential hazard before an accident can happen.

Facility policies relating to safety must be followed exactly. For example, at night all beds must be in lowest positon and all side rails must be up and secure in the locked position. Call bells should be left within easy reach and **gait belts** (safety belts) are to be used when transporting or transferring residents who are not able to fully assist, figure 7–5.

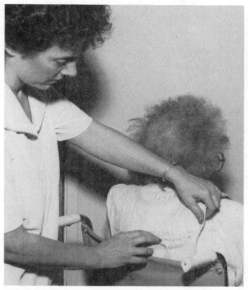

FIGURE 7–4. Check for frayed straps and replace.

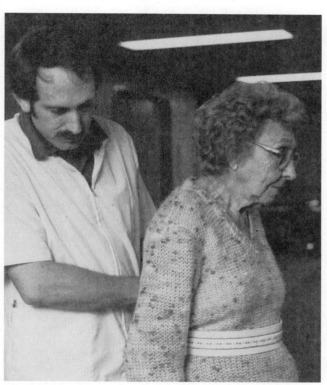

FIGURE 7–5. The gait belt offers a secure support during ambulation.

FIRES

Be alert to the danger of fires.

It is the responsibility of every staff member to know and practice the fire and evacuation plans for their facility, figure 7–6. Learn the location and operation of all fire control equipment such as fire alarms, extinguishers, sprinklers, fire doors, and fire escapes, figure 7–7. Fire drill procedures are conducted at least once each month according to each facility's plan, figure 7–8. Many residents could be injured during a fire because of their confusion and inability to help themselves. Keep alert to all possible fire hazards and report them immediately to the proper authorities.

Smoking in bed should never be permitted unless constantly supervised. Smoking should be strictly limited to specific smoking areas. This applies to residents, visitors, and staff alike. Ash trays should be large and the use of matches monitored. Smoking materials are usually stored at the nurses' station and should not be in the

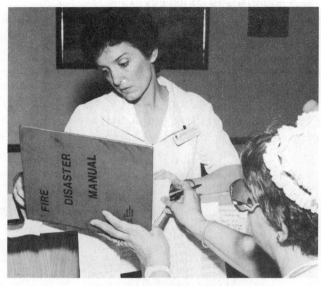

FIGURE 7–6. *Knowing the disaster and fire plan is the responsibility of the entire staff.*

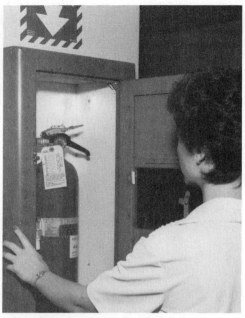

FIGURE 7–7. *Know the location of all fire alarms and fire fighting equipment.*

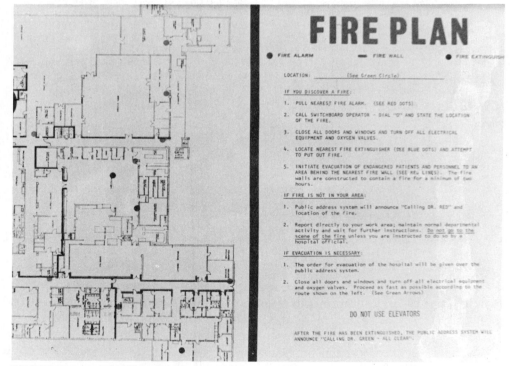

FIGURE 7–8. *The disaster plan is usually posted for ready reference.* (From Brooks, *The Nurse Assistant,* copyright 1978 by Delmar Publishers Inc.)

possession of any resident who does not have smoking privileges. If you notice someone with matches who doesn't have these privileges, collect the matches and inform the charge nurse.

The use of oxygen presents a specific hazard. When oxygen is in use:

1. Post a sign indicating that oxygen is in use.
2. Never permit smoking, lighted matches, or open flames in the area.
3. Do not use flammable liquids such as oils or alcohol.
4. Do not use electrical equipment such as radios or electric razors.

In case of fire, keep calm. Be sure those in danger are moved to safety and then sound the alarm or use the intercom. Follow the evacuation plan as you have practiced. Remember, the residents may be confused and frightened; therefore, the staff must be calm and in control. Remember:

- follow plan.
- keep calm.
- move residents to safety.
- sound alarm.
- close windows.
- shut off air conditioning.
- shut off oxygen.
- shut off lights.

REMEMBER:

R = Rescue
A = Alarm
C = Contain (Close doors, extinguish)
E = Evacuate

CHOKING

Residents who cannot chew their food well may have difficulty swallowing; because of this they are at risk for choking, figure 7–9. Gag reflexes and swallowing may be limited in post-stroke residents. Food may be hidden away (this is called **cheeking**) on the affected side of the mouth and forgotten. Residents should be seated upright when feeding. Be sure false teeth are in place.

Adjust feeding procedures to accommodate swallowing difficulties. For example:

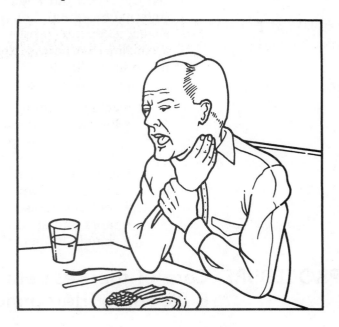

FIGURE 7–9. A choking resident.

1. Cut food into small pieces.
2. Feed slowly.
3. Offer fluids between solid foods.
4. Feed food to the unaffected side.

If choking should occur, your quick actions could save a life. If the food is visible, swab the mouth out with a crooked finger. If you have been certified to carry out the procedure for the Heimlich maneuver, you may have to perform this. Summon help using the intercom or call system. If the resident stops breathing, you may need to assist with **cardiopulmonary resuscitation** (**CPR**). CPR is a special skill that is not regularly taught in nursing assistant programs but can be learned through the American Red Cross and American Heart Association.

PROCEDURE: Assisting the Conscious Choking Person (Heimlich Maneuver)

1. Stand behind and to one side of the victim
2. If coughing does not dislodge the material:
   a. Clench fist, keeping thumb straight.
   b. Place fist, thumb side in, against abdomen between naval and tip of sternum.
   c. Grasp clenched fist with opposite hand.
3. Push forcefully with thumb side of fist against midline of abdomen, inward and upward 6 to 10 times (figure 7–10A). *Note:* If the victim becomes unconscious, place him/her flat on the floor and perform abdominal thrusts. Place the heel of one hand below the rib cage and above the umbilicus. Put the other hand on top as shown in figure 7–10B. Press inward and upward with a quick motion.

THE BLEEDING RESIDENT

Excessive bleeding is called **hemorrhage**. At times you will actually see the blood but sometimes bleeding occurs inside the resident (**internal bleeding**). You must be alert to the signs of possible hemorrhage. Keep the resident quiet, follow the emergency procedure according to American Red Cross guidelines, and inform the charge nurse immediately.

Signs and symptoms of hemorrhage include:

- actual bleeding
- low blood pressure
- weak, thready pulse
- pale to ashen skin color
- complaints of thirst
- low urine output
- cold and moist skin
- rapid and shallow respirations
- change in mental alertness

PROCEDURE: Care of the Resident Who is Bleeding (Hemorrhage)

1. Identify the location of bleeding.
2. Apply continuous, direct pressure over bleeding area with a pad or hand.
3. If seepage occurs, increase the padding and pressure.

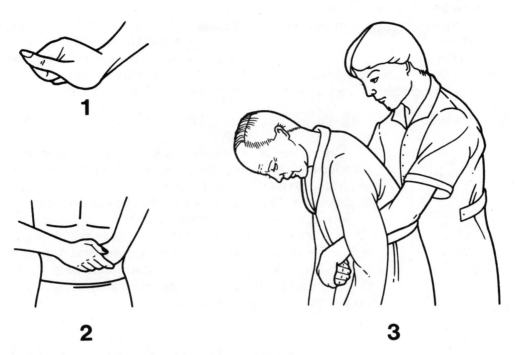

FIGURE 7-10A. *Heimlich maneuver*

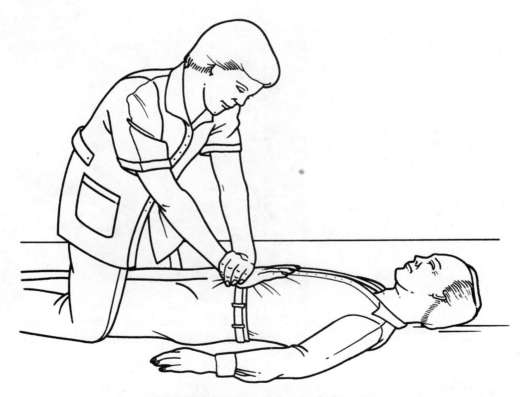

FIGURE 7-10B. *Abdominal thrusts.*

FIGURE 7-10. *If choking occurs, your actions could save a life.*

4. If there are no broken bones and no pain, raise, if possible, the wounded area above the level of the heart.
5. Support the elevated area.
6. If there is bleeding from more than one area, use binding of some kind to hold the padded pressure.
7. Apply pressure over the appropriate vessel to stem hemorrhage.
8. Keep the person comfortably warm and quiet until help arrives.
9. Signal for help but stay with the resident.

TRANSFER

Safe transfer procedures are everyone's responsibility. Before transferring a resident, check your assignment to learn which method of transfer to use. Determine how much help is needed and be ready to provide it. Remember that safety applies both to the resident and to yourself. Use proper body mechanics and avoid injury.

If you see that a resident is injured, do not attempt to move him or her. Stay with the resident, remain calm, and offer as much comfort as possible. Use the call bed light to summon help, figure 7–11. Briefly describe the situation to the person who answers the call. Remember—do not panic; help will come.

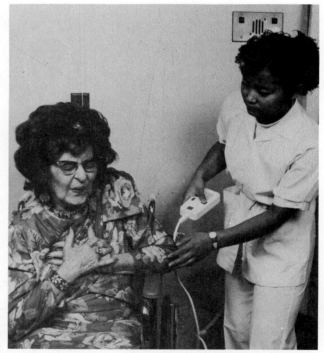

FIGURE 7–11. Use the call bell to signal for help but do not leave a resident who is injured or in distress alone.

INCIDENT REPORT

Despite the most watchful care, accidents sometimes happen. When this occurs, documentation of the event must be completed and included in the resident's health record. Forms also must be completed when the injury involves the staff or visitors. In your report:

1. Include the date and time of the incident or the time you first observed the resident.
2. Briefly describe the facts as you observed them. Do not offer opinions.
3. Include the action that was taken and the resident's reaction to it.
4. Include what action has been taken to prevent a recurrence of the event.
5. Record the name of the staff member who was notified. Sign your name.

STAFF SAFETY

It is important to carry out safe routines that protect your own health and that of other staff members as well as the health of the residents. Following the policy book and procedure manual is one way to do this.

Proper disposal of glass, broken equipment, and sharp articles such as needles can prevent serious injuries. Proper body mechanics can prevent many of the back injuries that are common to nursing assistants. Proper aseptic techniques protect both the residents and yourself from infection.

INFECTION CONTROL

Infections can occur when disease-producing organisms enter the body. Infectious diseases can cause distress in both residents and staff. Infections that occur while in the care facility are called **nosocomial**. Residents are particularly susceptible to infections of the urinary and respiratory tracts. Their **chronic** (long term) illness and/or advanced age can rob them of much of their natural resistance. Visitors and staff members may introduce infections that rapidly pass from resident to resident. Diseases passed this way are called **communicable**. The control of the spread (**transmission**) of these infections is based on three principles:

Infections are easily transmitted from person to person.

1. Keeping infected persons from visiting or working in the facility.
2. Interrupting the transmission of infectious agents, or **germs**, from one resident to another through medical aseptic techniques such as proper handwashing.
3. Separating those who are ill (isolation techniques).

Staff members who are infectious should not be on duty. Caring for your own health is vital in preventing yourself from becoming ill. Visitors should be encouraged not to visit when they do not feel well. Most visitors are cooperative, since they do not want their loved one put in danger. If a visitor is coughing or sneezing and obviously sick, refer the matter to the charge nurse. Residents who are infectious should be separated and placed into appropriate **isolation** until they no longer can spread the germs to others.

Asepsis

Asepsis means the *total* absence of microbial contamination. In real life this is difficult to obtain. We will be discussing *medical asepsis—*

specific procedures that you can carry out to prevent the spread of infection in the facility. Some knowledge of how infections are caused and spread is necessary if you are to understand the techniques used to control infection.

Pathogens are microbes which cause disease.

Causes of Infections. Infections are caused by germs known as **pathogens**. Pathogens, also called **microbes**, figure 7–12, are tiny living forms so small that they can only be seen with the aid of a **microscope**, which is an instrument that greatly magnifies objects. Pathogenic microbes increase their numbers rapidly and can do great injury to the body. There are many different kinds of microbes, and they are passed from the sick person to others in different ways.

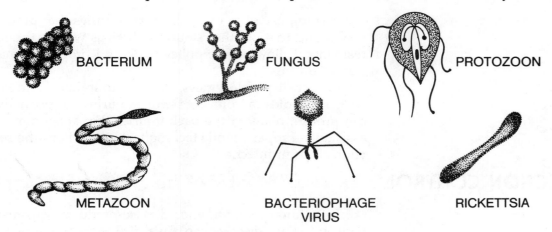

FIGURE 7–12. Samples of microbes.

Transmission of Infection. Viruses , bacteria and **fungi** are common pathogens that you will encounter. They can be transmitted or spread:

1. through respiratory secretions
2. through **excreta** (feces and urine)
3. through draining wounds
4. on instruments and equipment

Non-living objects, such as a drinking glass or an article of clothing, that carry germs are said to be **contaminated** and are referred to as **fomites**. Contaminated hands are a major source of germ transmission. Special techniques are used to prevent transmission through each of these routes. Handwashing is the single most important technique.

Handwashing

Transfer of germs from the sick person to the hands of the care giver and then on to other residents is controlled through proper handwashing. Proper handwashing is the keystone of medical asepsis, figure 7–13. Because nursing assistants realize this, handwashing is carried out:

- before eating
- after toileting
- after eating, drinking or smoking
- before carrying out procedures
- after caring for each resident
- any time the hands are soiled

Remember, microbes are so small that they may be present even though you cannot see them.

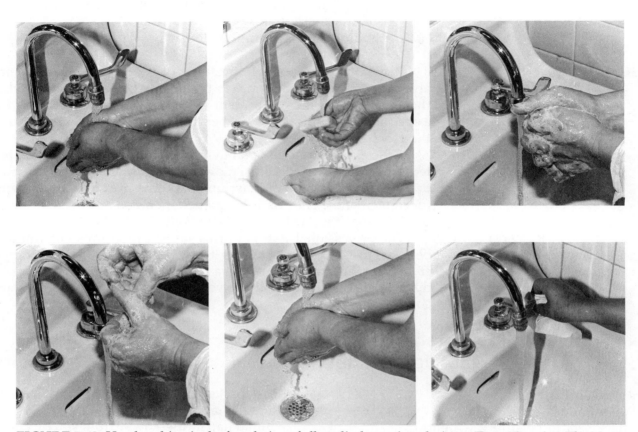

FIGURE 7–13. *Handwashing is the foundation of all medical asepsis technique.* (From Brooks, *The Nurse Assistant,* copyright 1978 by Delmar Publishers Inc.)

▓▓▓▓ PROCEDURE: Handwashing ▪▪▪▪▪▪▪▪▪▪▪▪▪▪▪▪▪▪▪▪▪▪▪▪▪▪

1. Assemble the following equipment:
   soap   paper towels   waste can
2. Turn on the faucet with a paper towel held between the hand and the faucet; drop the paper towel in the waste can.
3. Wet hands with the fingertips pointed downward.
4. Pick up the soap and rinse and lather the hands well. Rinse soap and replace in soap dish or apply liquid soap to hands and lather well.
5. Rub hands together in a circular motion and by interlacing fingers; clean fingernails. Rinse and repeat.
6. Rinse hands, fingertips down and dry them thoroughly.
7. Turn off the faucet with another paper towel; drop the paper towel in the waste can.

Natural Defenses____

Breaks in the skin are to be avoided since intact skin makes it more difficult for germs to enter the body and cause an infection. An unbroken skin is one of the body's natural defenses against microbes around us. Other natural defenses include:

- tears
- the mucus membrane of the respiratory, reproductive, and genitourinary tracts
- hydrochloric acid in the stomach

Aseptic Technique___

Remember, the possible presence of germs capable of causing an infection on an article makes that article contaminated. A glass that has been used by a resident with a cold should be handled in a special way (medical asepsis) because it has been contaminated by the resident's germs.

Articles that are free of all living organisms are **sterile**. **Aseptic technique** is used to handle sterile articles. Many articles such as gauze dressing, applicators, and instruments come prepackaged in paper for convenience. They must be opened, handled and used in special ways so that they will not become contaminated.

Sterile means no living organisms.

The professional staff performs sterile procedures but you may be asked to assist them. At times it may be necessary for you to apply sterile 4 × 4 gauze dressings to a resident. Study the procedure for opening sterile packages so that you can carefully carry it out without contamination.

 PROCEDURE: Opening a Sterile Package ■■■■■■■■■■■■■■■■■■■■■■■

Wrapped in Paper
1. Wash hands.
2. Check seal to be sure it is intact.
3. With two hands, grasp each side of separated end and gently pull apart, figure 7–14.
4. Do not open until the nurse or physician is ready to use the article.
5. If the article is to be taken by the nurse or physician, open only enough to expose the end sufficiently to be withdrawn without contamination.

Double-wrapped in Cloth
1. Wash hands.
2. Check tape seal to be sure color change indicating sterility has taken place.

3. Place package folded side up on a flat surface.
4. Remove tape.
5. Unfold flap farthest away from you by grasping outer surface only between thumb and forefinger.
6. Open left flap with left hand using same technique.
7. Open right flap with right hand using same technique.
8. Open final flap (nearest to you). Touch only the outside of flap. Be careful not to stand too close. Do not allow uniform to touch flap as it is lifted free. Be sure the flaps are pulled open completely to prevent them from folding back up over the sterile field.

Handling of Contaminated Articles _____

Infection control measures are special processing techniques used to control and destroy germs.

Special **aseptic techniques** must be used with all articles that might be carrying germs. Those articles which are not to be reused, such as dressings or tissues, should be tightly wrapped before discarding and disposing of them. Articles that are to be reused must be cleaned and processed to make them safe for reuse.

Disinfection. This is the process of destroying disease-producing organisms by using chemicals, figure 7–15. Chemical *disinfectants* do not kill *all* organisms that might be present on an article. Commonly used disinfectants include:

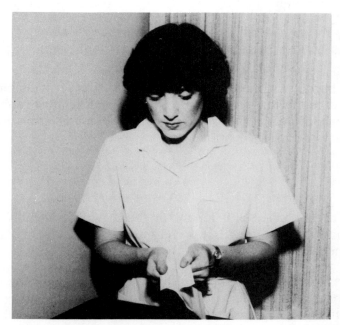

FIGURE 7-14. Never allow your fingers to touch the contents of the package.

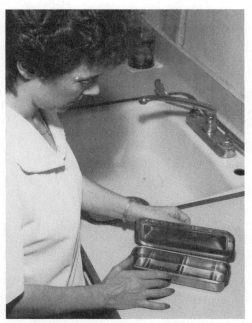

FIGURE 7-15. Soaking contaminated articles in a disinfectant solution enables them to be safely reused.

- alcohol
- aldehyde phenol
- chlorine

Disinfectants take time to be effective and must touch every surface of the article. To disinfect properly:

1. Read the directions carefully.
2. Completely cover articles and/or fill all tubings with the solution.
3. If necessary, take articles apart so that all surfaces may be in contact with the solution.

Antisepsis. This is the use chemicals on skin surfaces to destroy germs. Common chemical *antiseptics* include:

- alcohol
- iodine
- iodophor
- chlorhexidine

Sterilization

In some cases it may be desirable to completely destroy all microorganisms. This process is known as **sterilization**. Steam under pressure is the most common sterilization process in use. Many facilities have a machine called an **autoclave** that is used for this purpose. The autoclave operates in a way similar to a pressure cooker. Be sure you know how t operate the machine before you attempt to do so. Here again, time is an important factor in effectiveness. Remember, you are using very hot steam — never stand directly in front of the unit when opening the door at the end of the sterilization process.

UNIVERSAL PRECAUTIONS

Universal barrier technique is based on the simple principle that all residents have potential for spreading infection. Therefore, the health care provider should wear protective items when touching blood or body fluids of any resident. Protective barriers include:

- gloves
- gown
- mask

The use of these barriers will depend on the level of protection needed to carry out a procedure. Check with the charge nurse if and when barriers are necessary in the facility.

Isolation

The main purpose of **isolation** precautions is to prevent the spread of microorganisms among residents, personnel, and visitors.

To reduce the risk of spreading germs it is necessary to carry out adequate isolation technique.

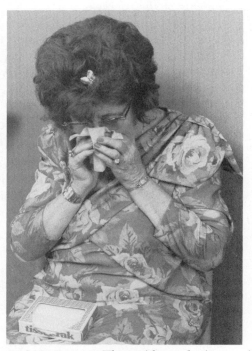

FIGURE 7–16. The resident who is sneezing and has flu symptoms should be isolated.

PROCEDURE: Isolation Techniques

Outside the Door

1. Place a "Barrier," "Isolation," or "Precaution" sign on the door.
2. Place a bedside table or cart beside the door and supply it with:
   a. isolation gowns, masks and gloves, if ordered
   b. waxed paper bags and/or plastic bags

Inside the Room

1. Line wastepaper basket with a plastic bag.
2. Supply a laundry hamper with a waterproof bag.
3. Check the supply of paper towels and liquid soap in a foot-operated dispenser.

Putting on and removing mask, gown, and gloves. To don clean mask and gown (figure 7–17):

1. Wash hands, following proper handwashing techniques.
2. Adjust mask over nose and mouth and tie securely.
3. Put on gown, slipping arms into sleeves.
4. Slip fingers under inside of neckband and grasp ties in the back. Secure in bowknot.
5. Reach behind and overlap the edges of the gown to cover uniform completely. Secure waist ties.
6. Don non-sterile disposable gloves.

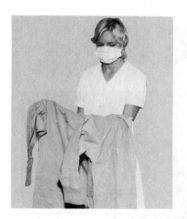 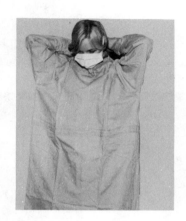 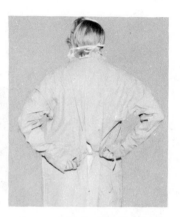

FIGURE 7–17. Gowning technique: A, Slip arms in sleeves; B, tie gown at neck; C, fasten at waist.

To put on gloves, if required, follow the procedure shown below.

▪▪▪ PROCEDURE: Donning Nonsterile Disposable Gloves, figure 7–18 ▪▪▪▪▪▪▪▪▪▪▪▪▪▪

1. Wash hands and dry thoroughly.
2. Open sterile package on a flat clean surface.
3. Make a cuff on each glove.
4. Grasp left glove with right thumb and fingers by the top of the glove.
5. Bring left thumb toward palm of hand.
6. Slip fingers into glove, easing glove over hand and fingers as you pull glove on with opposite hand.
7. Pick up right glove with left hand by slipping fingers of gloved hand under the cuff.
8. Curve fingers of right hand, bending thumb slightly forward and insert into glove.
9. Spread fingers slightly to slide into proper areas.
10. Adjust gloves by interlacing fingers.

To remove contaminated gloves, follow the procedure given on page 90.

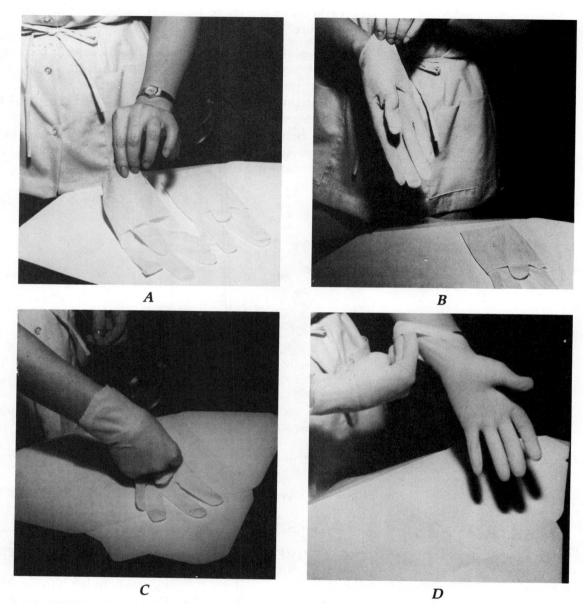

FIGURE 7–18. *Gloving technique: A, Grasp one glove by the cuff; B, lift the right glove clear of the package; curve your fingers and insert them into the glove, drawing the glove over your hand; C, slip gloved fingers under the cuff of the other glove; D, slip your left hand into the glove cuff and draw it over the hand and wrist.*

PROCEDURE: Removing Contaminated Disposable Gloves

1. Slip soiled gloved fingers of right hand under cuff of opposite hand, touching the glove only.
2. Pull glove down to fingers, exposing thumb.
3. Slip uncovered thumb into opposite cuff.
4. Allow glove-covered fingers of left hand to touch only the outer portion of soiled glove.
5. Pull glove down over right hand almost to fingertips and slip glove on to other hand.
6. With right hand touching only the inside of the left glove or hand, continue pulling left glove over right hand until only clean surface is outermost.
7. Dispose of gloves according to facility policy.
8. Wash hands thoroughly.

To remove contaminated gown and mask:

1. Undo waist ties and loosen gown at waist.
2. Turn on faucets, holding a clean paper towel. Discard paper towel in waste basket.
3. Wash hands carefully and dry with paper towels.
4. With a dry paper towel, turn off faucet; dispose of paper towel. Hands are not considered clean.
5. Undo mask. Holding by ties only, deposit in proper container.
6. Undo neck ties and loosen gown at shoulders.
7. Slip fingers of the right hand inside the left cuff without touching the outside of the gown. Pull gown down and over the left hand.
8. Pull gown down over the right hand with the gown-covered left hand.
9. Fold gown with contaminated side inward. Roll and deposit in laundry bag or waste container, if disposable.
10. Rewash hands using same technique.
11. Remove watch from clean paper towel. Touch only clean side of paper towel and deposit in the waste basket.
12. Open door with clean paper towel. Prop door open with foot and drop paper towel in waste basket.

Transferring Food and Disposable Items Outside the Isolation Unit. Two people assist in the transfer. One "dirty" person is inside the unit and a "clean" person is outside. Leftover liquids and food from the resident's meal are disposed of in the toilet. Be careful not to splash. Hard food such as bones should be wrapped in plastic (check facility policy regarding disposal of food).

For transfer of disposable items the following guidelines should be followed:

1. Door is opened with paper towel and propped with foot.
2. "Clean" person on outside holds cuffed plastic bag over hands to receive tray, or other items.
3. "Clean" person secures top of plastic bag tightly.
4. Disposable or expendable (throw-away) items such as dishes may be put in the waste container in the room.
5. Dressings should be sealed in a plastic bag and then deposited in a cuffed bag held by outside person.
6. The person outside the unit secures the second bag. The bag is then sent to the appropriate department (laundry, kitchen, central supply, or maintenance) where the items will be cared for according to department procedures.

Transferring Nondisposable Equipment Outside the Isolation Unit. Equipment that must be reused (nonexpendable) may be double-bagged in plastic, labeled "isolation," and sent to the central service for sterilization. Some equipment may also be washed and soaked in a disinfectant solution in the room for a prescribed length of time or sent for a higher level of sterilization.

Collecting a Specimen in the Isolation Unit. To collect a specimen in the unit:

1. Don non-sterile disposable gloves.
2. Place a clean specimen container and cover on a clean paper towel.
3. Place specimen in container without touching the container.
4. After properly disposing of the receptacle in which the specimen was collected, wash hands thoroughly.
5. Cover specimen and label. Place specimen in a plastic bag for transport, attach requisition and send to the laboratory.

Care of Laundry in the Isolation Unit (Double-Bagging), figure 7–19. Clean linen is brought to the unit as needed. Soiled linen is placed in a bag in the laundry hamper. When it is one half to two thirds full, the top is closed, and disposed of as follows:

1. A clean person cuffs and holds a specially marked laundry bag outside the room and receives the soiled laundry bag.
2. The cover of the outside bag is securely tied, and the linen is disposed of in accord with facility policy.

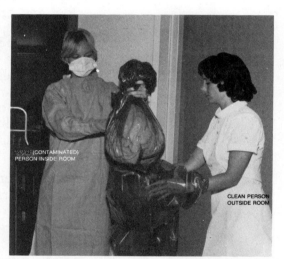

FIGURE 7–19. Double-bagging technique. Note that cuff of bag protects the clean person's hands.

Transporting the Patient in Isolation. Notify the charge nurse or others in the department where you will be transporting the resident that a resident from isolation is on the way. Identify the resident and tell what is planned and how the resident can be assisted. After reassuring the resident, you should:

1. Cover wheelchair or stretcher with clean sheets and wheel it into the room.
2. Put on clean gown, following proper technique, and assist the resident into the wheelchair or onto the stretcher.
3. Mask the resident if deemed advisable.

4. Wrap the resident in a sheet and instruct him or her not to touch the wheelchair or stretcher.
5. As unit is left, remove gown, following proper technique.

Nursing assistants can do much to limit the spread of infection. Keeping the residents and their environment clean is a basic step in limiting the development of infections and the transfer of infectious material to others.

VOCABULARY

antiseptic technique	disinfection	infection
asepsis	enteric	isolation
autoclave	excreta	medical asepsis
bacteria	fomite	microbe
cardiopulmonary resuscitation (CPR)	gait belt	nosocomial
	gavage	pathogen
cheeking	germ	sterile
chronic	gurney	sterilization
communicable	Heimlich maneuver	transmission
contaminated	hemorrhage	virus

SUGGESTED ACTIVITIES

1. Practice the procedures outlined in this unit until you and your instructor feel secure that you are adept in them.

2. Review the fire policy in your facility's policy manual.

3. Locate fire equipment in your facility.

4. Practice using a fire extinguisher.

5. Visit a facility and have a staff member or instructor demonstrate the safe operation of an autoclave.

6. Discuss ways in which you can help prevent the spread of infection.

REVIEW

A. Brief Answer/Fill in the Blanks

1. Who is responsible for safety practices?

    _____

2. List three reasons why residents in a long term care facility are vulnerable to accidents.

    a. _____

    b. _____

    c. _____

3. The major accident involving residents is _____.

4. Name two other common accidents among the elderly.

    a. _____

    b. _____

5. List three things you could do to decrease the possibility of accidental burns.

   a. _____

   b. _____

   c. _____

6. Equipment can be a source of danger. Describe five actions you could take to improve safety.

   a. _____

   b. _____

   c. _____

   d. _____

   e. _____

7. Residents are unlikely to be able to help themselves in a fire situation because of _____

   _____

   _____

8. The _____ has written guidelines for the Heimlich maneuver and for CPR.

9. Nosocomial infections are infections that are acquired in _____.

10. Proper medical aseptic techniques protect staff and residents from

   _____ .

CLINICAL SITUATION

You have just completed your morning duties, have reported to the charge nurse, and you are now on a coffee break. As you pass Mr. Ryan's room, you see he is lying on the floor unconscious. What should you do?

Answer: _____

_____

_____

A new section on isolation techniques follows on Page 94A.

ISOLATION TECHNIQUE

There are three key points to be remembered at all times for isolation technique.

1. Isolation technique is the name given to the method of caring for patients with easily transmitted diseases.
2. It is essential that every person take responsibility and use the proper isolation technique to prevent the spread of the disease to others.
3. All items that come into contact with the patient's excretions, secretions, blood, or body fluids containing the known or suspected microbe are considered contaminated. This potentially infective material must be treated in a special way.

Isolation Unit

The isolation area may be a unit or a private room. A room with handwashing facilities and an adjoining room with bathing and toilet facilities is best. A private room is indicated for patients who:

- are highly infectious
- have poor personal hygiene
- require special air control procedures within the room

Handwashing

Handwashing is basic to the practice of the isolation technique. Handwashing is the single most important means of preventing the spread of infection for all isolation precautions. Health care workers wash their hands as described earlier in this lesson, even when gloves are used.

Cover Gown

A gown (fabric or paper) should be used when soiling with secretions or excretions is likely. The use of the gown prevents self-contamination. It also prevents contamination of the uniform with the infective material. When using a gown, it should be worn only once. Discard gowns after use in an appropriate place.

Gloves

The use of disposable gloves (latex or vinyl) prevents contamination of the hands when touching the known infective material. For example, gloves should be worn when emptying the bedpan of a patient in enteric precautions. The patient's feces is the infective material that requires special handling to prevent the spread of disease.

Face Mask

Masks are to be worn when exposure to droplet secretions may occur. For example, a suspected tuberculosis patient who is coughing is releasing into the air moisture droplets containing the tuberculosis bacillus. When a mask is indicated, it is:

- used only once and discarded.
- discarded if it becomes moist.
- never left secured around the neck as it can contaminate the uniform and the environment.

A mask that covers both the nose and the mouth will give protection from the airborne spread of microbes.

Equipment_____

Disposable patient-care equipment is used widely. It is ideal for patients on isolation precautions. Frequently used equipment remains in the patient's unit. Most articles will not require special handling unless they are contaminated (or likely to be contaminated) with infective material.

Special precautions are not necessary for dishes unless they are visibly contaminated with infective material. An example of this would be dishes that have blood, drainage, or secretions on them. Disposable dishes that have been contaminated with infective material can be handled as disposable patient-care equipment.

Containment of Articles_____

Special handling of contaminated articles is called *bagging of articles*. It is important that contaminated equipment be bagged, labeled, and disposed of in accordance with the health care facility's policy for the disposal of infectious waste. Used articles are placed in an impenetrable bag (such as plastic) before they are removed from the room or unit of the patient. A single bag may be used if it is sturdy enough to confine and contain the article without contaminating the outside of the bag. Otherwise, the technique of double-bagging should be used.

In double-bagging, two bags are used to contain the contaminated items. Two people are needed for this procedure. One person works inside the patient's room. The second person is outside the door of the room. The person inside the patient's room places the contaminated articles in a plastic bag and seals the bag securely. This person opens the door of the patient's room and places the sealed bag into another bag held by the second health care worker. The outside of the second bag must not be contaminated by the first bag. The second health care worker then seals the second bag and labels it with an isolation tag. Separate bags are used for linens, equipment, and disposables.

▩▩▩ PROCEDURE: Putting On and Taking Off a Disposable Paper Face Mask ▩▩▩▩▩▩▩▩▩▩▩▩▩

1. Wash your hands.
2. Adjust the mask over your nose and mouth. Be careful not to touch your face with your hands.
3. First tie top strings of the mask behind your head. Then tie bottom strings securely.
4. Replace mask if it becomes moist during procedure.
5. When ready to dispose of mask, wash your hands first.
6. Untie bottom strings first.
7. Untie top strings. Remove the mask by holding the top strings. Discard in appropriate infectious waste receptacle, located inside the patient's room.
8. Wash your hands.

PROCEDURE: Putting On a Cover Gown

1. Remove your wristwatch and place on the clean side of an open paper towel.
2. Wash your hands.
3. Put on cover gown by slipping arms into sleeves.
4. Slip fingers under inside neckband and grasp ties in the back. Secure neckband with a simple bow, or fasten velcro strips.
5. Reach behind and overlap the edges of the gown so that your uniform is completely covered. Secure waist ties with a simple bow, or fasten velcro strips.
6. **Note:** The watch will be carried with you into the isolation unit. It will remain on the paper towel so it can be referred to without being touched.

PROCEDURE: Removing Contaminated Cover Gown, Gloves, and Mask

1. Remove gloves, turning them inside out. Dispose of gloves.
2. Undo waist ties of the gown.
3. Holding a clean paper towel, turn faucets on. Discard towel.
4. Wash your hands. Dry with paper towel.
5. Holding a dry paper towel, turn off faucets.
6. Undo mask (bottom ties first, then top ties). Holding by ties only, dispose of mask.
7. Undo the neck ties and loosen gown at shoulders.
8. Slip the fingers of the right hand inside the left cuff without touching the outside of the gown. Pull gown down over the left hand.
9. With the gown-covered left hand, pull the gown down over the-right hand.
10. Fold gown with contaminated side inward. Roll and dispose of in appropriate receptacle.
11. Wash hands using the technique described in steps 3—5.
12. Remove watch from clean side of paper towel. Holding clean side of paper towel, dispose of towel in wastepaper receptacle.

PROCEDURE: Double-Bagging to Transfer Contaminated Articles Outside the Isolation Unit

Key Point: this procedure is not always required. Check the policy of your facility.

1. Two people assist in the procedure. One person is inside the unit, and a ''clean'' person is outside the unit.
2. Inside the unit, place the item into an isolation bag (usually a color-coded plastic bag).
3. Secure with a tie.
4. The person on the outside of the isolation unit holds the cuffed plastic bag over hands to receive bagged item.
5. The clean person secures top of plastic bag tightly.
6. Clean person removes double-bagged item. Disposable items are routed as infectious waste.

PROCEDURE: Transferring Non-Disposable Equipment Outside the Isolation Unit

1. Equipment that requires reprocessing may be double-bagged and sent to the central service for sterilization.
2. Some equipment may not require sterilization. It can be terminally cleaned with an appropriate disinfectant in the patient's room.

PROCEDURE: Collecting a Specimen in the Isolation Unit ▪▪▪▪▪▪▪▪▪▪▪▪▪▪▪▪▪▪▪▪▪▪▪▪▪▪

1. Bring a clean specimen container and cover into the unit. Place them on a clean paper towel.
2. Put on gloves. Place specimen into container without touching the container.
3. Cover specimen and label.
4. Remove gloves and wash your hands.
5. Using a clean paper towel, pick up specimen and place it in a plastic transport bag. Have specimen transported to the laboratory.

▪▪▪ PROCEDURE: Caring for Linen in the Isolation Unit ▪▪▪▪▪▪▪▪▪▪▪▪▪▪▪▪▪▪▪▪▪▪▪▪▪▪

1. Bring clean linen to the unit as needed.
2. Handle soiled linen as little as possible.
3. Place soiled linen in leakproof laundry bag in unit.
4. The bag should be labeled or identified by color code.
5. Secure the bag and route linen according to facility policy. Many facilities use a plastic-type outer bag that dissolves in the washer, freeing the linen. With this type of bag, personnel do not have to handle the linen after it leaves the isolation unit.

▪▪▪ PROCEDURE: Transporting the Resident in Isolation ▪▪▪▪▪▪▪▪

1. Notify the department that the patient from isolation is being transported to their department. Identify the type of isolation technique required.
2. Cover transport vehicle with a clean sheet and wheel into the room.
3. Identify the patient and tell her what you plan to do and how she can assist you.
4. If required, put on appropriate barriers such as gown, mask, or gloves, Assist patient on-to transport vehicle.
5. Mask the patient, if required.
6. Wrap the patient in a sheet, if required.
7. Remove your gown and other barriers as you leave the unit, following the proper technique.
8. Upon return from the other department, return the patient to the unit. Follow appropriate barrier technique as requried and return patient to her bed.
9. Remove the sheet from transport vehicle and deposit in soiled linen hamper.
10. Wash your hands.

SUMMARY ▪▪▪

When patients have communicable diseases that are easily transmitted to others, special techniques must be used. The patient is placed in isolation. Everyone coming into contact with the patient must practice appropriate isolation techniques. The emphasis is on the infective material that carries the specific microorganisms. The goal of the health care worker is to interrupt the chain of infection by preventing the transmission of the microbes. By working toward this goal, the health care worker protects the patient, the environment, and self.

LESSON 8 Care of the Environment

OBJECTIVES

After studying this lesson, you should be able to:

- State the ways in which a clean, safe environment can be maintained.
- Describe concurrent and terminal cleaning.
- Demonstrate the safe operation of the bed and appliances.
- Demonstrate the proper way to make an unoccupied bed.
- Demonstrate the proper way to make an occupied bed.
- Define and spell all vocabulary words and terms.

Maintaining a safe, clean environment for the residents is a major responsibility of each nursing assistant. As a rule, since residents are up and dressed as much as possible, it will be necessary to make **unoccupied beds**; however, in some cases, you will need to make the bed with the resident in it—known as **occupied bedmaking**.

Each day you will care for the resident's personal belongings and ensure that the resident unit and the other areas are safe and clean. **Concurrent cleaning** activities go on daily. Concurrent cleaning is also known as *scheduled* or *routine cleaning*. Certain special cleaning procedures are carried out weekly. Others, known as **terminal cleaning**, are performed after a resident is discharged in order to prepare the unit for a new admission.

Proper handwashing, medical asepsis, and isolation are the foundation of methods used to control infectious germs. You may wish to go back to Lesson 7 and quickly review this material.

A safe environment is a clean environment.

ENVIRONMENTAL CONTROL

Environmental control should contribute to the comfort and safety of the residents. There is much you can do to create a safe, comfortable environment.

Eliminate drafts and keep the temperature fairly constant. Older people tend to feel chilly. Keep the temperature between 70 and 72 degrees Fahrenheit. A lap robe (figure 8–1), sweater, or shawl may add comfort. Screens and drapes can be used to shield the resident from drafts if deemed helpful.

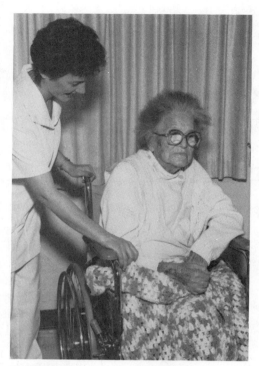

FIGURE 8–1. A lap robe adds comfort, keeping the resident from feeling chilly.

Make sure that there is adequate lighting. This is especially important at twilight and during the hours of dark. A night light near the floor will not be disturbing and is an added safety measure.

Prevent falls. Floors should be clean but not highly polished to the point of being slippery. Wipe up any spilled liquid immediately.

Return all equipment as soon as you finish using it. Clutter is very disturbing to the older person and is a safety hazard.

Keep all areas clean. Dust and dirt, crumbs from food, and dirty dishes and glasses harbor microbes and can contribute to the spread of disease. Food that is left around also draws insects, such as roaches and ants, figure 8–2. Remove all dishes as soon as they are no longer in use and clean up eating areas right away. Daily damp-dusting helps cut down on dust and the spread of germs. Housekeeping personnel will do much of the routine cleaning, such as the floors and bathrooms, but you are responsible for a safe and orderly environment, so do not neglect regular policing of all areas.

CONCURRENT CLEANING

Concurrent cleaning goes on every day as you damp-dust and straighten up the unit. Once each week, however, a more thorough cleaning is done. The mattress and bed frame are cleaned, using a disinfectant solution. The bedside stand, or table, is washed inside

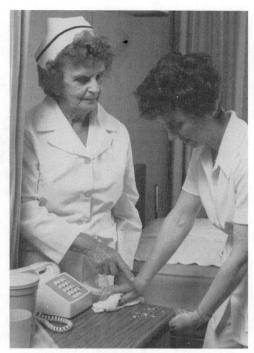

FIGURE 8–2. Food scraps draw insects and create an unhealthy environment.

and out, drawers are left open to dry. Equipment such as bed pans, emesis basins, and wash basins are also thoroughly cleaned and disinfected.

Many facilities encourage residents to retain personal belongings, but some articles are not permitted, figure 8–3. Although individual facility policy varies, usually uncovered food, matches, cigarettes, and razors are not permitted to be kept in the resident unit. Check the regulations in your facility and follow them carefully.

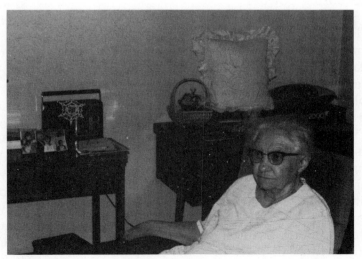

FIGURE 8–3. Residents are encouraged to bring personal items from their homes.

TERMINAL CLEANING

Terminal cleaning is done when a resident is discharged, figure 8–4. It is a complete cleaning.

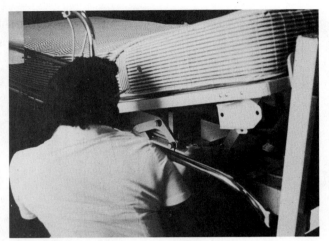

FIGURE 8–4. *After the resident leaves, a thorough terminal cleaning is performed.*

PROCEDURE: Terminal Cleaning of the Resident Unit

1. Assemble the following equipment:
   a. Basin of warm water
   b. Soap
   c. Brush
   d. Cleaning cloths
   e. Disinfectant solution
   f. Laundry hamper
   g. Newspaper for waste
   h. Scouring powder
   i. Stretcher
   j. Radiator brush
2. Remove any special equipment. Be sure it is clean and returned to the proper area.
3. Remove all disposable material from bedside table and wrap in newspaper to be burned. Do not discard anything that may be claimed by the resident or by members of his or her family.
4. Remove all basic equipment from bedside stand. Wash reusable equipment with hot water and detergent, and/or sterilize according to facility policy. If equipment is disposable, clean it and send the equipment home with resident or place in waste receptacle.
5. Strip bed and discard linen in laundry hamper. Place pillows on chair.

6. Take rubber drawsheet, if used, to utility room and wash with soap and water and rinse with disinfectant solution. Allow to dry thoroughly. Some facilities put plastic draw sheets in the laundry.
7. Move stretcher beside the bed. With help, lift mattress from bed to stretcher.
8. Dry-dust the coils of the bedsprings, using a long-handled radiator brush.
9. Using a cleaning cloth and disinfectant solution:
   a. Wash plastic cover on mattress with a damp cloth and damp-dust pillow surface.
   b. Wash bed frame, including the bedsprings. Remove parts for thorough cleaning, using scouring powder if needed.
   c. Wash bedside table inside and out. Leave drawers open to air.
   d. Wash bedside chair after placing pillows on mattress.
   e. Wash lamp and call bell cord.
10. Damp-dust all surfaces of mattress and pillows.
11. Place clean equipment in bedside stand and stock according to facility policy.

12. Air out bed as long as possible to be sure all moisture has evaporated.
13. Replace mattress and remake bed, (see procedure for unoccupied bedmaking).
14. Place bed in lowest horizontal position.
15. Place bedside table at head on right side of bed. Place chair at foot on same side. Place overhead table across from chair. Check the call bell and overbed lamp to be sure they are operating correctly. Line the waste basket with clean plastic. Try side rails to be sure they attach securely and then leave rails in the down position. Leave unit orderly.
16. Wash hands. Return cleaning supplies.
17. Report completion of task.

THE RESIDENT UNIT

Each resident is entitled to private space conveniently arranged.

The resident unit may be in a single room or it may be a space in a room shared with others and separated by curtains. The curtains may be drawn for privacy. Each unit consists of:

- bed
- bedside table, or stand
- chair
- overbed table
- storage space

All beds are equipped with adjustable side rails, and bed position is adjustable. The changing of bed position may be controlled electrically or by cranks found at the foot of the bed. Be sure cranks are returned to the non-use position so that no one will be injured by bumping into them, figure 8–5. Similarly, the large wheels often found on the beds should be locked to prevent the bed from rolling, and the wheels should be turned inward to prevent tripping over them.

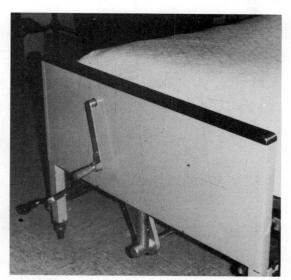

FIGURE 8–5. Cranks and handles can cause injury if not properly released.

Potential Hazards

Potential hazards in the resident units need attention; if overlooked, they could be dangerous.

Check for broken equipment. Make routine checks for frayed electrical cords, broken straps, and worn tips on canes and walkers. Make sure the intercom is always functional and that the signal button is operable and within reach of the resident. Electrical appliances should not be brought into the facility unless checked out by the maintenance department.

Arrange the furniture and equipment for the resident's convenience. A commode (bedside toilet) is of little value if a resident cannot reach it in time to use it.

Use bed rails properly. Bed rails are important safety features on all beds. They must be raised and lowered correctly and always checked for security. Bed rails must be up and secure at bedtime, when the bed is elevated from the floor, and at any other time that the condition of the resident makes it necessary.

Privacy

Remember, the resident's room or unit is his or her home. Be careful that you do not rearrange things without permission. Residents become used to the placement of their possessions, and a moved chair or table can be the cause of an injury. Even if a room is shared with others, a resident and his or her private space needs to be respected. Knock before entering a room and speak before drawing back a curtain. Draw curtains when carrying out procedures to assure privacy.

Beds

The bed is an important part of the resident unit.

Special adjustable **gatch beds** are used in the resident units. These can be raised in height to make giving care easier and lowered to make it safer and easier for the resident to get in and out of bed. The bed back can be elevated to different positions for comfort.

Linens

Bed linen should be changed as needed, but usually linen is changed completely, at least once or twice a week, on the days that

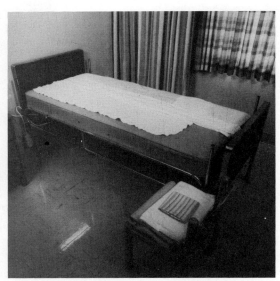

FIGURE 8–6. Note placement of bottom linens.

the resident is bathed. Pillow cases and cotton draw sheets (half sheets) are changed more often, usually daily. (The draw sheet may be changed frequently without needing to change the entire bedding.) Hospital mattresses that are treated with plastic do not require a moisture-proof sheet or cotton draw sheet. In some cases, the draw sheet may be used as a lifter to assist in moving the resident; it is usually used to keep the bottom sheet clean.

Since most residents are out of bed for long periods of time, the linen need not be changed as frequently as in an acute care setting. Nevertheless, soiled linen should be replaced right away.

It is essential that all bottom linens be smooth and tight, figure 8–6. Lying on wrinkles is uncomfortable and can lead to skin breakdown and the formation of bedsores (decubitis ulcers).

Dirty linens should be folded inward and never shaken, to prevent the spread of germs. Do not allow dirty linen to touch your uniform. Also, never allow clean linen to touch the floor, which must be considered a "dirty" area.

▪▪▪▪ PROCEDURE: Making the Unoccupied Bed ▪▪▪▪▪▪▪▪▪▪▪▪▪▪▪▪▪▪▪▪▪▪▪▪▪▪▪▪

1. Wash hands and assemble the following equipment:
   a. pillowcases
   b. spread
   c. blankets, as needed
   d. 2 large sheets (90 x 109) (substitute 1 fitted, if used)
   e. half-sheet (draw sheet)
   f. mattress pad and cover
2. Lock bed wheels so the bed will not roll and place chair at the side of the bed.
3. Arrange linen on chair in order in which it is to be used.
4. Position mattress to head of bed by grasping handles on mattress side.
5. Place mattress cover on mattress and adjust it smoothly.
6. Work entirely from one side of the bed until that side is completed, and then go to the other side of the bed. This conserves time and energy.
7. Place and unfold bottom sheet, smooth side (hem side) up with wide hem at the top, and center fold at the center of the bed or position and tuck in bottom sheet on one side.
8. Tuck 12 to 18 inches of sheet smoothly over the top of the mattress.
9. Make a mitered or squared corner.
10. Tuck in the sheet on one side, keeping it straight. Work from the head to the foot of

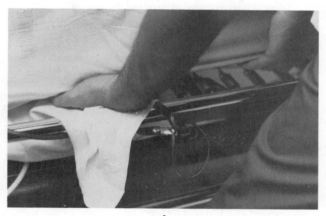

A

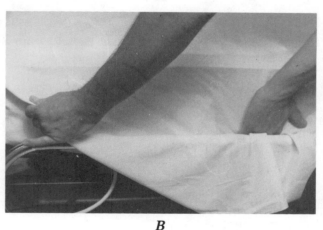

B

FIGURE 8–7. Making the unoccupied bed. A, Tuck top linen under mattress. B, Holding fold with one hand, tuck sheet in with the other hand.

the bed. Or adjust fitted sheet over the head and bottom ends of the mattress.

11. Unfold the top sheet and place wrong side up, top hem even with the upper edge of the mattress, and center fold on the center of the bed.
12. Spread blanket over the top sheet and foot of mattress. Keep blanket centered.
13. Tuck top sheet and blanket under mattress at the foot of the bed as far as the center only and make a mitered or square corner.
14. Place spread with top hem even with head of mattress.
15. Unfold to foot of bed.
16. Tuck spread under mattress at the foot of one side of bed and make mitered or square corner.
17. Go to other side of bed and fanfold the top sheet, blanket, and spread to the center of the bed in order to work with lower sheets and pad.
18. Tuck bottom sheet under head of mattress and make mitered or square corner. Working

from top to bottom, smooth out all wrinkles and tighten sheet as much as possible, or adjust fitted bottom sheet smoothly and securely around mattress corners (figure 8–8).
19. Tuck in top sheet and blanket. Pleat if it will help resident.
20. Fold top sheet back over blanket, making an 8 inch cuff.
21. Tuck in spread at foot of bed and make a mitered or square corner.
22. Bring top of spread to head of mattress.
23. Insert pillow in pillow case properly.
24. Place pillow at head of bed with open end away from the door.
25. Lower bed to lowest horizontal position.
26. Replace bedside table parallel to bed. Place chair in assigned location. Place overbed table over the foot of the bed opposite the chair. Be sure that signal cord or call bell is within easy reach of the resident.
27. Wash hands.
28. Report completion of task.

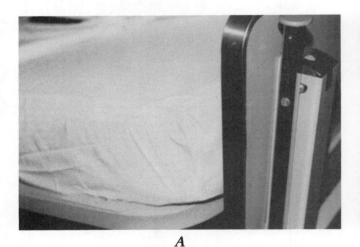
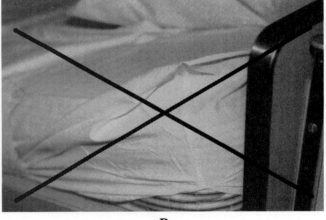

A   *B*

FIGURE 8–8. Properly fitted bottom sheet (A) and improperly fitted bottom sheet (B).

■■■ PROCEDURE: Making the Occupied Bed ■■■■■■■■■■■■■■■■■■■■■■■■■■■■

1. Wash hands and assemble the following equipment:
   a. cotton draw sheet or turning sheet for selected residents
   b. 2 pillow cases
   c. 2 large sheets (or 1 large sheet and 1 fitted one)
   d. laundry hamper
2. Identify yourself to the resident and explain what you plan to do.

3. Place bedside chair at the foot of the bed.
4. Arrange bed linen on chair in the order in which it is to be used.
5. Screen the unit for privacy.
6. The bed should be flat with wheels locked, unless otherwise indicated. Raise to working horizontal height.
7. Loosen the bedclothes on all sides by lifting the edge of the mattress with one hand and drawing bedclothes out with the other.
8. Never shake the linen because this spreads germs.
9. Adjust mattress to head of bed. Have patient bend knees, grasp bed head frame with hands, and pull on frame as you draw mattress to the top, or have another person help from the opposite side.
10. Remove covers, except for top sheet, one at a time. Fold to bottom and pick up in center. Place over the back of chair.
11. Place a clean sheet over top sheet. Have the resident hold the top edge of the clean sheet, if possible. If not, tuck the sheet beneath the resident's shoulder.
12. Slide out the soiled top sheet, from top to bottom. Discard in hamper.
13. Ask the resident to roll toward you and assist if necessary. Move one pillow with the resident and remove the other pillow. Pull up side rail.
14. Go to the other side of the bed. Fanfold the cotton drawsheet, if used, and the bottom sheet close to the resident.
15. Straighten out mattress pad. Place a clean bottom sheet on the bed so that the narrow hem comes to the edge of the mattress at the foot and the lengthwise center fold of the sheet is at the center of the bed.
16. Tuck top of clean bottom sheet under the head of the mattress.
17. Make a mitered or square corner.
18. Tuck side of bottom sheet under mattress, working toward the foot of the bed.
19. Position fresh turning sheet. If draw sheet is used, position and tuck it under the mattress.
20. Ask the resident to roll toward you and assist as needed. Move the pillow with the resident.
21. Raise side rail.
22. Go to the other side of the bed. Remove soiled linen by rolling the edges inward and place in hamper.
23. Keep soiled linen away from your uniform.
24. Complete the bed as an unoccupied bed. Make toe pleats in top sheet and blanket so that pressure is not exerted on the toes. (There are several methods of making toe pleats. One is to make a mitered or square corner but before making the final tuck, grasp the linen and make a 3-inch fold toward the foot of the bed. Then complete the corner.) Some residents prefer not to have the blanket, top sheet or spread tucked in.
25. Turn resident on back. Place clean case on pillow not being used. Replace pillow. Change other pillow case.
26. Adjust bed position for the resident's comfort.
27. Be sure side rails are up and secure. Lower bed to lowest horizontal position.
28. Place signal cord or call bell within resident's reach.
29. Replace bedside table and chair. Remove hamper.
30. Wash hands.
31. Report completion of task.

VOCABULARY

concurrent cleaning
draw sheet
environment
gatch bed

occupied bedmaking
terminal cleaning
unoccupied bedmaking

SUGGESTED ACTIVITIES

1. Practice carrying out the following procedures:
   a. terminal cleaning
   b. concurrent cleaning
   c. occupied bedmaking
   d. unoccupied bedmaking

2. Practice the operation of a bed side rail and attachments while making an occupied and unoccupied bed.

3. Make a list of disinfectant solutions used in your facility. Read the labels.

REVIEW

A. Brief Answer/Fill in the Blanks

1. The nursing assistant is responsible for maintaining a _____ environment.

2. The foundation of all cleaning procedures is _____.

3. List three things you can do to contribute to a safer environment.

   a. _____

   b. _____

   c. _____

4. Most residents prefer a room temperature of approximately _____ degrees Fahrenheit.

5. Side rails must be up and secured when:

   a. _____

   b. _____

   c. _____

6. A resident's unit is his or her _____.

7. Concurrent cleaning is done_____.

8. Terminal cleaning is done when _____ and

   _____.

9. The machine used in most facilities to sterilize equipment is called the

   _____.

10. This machine uses _____ to carry out the sterilization process.

B. True or False. Answer the following questions true (T) or false (F).

1. _____ The position of a gatch bed may be changed.

2. _____ In terminal cleaning, only the mattress needs to be thoroughly cleaned.

3. _____ Residents have linen completely changed about twice a week.

4. _____ Damp-dusting is an important part of concurrent cleaning.

5. _____ A draw sheet is a half sheet placed over the bottom sheet.

6. _____ When making an unoccupied bed, make one side completely before going to the opposite side.

7. _____ It is important that the bottom sheet be smooth.

8. _____ Pleats reduce pressure on the resident's feet.

9. _____ When making a bed, linens should be arranged on a chair with the top sheet on top.

10. _____ The mattress should be positioned to the top of the bed before fresh linen is applied.

CLINICAL SITUATION

A student visits the facility where you are employed and asks what is included in the resident unit. What is your response?

Answer: _____

_____

LESSON 9 Communicating Effectively

OBJECTIVES

After studying this lesson, you should be able to:

- State two ways in which people normally communicate.
- Identify situations that limit effective communication.
- Describe ways in which a nursing assistant can improve communication.
- Communicate in proper medical terms.
- Define and spell all vocabulary words and terms.

THE COMMUNICATION PROCESS

Messages may be verbal or nonverbal.

People communicate with one another in a variety of ways: some messages are verbal; others are non-verbal. The look in the eyes can flash a message of anger, a smile of the lips can indicate pleasure. Words are a major way of communicating, but the tone of voice, the emphasis, tell a story of their own, (figure 9–1). **Body language** and **symbols** are non-verbal signs that give directions and sometimes replace words in our understanding.

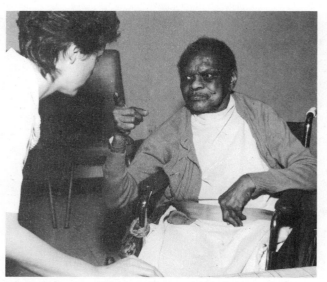

FIGURE 9–1. This resident's body language leaves little doubt that she is angry.

Body Language_____

Body language refers to messages we send through body movements. For example, a raised eyebrow indicates a question, a gentle back rub signals caring, and a turned back may signify rejection.

Symbols_____

Symbols can take the place of a word or even an entire thought. See if you can identify the meanings behind each of the symbols in figure 9–2. Symbols are non-verbal signs that communicate a message effectively. You must know and follow directions that are given through symbols. If you are unsure what an abbreviation, term or symbol stands for, be sure to ask before proceeding.

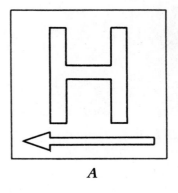
A

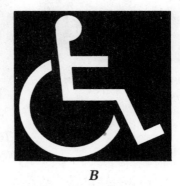
B

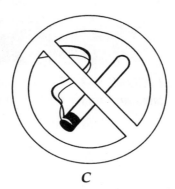
C

FIGURE 9–2. Symbols. A, Hospital in this direction; B, handicap; C, no smoking.

For successful **communication**, you must have:

- a message
- a sender
- a receiver

There are three specific groups of people in your work situations with whom you will need to effectively communicate: visitors, co-workers, and residents.

COMMUNICATING WITH VISITORS

Visitors may be family members or friends of the resident, figure 9–3. Members of the clergy may make visits, and often community groups come to cheer the residents, especially at holiday times, figure 9–4. In each case, the visitors will be observing the physical facility and how you and your co-workers interact with the residents, with each other, and with the visitors themselves.

Remember, you represent both yourself and the facility to visitors, figure 9–5. What you do and say, as well as your appearance, shows how much pride you have in yourself and your work and how much respect you have for those in your care.

Always remember that the ethical code forbids discussion of personal information; however, general information is permitted. For example, if a resident's daughter asks how her mother seems today, a general, truthful response such as "she seems more responsive" is permitted. If more specific information is required or asked for, refer the matter to the charge nurse.

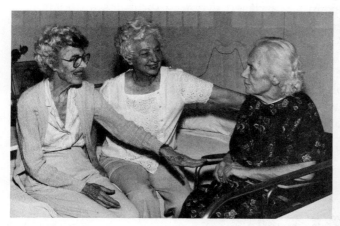

FIGURE 9–3. The love and concern are shown in the faces and touch of these visitors.

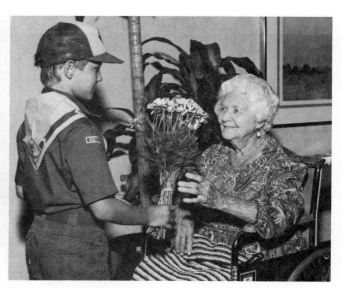

FIGURE 9–4. Community groups often visit the residents to bring cheer.

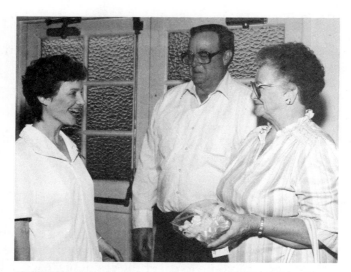

FIGURE 9–5. Remember that you represent the facility in the eyes of visitors.

Treat visitors with the same courtesy that you would extend to guests in your own home. Provide privacy as requested. If you must interrupt to provide care, excuse yourself.

Even though the resident is your primary responsibility, visitors sometimes also need support when they are stressed. A kind word or sympathetic gesture can ease the sadness a family member is feeling when the loved one is ill or fails to respond to them. Allow the family to help when possible. Above all, your assurance through words and manner that the resident is receiving the very best of care is helpful.

CO-WORKER COMMUNICATION

Words and written language are major ways that we use to communicate with co-workers. To ensure accurate communications, it is important that words are correctly used and, when written, that they are correctly spelled.

Some of the messages between co-workers are oral, directly from person to person. Think before you speak so that your ideas will be centered on the topic, figure 9–6. Try to avoid slang expressions that not only reflect poorly on your education, but also do not aptly convey your message.

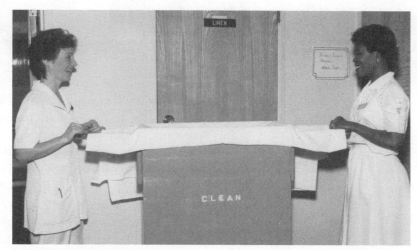

FIGURE 9–6. Think before you speak so that the message you send will be properly received.

Remember to use only accepted symbols, abbreviations, combining forms.

Listen carefully to what is being said and be observant of words that are stressed. Watch facial expressions, hand movements, and other body language for clues or meanings.

Written communications may be in the form of assignment sheets, nursing care plans, and other health record forms. Be sure to use the proper terms, printing or writing clearly and spelling accurately, so that there will be no confusion as to your meaning. Use only accepted initials and **abbreviations** (shortened forms), and use combining forms correctly. Review initial forms and abbreviations learned in Lesson 3.

COMMUNICATING WITH RESIDENTS

Communications travel in two directions. Being a good listener is as important to proper communication as being able to choose the proper words, expressions, and gestures, figure 9–7. A good listener:

- pays attention and remains centered on the conversation even though there are distractions.
- is patient with the speaker, especially if there is difficulty in communicating.
- asks questions, figure 9–8.
- reframes statements until the message is clearly understood.

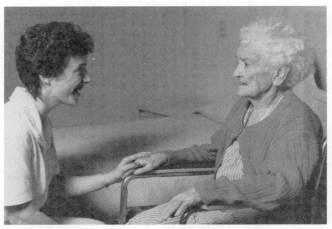

FIGURE 9–7. Hold conversations with residents whenever possible.

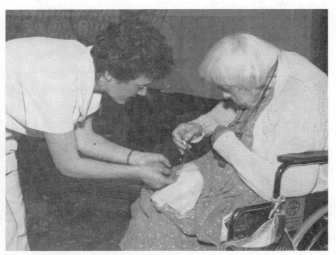

FIGURE 9–8. Show interest in the resident's activities.

Talking with residents is an important part of your work. Through your words and body language, you let the resident know that you like him or her and really care.

Each time that you contact the resident, you should converse with him or her, even if the conversation is brief. You might:

- communicate with the residents while you give care.
- briefly smile and speak as you pass in the hall.
- touch when appropriate (residents often welcome a pat on the hand or a hug, figure 9–9).
- hold longer conversations when time is available.
- let residents know when you will be able to sit and talk with them.

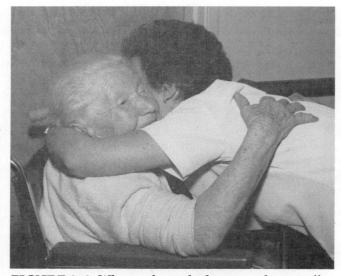

FIGURE 9–9. When welcomed, show your honest affection with a hug.

It is sometimes difficult to end a conversation without making the other person feel rejected. You can prevent this by:

- letting the resident know how much time you have.
- explaining the need to finish your assignments.
- telling the resident when you can come back.

Talking with residents is the same as conversing verbally with visitors or co-workers, except that residents may have a physical problem that slows or inhibits the usual two-way flow of conversation. For example, language skills of a resident may be hampered by a stroke, and deafness or blindness may limit the full extent of verbal exchange. **Comprehension** (understanding) may be diminished by nervous system changes that occur in some elderly persons. If the mechanics of the receiver or sender is not in perfect order, even a wireless message may turn out wrong.

The day-to-day contact you have with residents gives you an inside track in understanding and communicating effectively. The stronger the interpersonal bonds, the easier it is to overcome the handicaps. Good interpersonal relationships help promote positive reception of the message.

OVERCOMING BARRIERS TO EFFECTIVE COMMUNICATIONS

Successful communication depends on the ability to:

1. develop information to be expressed.
2. translate the information correctly into spoken, understandable words.
3. process and respond appropriately to the information coming back.

Any impairment of the senses diminishes the communication process. The post-stroke resident may have difficulty framing thoughts in a logical manner, may not be able to find the correct words to express an idea, or may have difficulty, because of lost muscle control, in being able to **articulate** (put into words) logical thoughts. A blind person cannot receive the information that body language and facial expressions convey, and the person who is deaf, because he or she cannot hear, is unaware of verbal emphasis, or the stressing of certain words.

Pretend that you are separated from someone else by a thick piece of glass and therefore unable to hear any sounds, or blindfolded, and you can better appreciate the frustration experienced by residents with these disabilities. Try to speak with a limited vocabulary at your command and without moving one side of your tongue or lips and you will better understand the plight of the post-stroke resident.

To help overcome communication barriers with the residents you are caring for, begin by determining what handicaps exist. This information can be found:

1. in the nursing assessment
2. in the nursing care plan
3. by your own observation

Comprehension Difficulties_____

Use simple words, speak slowly, stay calm. Center on one subject. Keep contacts short but frequent.

If a resident has difficulty saying words, encourage all attempts at conversation between yourself and the resident and between the resident and others. Do not critize, but be honest if you do not understand. Use simple words or short sentences and do not raise your voice. Speak slowly, saying the words carefully. Sometimes picture cards (figure 9–10) can be used to help express the ideas. Try to stay on one subject, and keep calm. Do not overtax the resident by prolonged conversations. Frequent, shorter interactions are less frustrating and less fatiguing.

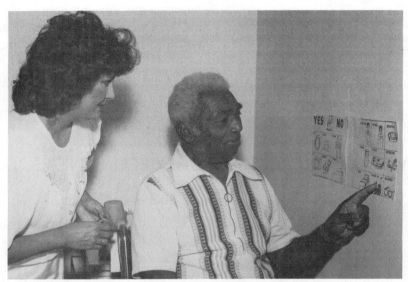

FIGURE 9–10. This post-stroke resident is using picture cards to communicate.

If the resident has difficulty understanding what you are saying, speak slowly. Time may be needed for the resident to process the information and give an appropriate response. If the resident can see them, use hand gestures and facial expressions to enhance the meaning of your words. Realize that the resident may not always respond in a correct or expected way and that the ability to respond varies from day to day. Even if you think that the resident does not understand you, always act as if he or she does. Do not start conversations that you may not have time to finish, since the resident may not only feel frustrated but he or she may also think that you are impatient and do not understand that a problem exists.

Hearing Aids_____

If a resident uses a hearing aid, make sure that it is properly placed. A well-fitting hearing aid can be invaluable. Face the resident so that your face and lips are well-lighted and on a level with his or her own.

A gentle touch can focus the resident's attention on what you are saying. Most residents welcome the touch of another, but if there is resistance, never persist. Again, use your face and hands to reinforce the message. When conversing with a resident with a hearing aid, you should:

1. Speak slowly and distinctly.
2. Form words carefully; keep sentences short.
3. Rephrase words as needed.
4. Face the listener.
5. Make sure any light source is behind the listener.
6. Use facial expressions or gestures to help express meaning.
7. Encourage lip reading.
8. Diminsh outside noise or distractions.

PROCEDURE: Care of Hearing Aid

1. Keep hearing aid in a safe, dry place when not in use.
2. Keep ear mold clean by disconnecting the mold from the hearing aid.
3. Insert a needle or pipe cleaner gently into the opening of the hearing aid and rotate to remove wax.
4. Wash ear mold gently in warm, soapy water.
5. Rinse and allow mold to air-dry thoroughly before reconnecting to hearing aid.

PROCEDURE: Applying and Removing Behind-the-Ear Hearing Aid

Applying Hearing Aid (figure 9–11)
1. Wash hands and explain to resident what you plan to do.
2. Assist resident to a comfortable position with head turned so that the ear needing the hearing aid is closest to you.
3. Check that the hearing aid is off or that volume is at lowest level.
4. Make sure that there are no chips or breaks in the equipment, and check tubing for bends or kinks.
5. Place the aid over the resident's ear, allowing the ear mold to hang free.
6. Adjust the hearing aid behind the resident's ear.
7. Grasp the ear mold and gently insert the tapered end into the ear canal.
8. Gently twist the ear mold into the curve of the ear, pushing upward and inward on the bottom of the ear mold, while pulling on the ear lobe with the other hand.
9. Turn on control switch to comfortable level.
10. Wash hands and record procedure.

Removing Hearing Aid:
1. Wash hands and explain to resident what you plan to do.
2. Turn off the hearing aid.
3. Loosen the outer portion of the ear mold by gently pulling on the upper part of the ear.
4. Lift the ear mold upward and outward.
5. Store in safe area.
6. Wash hands and record procedure.

Lip Reading and Signing

Some hard-of-hearing residents who cannot be helped by a hearing aid may rely on **lip reading** or **signing** as forms of communication. Lip reading is not easy, since many sounds are formed in the throat and mouth without moving the lips. In addition, many sounds are formed with similar mouth movements. When using lip reading to communicate, remember to:

- speak slowly and form words carefully.
- be patient and try a different word to express the thought if necessary.
- use body and hand language to amplify your meanings.

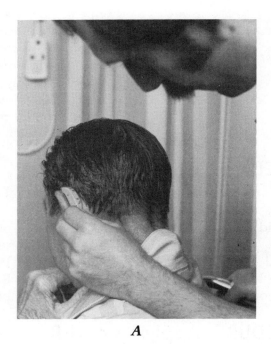

A

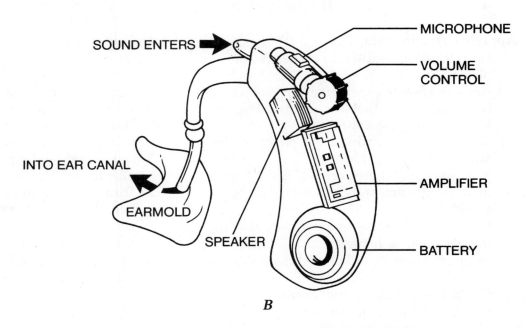

SOUND ENTERS ➡

MICROPHONE

VOLUME CONTROL

INTO EAR CANAL

EARMOLD

SPEAKER

AMPLIFIER

BATTERY

B

FIGURE 9–11. *A, Position the hearing aid carefully behind the ear; B, the ear mold fits into the resident's ear canal.*

Signing is the way in which deaf people communicate with one another without words. It is a language used throughout the world. Signing depends largely upon hand movements, eye movements, and facial expression to convey the message.

Learning to sign requires practice and skill but you might wish to familiarize yourself with some of the basic signs. A few are shown in figure 9–12.

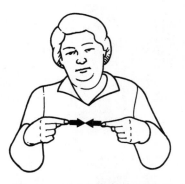

A. HURT, PAIN, ACHE, SORE

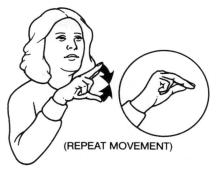

(REPEAT MOVEMENT)

B. NO

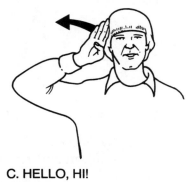

C. HELLO, HI!

D. GOOD MORNING

FIGURE 9–12. Signing. *A, Palms facing chest, index fingers extended toward, but not touching one another. Thrust them toward one another several times: Hurt, pain, ache, sore; B, Extend index and middle fingers bringing them down to meet the thumb in two quick movements: No; C, Start with the index finger of the right hand at the right temple, palm forward and fingers pointing up. Bring the hand outward to the right: Hello, hi; D, Start with fingertips of right open hand toward face. Touch lips and bring hand down bending elbow. Touch inner elbow with left open hand as the right hand is brought upward: Good morning.*

Vision Impairment___

Touch and word selection become important when communicating with someone who has limited vision, figure 9–13. If the resident wears glasses, they should be clean and placed where they are easily accessible to the resident. When speaking, make sure to position yourself directly in front of the vision-impaired resident so that the light falls on your face and lips.

Choose descriptive words and phrases. Whenever possible, relate your conversation to the orientation which the resident has already established. For example, when describing the position of the call bell, relate it to an article of furniture such as on the beside table. Since the resident is familiar with the location of the bedside table, he or she will have an easily identifiable frame of reference.

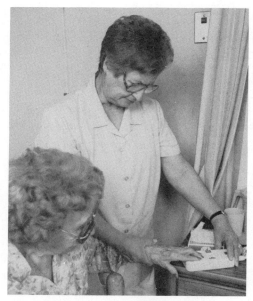

FIGURE 9–13. Always be sure the vision-impaired resident knows how to signal for help.

PROCEDURE: Care of Eyeglasses

1. Wash hands and assemble the following equipment:
   a. resident's eyeglasses
   b. cleaning solution
   c. clear water
   d. soft cleansing tissues
2. Explain to the resident what you plan to do.
3. Handle glasses only by frames.
4. Clean with cleaning solution and rinse with clear water.
5. Dry with tissues.
6. Return eyeglasses to case and place on bedside table or return to resident.

EMOTIONAL WITHDRAWAL

The resident who is depressed or withdrawn presents a special challenge. Do not assume that what you are saying is not being taken in just because there is no immediate response. Touch may not be welcome, so approach the resident slowly. Positioning yourself at a little lower level and not too close presents a less threatening profile. Talk in a calm manner. Do not raise your voice. Again, frequent, short contacts are usually more effective.

VOCABULARY

abbreviation	comprehension
articulate	lip reading
body language	signing
communication	symbol

SUGGESTED ACTIVITIES

1. Work in pairs. Put a blindfold on your partner and practice communicating. Exchange places and repeat.

2. Working with your partner, place cotton in your ears and try to communicate the following words:
   a. jade/shade
   b. pale/male
   c. put/but
   d. side/sight
   Exchange places and repeat.

3. When visiting a long term facility, look for non-verbal forms of communication.

REVIEW

Brief Answer/Fill in the Blanks

1. Verbal communication uses _____ to convey a message.

2. As a nursing assistant, you will need to communicate effectively with:
   a. _____
   b. _____
   c. _____

3. How well you interact with visitors reveals how much _____ you have in the work you do.

4. All written communication should be _____ correctly and the _____ terminology should be used.

5. _____ can take the place of a written message.

6. Communication requires:
   a. _____
   b. _____
   c. _____

7. The resident who has had a stroke may not be able to _____ ideas and may have difficulty expressing them.

8. If the resident has a hearing aid, be sure it is _____ correctly.

9. An important way of getting and maintaining the resident's attention is _____.

10. List three things you can do to heldp the post-stroke resident communicate more effectively.
    a. _____
    b. _____
    c. _____

11. List three things you can do to help the vision-impaired resident to communicate more effectively.

    a. _____

    b. _____

    c. _____

12. List three things to keep in mind when communicating with an emotionally stressed resident.

    a. _____

    b. _____

    c. _____

13. Identify the following messages.

    a.

    b.

    c.

A

B

C

CLINICAL SITUATION

Mrs. Wells is completely deaf, and so communicating with her is sometimes quite difficult. How might you improve your ability to make her understand you?

Answer: _____

_____

_____

SECTION II Achievement Review

A. Brief Answer/Fill in the Blanks

1. Twilight hours are particularly dangerous because poor lighting casts _____ which can be misleading.

2. The situation in question 1 can be corrected by _____.

3. A gait belt is a _____ which is used in ambulating or transferring residents who cannot fully assist.

4. Smoking can cause fires; therefore all smoking must be limited to _____ areas.

5. A resident who is pale, has a weak thready pulse and low blood pressure, and is complaining of pain should be checked for _____.

6. When carrying out isolation techniques, the "clean" person stands_____ the resident's room.

7. When entering an isolation room, you should take care of your watch by placing it in _____ or laying it on a _____.

8. When turning faucets on or off in an isolation unit, always use_____.

9. When double-bagging, the person outside the isolation room protects his or her hands from contamination by a _____ on the outside bag.

10. Sealed isolation bags should be delivered to the _____ room.

11. For communications to be successful, three parts are necessary. They are:

    a. _____

    b. _____

    c. _____

12. Problems associated with lip reading in communicating include

    a. _____

    b. _____

13. Your resident wears glasses to improve her vision. What can you do to help her?

    a. _____

    b. _____

    c. _____

14. Visitors who come to your facility are evaluating _____,
_____, and the kind of care being given.

15. When communications are successful, the _____ message passes from sender
to receiver.

B. **Matching.** Match the correct word or term on the right with each statement on the left.

1. _____ failing to perform a task competently and safely

2. _____ name given to a long term care facility

3. _____ microorganisms that cause disease

4. _____ placing yourself in another's position

5. _____ articles that can act in the transfer of germs

6. _____ position of body parts

7. _____ a moral code of behavior

8. _____ chemical that destroys pathogens on living tissue

9. _____ hospital-acquired infection

10. _____ harmful, inaccurate written information

Choices:
a. Empathy
b. Ethics
c. Slander
d. Libel
e. Negligence
f. Contractures
g. Alignment
h. Nosocomial
i. Chronic care
j. Acute care
k. Fomites
l. Antiseptic
m. Disinfectant
n. Pathogens

C. **Multiple Choice.** Select the one best answer and circle the correct letter.

1. Your resident is slowly feeding himself. You should
   a. pick up the fork and feed him yourself
   b. rewarm the food if it gets cold
   c. remove some of the food since he doesn't need as much anyway
   d. tell him to hurry up

2. You can let a resident know how you really feel by
   a. the words you choose
   b. your tone of voice
   c. the way you touch him or her
   d. all of the above

3. When wearing your uniform, you
   a. may smoke
   b. must follow the facility policy
   c. do not need to have clean shoes and laces
   d. may wear strong perfume or shaving lotion

4. Information about a resident can be shared
   a. with visitors
   b. with all co-workers
   c. with other residents
   d. with the charge nurse under special circumstances

5. If you observe someone stealing equipment and fail to report it, you are guilty of
   a. negligence
   b. libel
   c. aiding and abetting
   d. slander

6. Following proper body mechanics, you should
   a. avoid twisting your body
   b. keep your feet close together
   c. bend from the waist
   d. use your less strong muscles

7. The work an assistant will perform is outlined in the
   a. policy book
   b. job description
   c. organizational chart
   d. physician's orders

8. You notice a resident who is not part of your assignment has slipped down in his geri chair. You should
   a. reposition him
   b. report the fact to the supervisor
   c. find the assistant who is assigned to his care
   d. ignore him, because someone else will take care of him

9. A special procedure you might perform is
   a. taking a blood pressure
   b. putting a sterile tube into the resident's bladder
   c. starting an intravenous feeding
   d. changing a sterile dressing

10. Falls are common in the elderly because of
    a. good distance judgment
    b. confusion
    c. too-bright lighting
    d. rapid reflexes

11. You can prevent resident burns by
    a. telling resident the placement of hot liquids on trays
    b. never leaving the resident alone in the tub
    c. being sure that foot soaks are the proper temperature
    d. all of the above

12. Which of the following could contribute to an accident?
    a. Improperly secured carpeting
    b. Inadequate lighting
    c. Highly polished floor
    d. All of the above

13. A resident in your care starts to choke. You should
    a. pound him vigorously on the back
    b. not interfere if he is conscious and coughing
    c. have him lie down so that he won't get tired
    d. start cardiopulmonary resuscitation

14. When an accident occurs, you should document the event by
    a. completing an incident report
    b. giving a verbal report to other assistants
    c. making a notation on the physician's orders
    d. calling the resident's family

15. The keystone of medical asepsis is
    a. proper burning of disposables
    b. proper disposal of broken glass
    c. proper handwashing
    d. proper washing of used equipment

16. When communicating with a resident who has a hearing aid, you should
    a. speak very loudly
    b. use only sign language
    c. stand above the resident
    d. check to be sure the hearing aid is in place and turned on

17. A turned back, in body language, may indicate
    a. happiness
    b. interest
    c. rejection
    d. sadness

18. You apply an ointment to a resident's bed sores, contrary to facility policy order. You are guilty of
    a. malpractice
    b. negligence
    c. libel
    d. slander

19. You must reposition a very heavy resident in bed. You had best
    a. do the job alone and not bother others
    b. use a lift sheet
    c. ask for help
    d. use your strong back muscles

20. Another staff member asks you to perform a task for which you have had no previous experience. You had best
    a. tell the staff member and ask for help
    b. pretend you can do it and try anyway
    c. get another assistant to help you
    d. just forget the whole request

21. Which of the following are nursing assistant responsibilities?
    a. Answering lights
    b. Applying an ace bandage
    c. Cleaning the utility room
    d. All of the above

D. **Identification.** Look at each picture and explain what safety factor is involved.

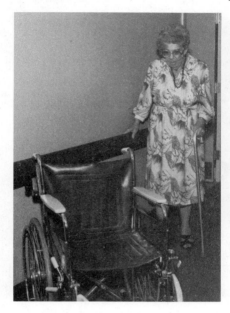 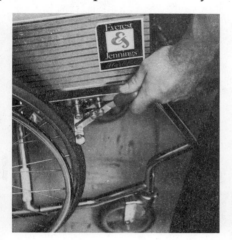 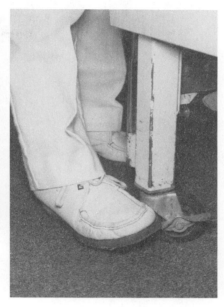

E. **Word Search.** Words appear horizontally, vertically and diagonally. Circle correct word.

1. Shortened form.

2. Combining form that appears at the beginning of a word.

3. Word that means to understand the message.

4. Word that means to send and receive a message.

5. A picture that sends a message.

6. A way of sending a message using the hands and fingers.

D	O	Q	R	C	S	F	L	X	K	U	I	N
G	A	P	V	T	I	B	M	Q	F	Y	O	X
B	U	X	Q	N	G	D	A	E	W	I	T	B
C	O	M	M	U	N	I	C	A	T	I	O	N
T	S	N	R	Y	I	E	B	A	X	P	M	E
U	Y	Y	V	W	N	R	I	N	C	R	U	M
S	M	M	T	U	G	V	C	R	T	E	Y	I
N	B	O	A	D	E	U	T	E	C	F	P	X
C	O	M	P	R	E	H	E	N	S	I	O	N
A	L	U	B	K	L	O	Q	X	T	X	V	E
Q	U	B	T	O	N	V	Y	A	C	D	E	R
C	A	B	B	R	E	V	I	A	T	I	O	N
T	U	B	W	V	C	O	R	N	A	X	Q	O

SECTION III
The Resident

LESSON 10 Characteristics of the Resident

OBJECTIVES

As a result of studying this lesson, you should be able to:

- State the average life span of men and women in 1987.
- List terms used to describe different age groups beyond 60 years.
- Identify normal physical changes that occur in the aging process.
- List five common physical impairments affecting the elderly.
- Define and spell all the vocabulary words and terms.

THE PROCESS OF NORMAL AGING

As aging progresses a unique individual is fashioned.

Aging is a process that begins at the time of birth and continues in a progressively **debilitating** (weakening) fashion until death. It is a normal process experienced by all human beings. During this life span, a unique person of great value emerges and makes contributions to society. When elderly, this same special person still has great value and needs and deserves respect, support, and care. The elderly can and do make valuable contributions to society.

The average life span today is about 67 years for men and 75 years for women. Most elderly people are able to remain independent, living out their lives in their own homes or in homes they share with others, figure 10–1. Only 5 percent require custodial care, and only 1 percent are confined to hospitals for the mentally ill. Remember, however, that these ages are averages. Some people die at an earlier age and some live much longer.

Care is needed by frail seniors and those who are sick or infirmed.

So many people are living into the eighth and ninth decades (80s and 90s) that new ways of describing the age groups have been devised. Those persons between 65 and 75 years of age are considered in the **late mature stage** of their lives. Those between 75 and 85 are considered **elder adults** and are classified as **old-old**. Those beyond 85 years of age are considered **frail seniors**.

124

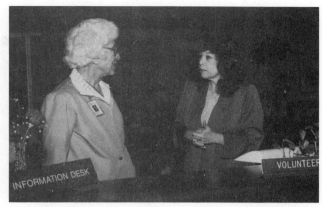

FIGURE 10–1. Most older persons continue to live active, productive lives, giving service in the community.

The population of long term facilities is composed of impaired and sick elder adults and frail seniors. The greater number of these residents are women, and have multiple health problems. Services to the elderly through federal and state agencies have helped finance care for these people. Such care is more available today than ever before.

As the aging population increases, more and more frail elderly individuals will need the support and care of the long term care facility. The role that skilled nursing assistants play in this care will become increasingly important.

Physical Changes

The rate of aging varies even with the individual.

Aging changes occur in all parts of the body, figure 10–2. Some are more obvious than others. It is important to recognize that aging doesn't occur at exactly the same rate in all persons or at the same rate in all parts of the body. Aging is both a physical and a psychological process. One person may feel and act old at 60, and another may be spry at 80; yet both will show physical evidence of their ages. In general, with increasing age:

1. The body's systems become less effective.
2. Disease processes begin to cause increasing stress.
3. The incidence of disease and disability increase.

Common disabilities include:

- cardiovascular disease such as heart attacks and strokes
- diabetes mellitus
- sensory losses
- cancer

However, remember that most of the elderly continue to live outside of care facilities.

Normal aging changes are called **senescent** changes, figure 10–3. Some of these changes are seen in all older persons. For example, hair begins to turn grey, the skin becomes dry and wrinkles develop, and vision becomes less acute so glasses are often needed. As a rule,

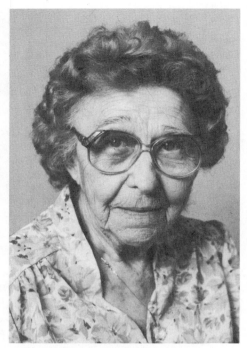

FIGURE 10–2. Note the physical signs of aging.

frail seniors are less heavy than when they were younger. They have less strength in their muscles and there are postural changes. They become shorter as hips and knees become slightly bent (**flexed**), although most of the loss in height is due to changes in the **spinal column** (backbone).

Changes also take place in the nervous system of the elderly. A major change is that sensory awareness diminishes. For example, pain is not felt as strongly and the senses of taste, vision, and hearing are less acute. Response time to internal stimuli affecting muscles and joints is increased, contributing to loss of balance and poor ability to recover balance if a fall is started.

Changes in brain function may cause memory loss, particularly short term memory loss. Long term memory and intellect are not necessarily affected. For example, a resident might not recall if she ate breakfast (short term memory), but can describe every house on the street where she lived when she was ten years old (long term memory).

As a person ages, his or her voice is not as strong and is higher pitched. Breathing capacity, though adequate when no disease is present, is somewhat lessened.

Changes in the urinary and cardiovascular systems result in less urine production and a decreased ability to concentrate urine at night. Residents may need to get up more often to go to the bathroom at night (**nocturia**). Men may find it more difficult to empty their bladder completely because of enlargement of the **prostate gland** (small gland at the exit of the bladder). Blood pressure may rise, and the heart becomes generally less efficient and frequently enlarges (**hypertrophy**).

Body System	Physical Changes of Aging
Integumentary	Hair loses color Hair may be lost Skin dries Wrinkles develop Skin is less elastic Fingernails and toenails thicken Areas of pigmentation develop Itching is common
Nervous	Loss of nerve cells Vision changes; glasses may be required Nerve endings are less sensitive Pain is not perceived as strongly Decrease in senses of taste, vision, hearing, and smell Memory changes occur, especially short term
Musculoskeletal	Muscles lose strength and tone Energy reserves are diminished Rib cage becomes more rigid Joints are less flexible Bones become more porous and brittle Sense of balance is less sure
Respiratory	Breathing capacity drops Lung tissue thins out and becomes less elastic Gaseous exchange is reduced Voice becomes weaker and higher pitched due to changes in the larynx
Excretory	Sweat glands are less active Kidneys decrease in size Urine production is less efficient Emptying bladder may become more difficult Poor urine concentration may lead to nocturia Elimination is less efficient
Cardiovascular	Blood vessels are narrowed and less elastic Blood pressure is elevated Heart muscle is less efficient Cardiac output diminishes
Endocrine	Decrease in the levels of some hormones such as estrogen, progesterone Higher levels of parathormone and TSH Uptake of iodine by thyroid is slower, so thyroxine production slows Thymosine, insulin, and aldosterone production is less effective
Digestive	Lowered level of digestive enzymes Decreased chewing capacity Loss of muscle tone Slower peristalsis

FIGURE 10–3. Summary of senescent changes.

Senescent changes also affect the digestive system. The gag reflex becomes less active, and foods that once were easily digested now cause indigestion and **flatulence** (gas).

Aging brings changes in the endocrine system that alter the level of **hormones**, which are chemicals that regulate body functions. When the activity of these body functions are lowered, all the body's systems

Aging affects all body systems.

are affected, including the reproductive and the integumentary systems. The **integumentary system** is composed of the skin, nails and hair. In addition to the changes already mentioned, the nails become thickened, the skin loose, some elasticity is lost and dark colored spots called **senile lentigines** appear. These spots are sometimes called "liver spots" but have no relationship to liver function at all.

Gradually, the normal physical changes are intensified, and the body is further altered and impaired by disease. The elderly are more susceptible to any disease that affects other age groups. Because natural resistance is decreased with the aging of the protective immune system, infectious diseases can have devastating effects. Heart disease, cancer, diabetes mellitus, strokes, and falls take a great toll on the well-being of the elderly, increasing their need for care and support.

In later chapters, you will learn more in detail about the specific physical impairment and diseases common to the elderly people in your care.

PSYCHOSOCIAL ADJUSTMENTS

Throughout life, people make adjustments, emotionally and socially, to changes in their circumstances. These adjustments are referred to as **psychosocial**. Successful adjustments require an accurate assessment of reality based on the information brought in by the senses. If the senses are functioning poorly, the messages brought in will be faulty. For example, when a person is deaf, only part of a message may be heard, so the full intent of the message may be misinterpreted or misunderstood. To be of value to the adjustment process, the message must be understood and a proper response formulated.

More time is needed to process information.

After age 70, many people need more time to process the sensory information they receive, figure 10–4. This doesn't mean that they are not as intelligent as they were, although the slowness of response might lead us to believe so. In addition, remember that the eyes and ears are the major way that we learn about what is going on around us, and as eyes and ears age, they may become less functional.

A sense of self worth and independence are closely linked.

A large number of residents in your care will suffer both from decreased sensory awareness and from slower processing ability, which makes social and emotional adjustments more difficult.

Another factor that influences mental health and emotional stability is a sense of personal worth. Elderly people, confined to long term care facilities can, without proper care, gradually lose more and more independence and suffer from a sense of lowered personal worth. It is our job to keep this from happening.

All of these factors combined together make psychosocial adjustment very difficult for the elderly.

EMOTIONAL RESPONSE

Early in life, people develop a characteristic way of responding emotionally to life's circumstances. When a response is found to be successful, it becomes a part of a pattern of responses that becomes integrated with the resident's personality. As a person ages, these responses become more and more ingrained, figure 10–5.

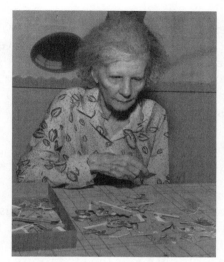

FIGURE 10–4. As a person ages, it takes longer to process information.

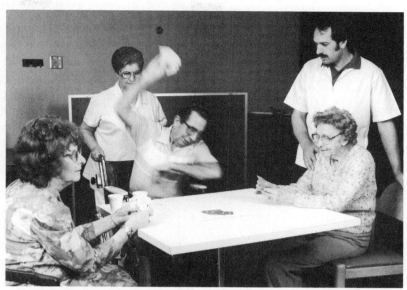

FIGURE 10–5. When frustrated, this person's usual response is anger. As he has aged, this response has become more and more ingrained.

Aging intensifies the basic personality traits.

The stress of growing old does not alter the basic personality. However, certain characteristics become more pronounced, and this can sometimes bring the resident into conflict with others in the care setting. When conflict does occur, frustration and tension can cause a breakdown in the ability to use responses that have been successful in the past. For example, a resident who has spent a lifetime handling conflict by simply walking away from it (that is moving himself physically out of the area) is now confined to a geri chair which he or she cannot leave. A nursing assistant wants him to go into music time and he wishes to stay where he is—a conflict develops. As the resident is unable to follow his usual response, he becomes hostile and combative.

Emotional health is promoted when basic psychological needs are met. These needs include:

- the need to love
- the need to be loved
- the need to feel a purpose to life
- the need to express and share feelings with others

Because elderly people living in long term care facilities tend to be isolated or set apart to some degree from the community, their ways of satisfying these important emotional needs are limited. Because residents have similar needs and degrees of limitations, they are not always able to be of much help to one another. Therefore, they often turn to members of the staff for emotional support.

Care must be taken not to encourage excessive dependency that will further downgrade a resident's sense of self-esteem. Encourage as much independence and interaction as possible. Allow time for the elderly to mentally process the details of the situation and the intent of your communication.

To prevent problems relating to stress:

Intervene before the situation gets out of hand.

- Be on the alert for stressful situations developing between residents or between a resident and yourself and intervene before the situation gets out of hand (figure 10–6).
- Try to determine the source of the stress and eliminate it.
- Speak slowly and calmly.
- Look directly at the resident.
- Use very simple terms.
- Try to get residents away from one another.
- If necessary, get help.

Protect residents' self-esteem by being tactful. For example, if you notice that Mr. Hughes has not zipped up his trousers, call this to his attention tactfully. If he does not respond or react, repeat the suggestion using fewer words. Don't impatiently do the task yourself just to save time. Remember, he probably needs time to process your request.

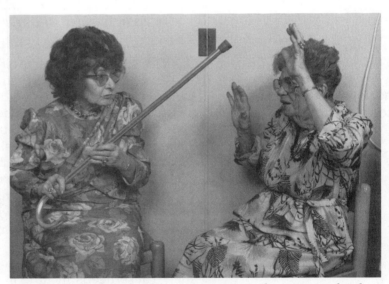

FIGURE 10–6. Be quick to intervene when stress develops between residents.

VOCABULARY

debilitating	hormones	prostate gland
elder adults (old-old)	hypertrophy	psychosocial
flatulence	integumentary system	senescent
flexed	late mature stage	senile lentigines
frail seniors	nocturia	spinal column

SUGGESTED ACTIVITIES

1. Visit the residents of a care facility. Note the obvious changes associated with aging. After your visit, discuss these changes with your instructor and classmates. Identify any that you recognize in yourself.

2. What conclusions can you draw as to the population distribution of the residents at the facility you visited?

3. Discuss reasons why psychosocial adjustments are difficult for elderly people in a long term care facility.

REVIEW

A. **Brief Answer/Fill in the Blanks**

1. In 1987, the average life span was _____ years for a man and _____ years for a woman.

2. People between the ages of 65 and 75 are described as being in the _____ stage.

3. List three major health problems that afflict the elderly.

    a. _____

    b. _____

    c. _____

4. Elderly people lose height because of changes in:

    a. _____

    b. _____

5. List three areas of sensory loss experienced by the elderly.

    a. _____

    b. _____

    c. _____

6. Hormones are chemicals that _____ body functions.

7. List three changes in the integumentary system associated with aging.

    a. _____

    b. _____

    c. _____

B. **True or False.** Answer the following questions true (T) or false (F).

1. _____ Most people who have reached the age of 85 will require custodial care.

2. _____ Illness complicates the aging process.

3. _____ All body systems age at the same rate.

4. _____ Heart disease is a common health problem of the aged.

5. _____ Senile lentigines are related to a poorly functioning liver.

6. _____ Psychosocial adjustments are easier when the elderly are confined to long term care facilities.

7. _____ Improper sensory input can confuse the intent of the communication.

8. _____ Older people tend to respond emotionally much as they have responded throughout their lifetime.

CLINICAL SITUATION

Mrs Frazier, age 82, is ambulatory and very spry. You notice that her dress is unbuttoned and when you call this to her attention, she just looks at you, making no move to button up. What is the best way to handle this situation?

Answer: _____

_____

_____

LESSON 11 Stereotypes and Myths

OBJECTIVES

After studying this lesson, you should be able to:

- Explain the difference between a myth and a stereotype.
- List at least two ways that myths and stereotypes limit the elderly.
- Describe two positive stereotypes about the elderly.
- Define and spell all the vocabulary words and terms.

STEREOTYPES

Stereotypes of people are rigid, biased ideas about people as a group. Although a stereotype may partly be true, all members of a group are falsely seen as being alike and having the same characteristics. Beliefs of this kind that are not even partly true are **myths.**

Myths are stereotypes which are untrue.

Imagine someone asking you to describe a cat if you had only seen two small, black, short-haired cats in your life, figure 11–1. You would undoubtedly say that cats are small, black, and short-haired. As you know, this does not even begin to describe all the different cats throughout the world. Describing all cats with only one narrow set of characteristics establishes a stereotype for cats: it is only partly true. It is easy to form stereotypes, because limited experience tends to make us think that everyone in a certain group has the same characteristics as those few people we know in that group.

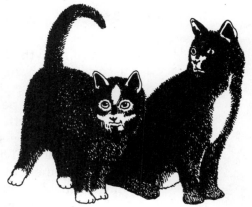

FIGURE 11–1. Cats have similar characteristics, but they are not exactly the same.

133

The Dangers of Stereotyping_____

Stereotypes about the elderly are limiting both to the people who believe them and to the elderly themselves. This is true for several reasons.

Stereotyping does not take into consideration the uniqueness of the individual. Although they have certain characteristics in common, the elder members of society have been fashioned by their own special life experiences, and this makes each person different, in some ways, from all others.

Stereotyping may make people devalue themselves as they see themselves as a reflection of what others think. If others treat us with respect, we feel respectable and behave in respectable ways. If, on the other hand, we are viewed as helpless and unable to make our own decisions, we quickly lose confidence in our ability to handle our affairs and become increasingly dependent on others.

Ninety-five percent of the elderly live in the community.

As you can see, it is unwise and unfair to take stereotypes at face value, accepting what might be myth as truth, and apply them to the entire older population. It is especially important for those who work in long term care facilities to realize that those in their care are not representative of all the people in that particular age group. Only 5 percent of the elder members of society are unable to care for themselves and require the support of long term care. Most live independent lives in the community supported by family and friends.

It might be easy to believe the stereotype of the helplessness of the elderly if the only older persons we knew were those in our care facilities; however, even here there are great differences. Residents are not representative of the elderly population as a whole, and no single resident is exactly like another resident.

How You Can Help__

Treat each person as special and unique.

You can best help the residents by:

- resisting the temptation to stereotype.
- accepting them as individuals.
- giving them as much control over their lives as possible.
- supporting their efforts to remain as independent as possible.

MYTHS ▪▪▪▪▪▪▪▪▪▪▪▪▪▪▪▪▪▪▪▪▪▪▪▪▪▪▪▪▪▪▪▪▪▪▪▪▪▪

It is a myth that age alone causes the diseases that are often associated with the residents. Although it is true that many residents suffer from cancer, heart disease, diabetes mellitus, emphysema, and strokes, younger people also suffer from these conditions, figure 11–2.

Another myth is that age alone determines the value of the contributions a person can make to society. Nothing could be further from the truth. Civic groups and charities could not survive without the involvement of older people, and many people have made their most valuable contribution to society in their later years.

As you can see, myths are stereotypes that are not even partly true. Let us explore some of the more common stereotypes and learn if they are true of the majority or only myths to be investigated and ignored.

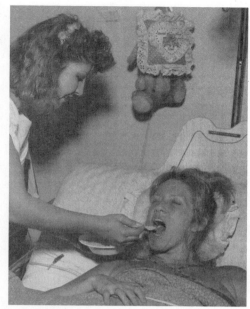

FIGURE 11–2. It is a myth that only the elderly become ill with chronic disease and require long term care. This young woman suffers from multiple sclerosis.

COMMON STEREOTYPES AND MYTHS

As people age, they experience the same characteristic changes in the structure and function of their bodies. This stereotype is partly true. Aging is usually evidenced by graying of the hair, glasses are usually needed to improve eyesight, and reaction time is usually delayed. However, the hair of some older people does not turn gray, and others do not need to wear glasses. The rate and type of changes that accompany aging are different for different people. In general, the functioning of the body is slowed but still is usually adequate to meet the needs of the older life-style.

Older people are incompetent and unable to make correct judgments and decisions. This is a myth. Sensory losses occur with aging, but most older people remain mentally sound until they die. They manage their own affairs and, when properly stimulated, can learn new skills and process new information, figure 11–3.

Older people are unhappy, without focus to their lives, and have little interest in sexual matters. In general, the older population is no less and no more content with life than younger persons. They fill their lives with activities suitable to their needs. Their view of life in later years is usually a reflection of the attitudes they had in younger years. Reading, watching television, playing cards, conversing with others, or just carrying out the activities of daily living can be quite satisfying. They are still sexual beings, but with more limited opportunity to express sexual feelings and to fulfill sexual needs, figure 11–4.

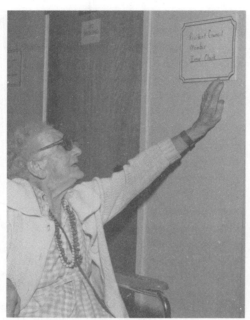

FIGURE 11–3. This resident is proud that she is an active member of the facility resident council.

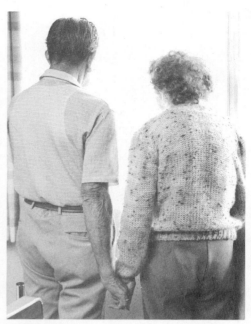

FIGURE 11–4. Sexual attraction is maintained throughout life.

Old people are sent to homes because society doesn't want to be bothered with them. Admission to a long term care facility is often a very difficult decision for the resident and his or her family. Usually, it is a decision based on the fact that a person needs the type of care available only in a long term care facility. Society helps to pay for this care through government subsidies in the form of social security payments, federally-funded Medicare and state-supported Medicaid financing. This is *not* charity. Residents have earned this support through their own contributions, or those of their spouse, during their working years.

Being "old" is determined solely by the number of years a person has lived. This is not necessarily true. The term *old* is both indefinite and relative. To a child 5 years old, someone age 35 is old; to someone who is 80, the 35-year-old seems very young. In the minds of some people, the age of retirement is the beginning of the "old" period. This is an arbitrary time since some people retire at 60 or 65 while others are gainfully employed until many years later. The mandatory retirement age keeps moving up. It was 65, and now it is in the area of 75, according to the U.S. government data.

Remember that the 85-year-old person of today was a senior citizen 20 years ago, a productive member of the work force 5 years before that, and a respected, dynamic husband or wife and parent for many years prior to that. He or she is the same person, gradually changing and growing through life's experiences.

Sometimes the past retirement years are referred to as the **sunset years**, a somewhat negative reference to the fact that the elderly are at the end of life. Being old is related more to the way a person thinks, feels, and behaves than to the actual number of years lived.

Other names applied to the elderly that promote this negative point of view include *senior citizen*, *aged* or simply, *seniors*.

MYTHS VERSUS FACTS ABOUT THE AGED

The following lists of ideas about the aged contain common negative stereotypes. The first list is made up of myths; the second is based on facts.

List 1: Myths_____

Many people believe that all older persons:

- cannot care for themselves
- are unable to learn
- have no interest in life
- are neglected by family, friends, and society
- are all living in poverty
- no longer contribute to society
- have no interest in sex
- become "old" at a certain age (e.g., 65)
- are incompetent to make decisions

List 2: Facts_____

It is true, in general, that the elderly:

- have sensory losses (e.g., vision, hearing)
- have changes in sleep patterns
- have slower sexual responses
- are more prone to certain chronic conditions
- undergo postural changes
- have less efficient elimination
- have less tolerance to glucose
- experience graying of the hair
- have short-term memory loss

POSITIVE STEREOTYPES

Although many stereotypes are negative, some may be positive. For example, some positive stereotypes are that older people:

- are more peaceful
- get into fewer verbal arguments (fights) with others
- are less pressured and more generous

Again, these ideas apply to some older people, but not all older people can be described this way.

VOCABULARY

golden years   stereotype
myth   sunset years
senior citizen

SUGGESTED ACTIVITIES

1. Ask a librarian to help you select a biography of a person who continued to make significant contributions to society after the age of 60. After reading the biography, share what you have learned with classmates.

2. Write an imaginary, brief description of a woman or man older than age 70. Discuss your description with other classmates. Consider the following:

   a. How many "facts" in your description are partly true of elderly persons you know?

   b. How many are not true at all about elderly persons you know?

3. Think about the older members of your community or church. Try to list ways they still contribute in a positive way.

4. With your classmates, discuss possible stereotypes of people in the 65- to 75-year-old age group.

5. Shut your eyes and try to imagine yourself at the age of 80. Do you think you will fit the common stereotypes?

REVIEW

A. Brief Answer/Fill in the Blanks

1. Name four reasons why stereotyping is unwise.

   a. _____

   b. _____

   c. _____

   d. _____

2. How others view us often determines how we _____.

3. _____ percent of the older population live independent lives in the community.

4. _____ alone is not responsible for many of the illnesses seen in residents.

5. Many older people continue to make _____ to society.

6. Carrying out the _____ often keeps older people occupied and contented.

7. Name four activities that the elderly engage in to meet social needs.

   a. _____

   b. _____

   c. _____

   d. _____

8. Older people are still sexual beings, but the opportunities for expression are _____.

9. Older persons prefer to be called _____.

10. Positive stereotypes of the elderly are that the older person

    a. _____

    b. _____

    c. _____

    d. _____

B. True or False. Some of the statements below are *stereotypes* (partly true) and some are *myths* (not true). Mark those that are stereotypes and partly true (T) and those that are myths (F) for false.

1. _____ Aging is evidenced by a slowing of body processes.

2. _____ Older people are unable to make sound judgments.

3. _____ Older people cannot learn new skills.

4. _____ Most older people are unhappy.

5. _____ Society has abandoned the elderly.

6. _____ The elderly usually need glasses to improve their vision.

7. _____ People are old by the age of 60.

8. _____ Older people are all pretty much alike.

9. _____ All older people who reach the age of 80 require admission to a long term care facility.

CLINICAL SITUATION

Another nursing assistant tells you that a resident who is 79 is interested in the new programs that the local community college is bringing to the residence. She cannot understand why the resident would want to study at his age. She thought that old people's minds didn't function that well. How do you respond?

Answer: _____

_____

_____

_____

_____

_____

LESSON 12 Special Needs of the Geriatric Person

OBJECTIVES

As a result of studying this lesson, you should be able to:

- list the activities of daily living (ADL).
- describe ways in which the nursing assistant can help residents carry out ADL.
- recognize unusual responses to common drugs that need to be reported.
- explain ways that nursing assistants can assist in the rehabilitation process.
- list recreational and occupational opportunities for residents in a long term care facility.
- define and spell all the vocabulary words and terms.

Residents have special needs just because they are older and are, in many cases, not well. Basic human needs, described in Lesson 9, remain the same. It is the means of satisfying these needs that must be altered, figure 12–1.

People become residents, entrusted to your care, because they are unable to do all or some of these things for themselves without help. It is your responsibility as a nursing assistant to ensure that all activities of daily living are carried out by or for each of the residents assigned to you.

PROMOTING INDEPENDENCE

Residents need to be encouraged to do as much as they possibly can for themselves, figure 12–2. It may take them longer and they may not accomplish the task as neatly or efficiently as you might; however, independence must be protected. Loss of independence lowers the resident's self-esteem. A resident's sense of independence is threatened when he or she gives up personal control of his/her life and is admitted to the care facility. The less a resident is permitted to do for himself or herself, the less independent he or she becomes. Gradually, as confidence in their own ability to care for themselves slips away, the residents participate less and less in their own care. Remembering this important fact will help you exercise patience and tact as you assist residents in carrying out the ADL.

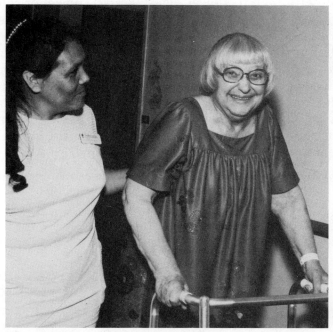

FIGURE 12–1. *This resident needs help in meeting the basic need to exercise.*

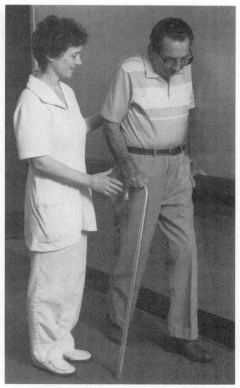

FIGURE 12–2. *Encourage residents to remain as active and independent as possible.*

ASSISTING THE ACTIVITIES OF DAILY LIVING (ADL)

The physical changes that occur with aging make carrying out the usual activities associated with caring for one's self more difficult. Let us briefly review these functions called the activities of daily living (ADL). They include:

Basic human needs must be met in new ways as aging progresses.

- being able to breathe (exchange gases)
- taking nourishment
- eliminating wastes
- getting adequate rest and activity
- maintaining proper hygiene
- having a purpose in living
- fulfilling mental, spiritual, and sexual needs

Now let us look at each of the ADL and the kind of assistance that a resident might need which you could provide. The activities related to nutritional needs require a background in general nutrition and are covered in Lesson 13. Those activities related to mental, spiritual, and sexual needs are discussed in Lesson 14 under *meeting psychological needs.*

Eliminating Wastes___

Residents need to take in adequate fluids and to eliminate waste products that are formed in their bodies. Wastes are eliminated from

Wastes to be eliminated include feces, urine, perspiration, carbon dioxide.

the body through the lower digestive tract (**bowel** or **colon**) and the urinary system, through the skin, and through the lungs. The colon eliminates solid wastes as **feces**. Perspiration is eliminated through the skin, urine is eliminated through the kidneys and bladder, and the gas carbon dioxide is eliminated through the lungs.

Elderly people may need assistance in reaching the proper facility for elimination, figure 12-3. Bedside **commodes** (portable toilets) eliminate the need to make long trips to the bathroom. Bed pans and urinals can be used for those who must remain in bed. When the resident is using a bed pan, make sure that:

- the resident is properly positioned
- the resident is as comfortable as possible
- bathroom tissue is readily available
- the call bell is close at hand
- the resident has privacy

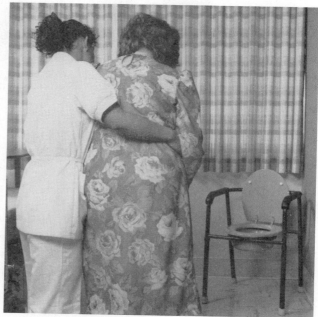

FIGURE 12-3. Elderly persons may need help reaching the commode in time.

Cleansing oneself after using a toilet, commode, or bed pan can be difficult for the elderly. Be ready to do this task yourself. Be gentle but thorough. Note the amount and characteristics of the elimination and report anything unusual. Aids to bowel elimination include **enemas** and **suppositories**. Enemas consist of an introduction of fluid into the bowel. Suppositories are small, bullet-shaped bowel aids composed primarily of glycerine. Nursing assistants give enemas and, in some facilities, may insert suppositories. If the resident has an artificial opening (**colostomy**) in the abdominal wall for the elimination of feces, it may be your responsibility to assist in the periodic irrigation of the colostomy. (The specific procedures are presented in Lesson 22.)

Exercise and a diet that includes plenty of liquids, fruit, and vegetables aids in maintaining regularity.

Urine may be collected through a **catheter** (small tube) inserted into the bladder and attached to constant, closed drainage; catheters may be used when there is a specific complicating medical problem. Emptying the drainage bag, measuring the contents and keeping the catheter clean are your responsibility. (The procedures for catheter care are presented in Lesson 23.)

Rest and Exercise____

Rest and recreation must be balanced.

It might seem that residents have plenty of opportunity to rest. However, sitting all day or being confined to bed doesn't assure that real rest and relaxation are being achieved.

Rest and sleep patterns change as we grow older. More frequent but shorter rest periods are needed, figure 12–4. Elderly people tend to sleep less deeply. Residents may nap during the day, fall asleep earlier in the evening, and awaken during the night and early in the morning.

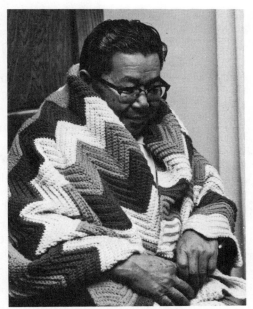

FIGURE 12–4. Frequent rest periods are needed.

Provide quiet periods for napping. If residents awaken in the night, use simple nursing measures to encourage relaxation. A back rub, warm milk, a position change or just a few minutes of conversation may be all that is needed to help the resident relax and go back to sleep. Try to plan your care *around* the times that a resident prefers to rest. Remember that the elderly often have little energy reserves and need to conserve them as much as possible.

Exercise may be random or planned. In most facilities, special times during the day are set aside for group exercise, figure 12–5. You can help by participating in the exercise periods and making sure that the residents in your care are ready at the proper time. If necessary, exercising can be carried out sitting in a chair or lying in bed. Carrying out range-of-motion exercises for those unable to perform them for themselves and assisting residents to ambulate are other ways that you can help.

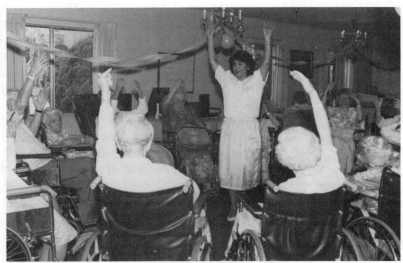

FIGURE 12–5. The activity director leads a group of residents in an exercise program.

The position of a resident must be changed every one to two hours. Give particular attention to chair-bound residents. Proper exercise improves circulation and maintains optimum mobility and respiratory functions.

Personal Hygiene

General hygiene includes cleanliness of body, hair, and teeth. Several methods of bathing are employed to carry out cleanliness routines. Bed baths, either full or partial, can be refreshing, but a tub bath, shower, or whirlpool bath are more stimulating. Use the method that is best for each particular resident. Complete baths are not given daily. Not only is it unnecessary, but it is drying for the elderly person's skin. Baths are given one to three times a week, depending on the resident's condition and facility policy.

When bathing a resident, make sure that bath water is a comfortable temperature (about 105° to 110° F), rewarming it as necessary. You must wash those areas the residents cannot wash themselves, figure 12–6. Carefully transfer the resident into the tub or whirlpool (help will probably be needed). Never leave the resident alone in the bath or shower. Be sure the resident's room or the tub room is warm and draft-free. Bathing is fatiguing, so allow an adequate rest period before and after the procedure.

Personal care includes attention to teeth, hair, nails.

Cleaning of teeth is part of general hygiene. If a resident has his or her own teeth, assist him or her to brush them in the usual manner and floss at least twice daily. Many older people have dentures. These must be cleaned regularly and stored safely when not in the resident's mouth.

Fingernails and toenails should be kept trimmed and clean. Trim toenails straight across. The toenails of the diabetic resident and those with poor circulation or on special drugs such as Coumadin or heparin should be cared for by professionals. Very thick or unusually shaped nails should be reported. When in doubt, never cut nails; get help. A podiatrist may be required to provide proper care; some facilities have a podiatrist to do all toenail cutting.

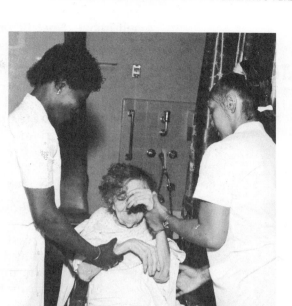

FIGURE 12–6. Residents may need help in meeting cleanliness needs.

Most facilities have hairdressers shampoo and style the resident's hair, figure 12-7. If a hairdressing area is not a separate room, often hairdressers will visit the resident unit to perform these services. If these services are not available, and in between hairdresser appointments, you must see that the resident's hair is clean, combed, and neatly arranged. Medicated shampoos are frequently ordered.

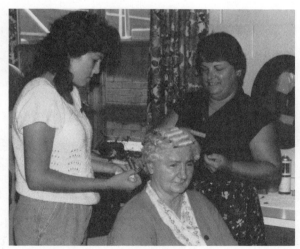

FIGURE 12–7. Most extended care facilities provide beauty salon and barber shop services.

Men residents need to have their hair trimmed, and to be shaved regularly, if they cannot do this themselves.(Women residents may also need regular shaving as well.) Shaving may be done by a barber who regularly visits the residents or by the nursing assistant, depending on facility policy. Having their hair combed and shaving regularly makes residents feel well-groomed which in turn promotes a positive self-image. Specific procedures for carrying out personal hygiene are found in Lesson 20.

MEDICATIONS ▪▪

There is a special geriatric need for drugs to support failing body systems. Drugs are broken down in the body in ways that are similar to that in which nutrients are handled. Reduced metabolism will affect not only the digestive process of foods but will alter the assimilation of drugs. Older people do not respond to drugs as well as young persons, figure 12–8. Drugs frequently given to residents include:

- cardiac stimulants
- diuretics
- blood pressure regulators
- laxatives and suppositories
- mood-altering drugs
- medications to fight infections

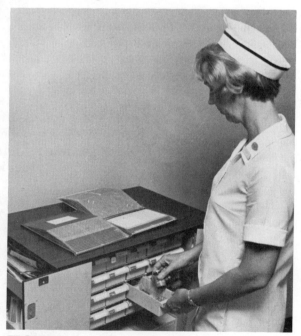

FIGURE 12–8. The professional nurse gives the medications but you must be on alert for reportable changes in the resident's behavior.

Cardiac Stimulants___

Cardiac stimulants improve heart function. One of the most commonly given of these is digitalis. This drug slows the heart rate but increases the strength of contractions. Digitalis builds up in the body and sometimes causes undesirable effects, such as toxicity. Changes or signs to watch for include:

- nausea
- vomiting
- mental confusion
- changes in heart rate or rhythm

Be on guard for these changes and report any to the charge nurse.

Diuretics

Medications can affect older persons differently.

Diuretics are drugs that increase urine output (**diuresis**). Residents receiving diuretics such as Lasix must be carefully observed for too much fluid loss (**dehydration**) and an upset in the normal balance of certain chemical elements found in the body. One of these elements is *potassium*. Carefully measure the amount of fluid taken in by the resident and the amount of urine eliminated. Watch also for signs of excessive **potassium loss**. These signs include:

- weakness
- slow heart rate
- apathy

Apathy is indicated by a lack of interest and a slow response. Any changes should be reported.

Blood Pressure Regulators

Drugs that regulate blood pressure include **antihypertensives** and **vasodilators**. These two types of drugs reduce blood pressure in different ways. Residents receiving them should have their blood pressure carefully monitored. Watch for signs of **hypotension** (lowered blood pressure), which include:

- dizziness
- weakness
- **disorientation** (confusion)
- light-headedness

Be sure to report any of these signs.

Laxatives and Suppositories

Laxatives and suppositories are given to promote bowel regularity. Some add lubrication to the bowel while others increase the bulk of the stool or increase the strength of bowel muscular contractions. The muscular contractions of the bowel that move food along the digestive tract is called **peristalsis**.

Because residents can begin to rely excessively on these aids to elimination, you must do all you can to promote natural bowel evacuation. You can help by encouraging the resident to be as active as possible, to eat fruits and high-fiber vegetables, and to drink fluids freely. Your constant reminders and encouragement can sometimes eliminate the need for laxatives and suppositories.

Mood-Altering Drugs

Mood-altering drugs include **tranquilizers** and **antidepressants**. These may be given to make residents feel more relaxed and cheerful, but they may have the opposite effect in some residents. Watch for signs of:

- excessive response (e.g., resident sleeps all the time)
- mental confusion or depression
- inappropriate behavior such as mood swings (e.g., happy and bright one moment, depressed and withdrawn the next)

As an example of inappropriate behavior, a resident may laugh as another resident talks about her sick granddaughter; or a resident who is normally cooperative and friendly may become withdrawn and barely answer your questions. Residents receiving these drugs must also be watched for faintness and drops in blood pressure.

Many changes due to drugs or their interactions occur gradually; your current judgment must be based on your original assessment of the resident as well as your ongoing observations.

Medications to Fight Infections_____

When a resident is ill with an infection, **antibiotics** and **sulfa drugs** (to destroy germs) and **expectorants** (to clear air passageways) may be ordered. Since the elderly tolerate such drugs less well than younger individuals, watch for any unusual changes. If you know that one of your residents is receiving such drugs, ask your charge nurse what particular changes might occur. In general, watch for:

- signs of dizziness
- ringing in the ears
- changes in color of urine that might indicate **hematuria** (blood in the urine)

Nutritional supplements in the form of vitamins and minerals may be needed.

REHABILITATION ▪▪

Helping elderly persons to do as much as they can to care for themselves, as well as they can, for as long as they can, is the principle upon which **rehabilitation** goals are based. Rehabilitation is an ongoing process that is a special geriatric need, and it is one that all staff members must support. The goals for rehabilitation are both short term and long term, designed individually for each resident during the care conference. These are not static goals but are ever-changing as the resident's condition changes.

The goals of rehabilitatoin should be realistic and should reflect the physical and emotional needs of the individual resident. Whenever possible, the resident should help to determine these goals. In general these goals should take into consideration:

- the need for frequent rest periods
- the physical limitations of aging
- the involvement and motivation of the resident
- the resident's view of his or her disability

For example, Mrs. Sweeney, who is recovering from a stroke, is unable to use her right arm or leg and has difficulty speaking; consequently she is depressed and cries quite a bit. She will not even try to communicate with the woman who shares her room. This resident has many rehabilitative needs, figure 12–9. A long term goal would involve improving Mrs. Sweeney's ability to help care for herself. To reach that goal, many small steps must be taken. These small steps are a series of short term goals, such as recovering some form of communication and an increase in socialization. Still another short term goal might be related to Mrs. Sweeney's motivation.

Independence must be encouraged.

You, as nursing assistant, play an important role in the rehabilitation process. You are in constant contact with the resident and are in a position to offer support and encouragement — two vital parts of the process. Remember that you are dealing with adults and:

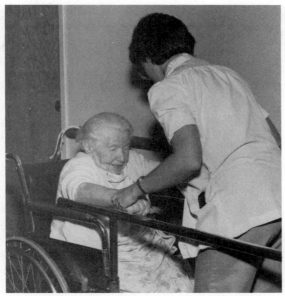

FIGURE 12–9. A rehabilitation goal for this resident is to improve her ability to walk.

- never push too hard or the resident will resist.
- acknowledge success, however slight.
- be there to support the times of frustration and discouragement.
- accept the fact that failures are expected and natural.

The most important contributions you can make are:

- carefully follow the nursing care plan (evaluating and reporting on difficulties and progress).
- let the resident know that you genuinely care and that you have confidence that he or she can succeed.

RECREATIONAL AND OCCUPATIONAL OPPORTUNITIES

For all individuals, each day must offer both a purpose and quality to life; otherwise the desire to continue living ceases, figure 12–10. Confined to a care facility, with many unresolved problems facing them, some residents see little purpose to their existence and some simply give up trying. Recreational and occupational activities can improve the quality of life by:

- filling long hours
- providing entertainment, figure 12–11
- promoting relaxation and a sense of accomplishment
- giving purpose to living

In addition, many activities can promote rehabilitation goals.

Watching television, playing cards, writing a letter, reading, and conversation are the major sources of recreation for residents in the long term care facility. Planned recreation periods may include chair exercising, group singing, dancing, and hand-clapping to music.

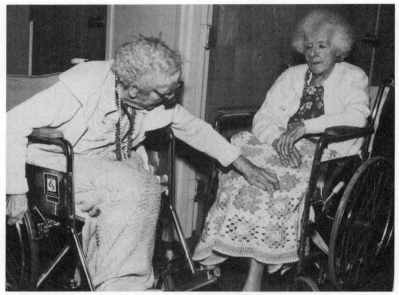

FIGURE 12–10. *Residents learn to care for one another and try to help each other, becoming very much like family members.*

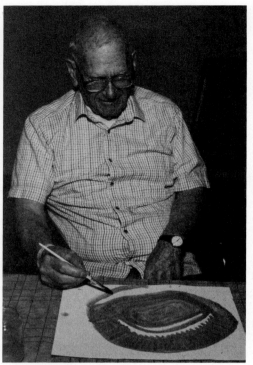

FIGURE 12–11. *Recreational activities provide enjoyment and help to fill long hours.*

Recreational activities must be adapted to the abilities and desires of the resident.

Community groups often entertain the seniors and sometimes bring gifts. Scout troops, schools, and other service-oriented groups may "adopt" the residents and visit regularly, particularly on special holidays, figure 12–12. They may perform skits or songs to entertain the residents. Residents may do many of these same activities themselves, sharing personal talents and skills.

For those residents who are able, handicraft materials are available. Instruction in new skills and practice in old are productive and help maintain small muscle tone. Educational opportunities are organized for those residents who are interested. Elderly people are still capable of learning, and the challenge can be both stimulating and satisfying. Although gainful employment is not a primary goal, all activities contribute to the sense of purpose that each resident needs to make living worthwhile.

You can best help by encouraging residents to participate in the activities available, by making sure that residents are transported to activity areas, and by assisting in activities as needed. Also, if you consider these activities important, residents will note your attitude and be positively influenced by it.

PET THERAPY

If you have ever held a kitten or puppy or heard the bright song of a canary, you know what warm, happy feelings this can bring. Pets help overcome loneliness and bring much pleasure to their owners, figure 12–13.

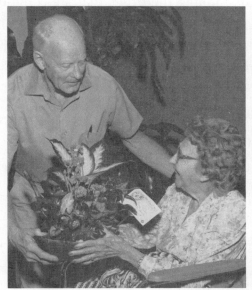

FIGURE 12–12. Scout groups and other community groups bring cheer to residents.

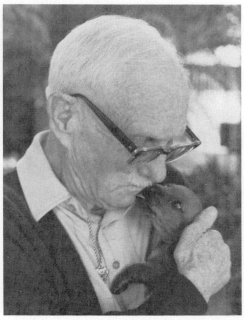

FIGURE 12–13. Pets can bring a real measure of happiness to the elderly.

We are only beginning to understand the real value of a pet to the elderly. Although we are not sure how the process works, having a pet to care for and relate to has a positive effect on the well-being of the older person.

Caring for a pet such as a cat or bird or turtle in private homes is much easier than in a long term care facility; yet with a little planning, residents also can have this benefit. A single cat, living in the facility, can provide much affection for all the residents. Residents in largely self-care facilities can provide much of the ongoing care themselves. With assistance, this form of therapy could be made available to many more of the elderly.

VOCABULARY

antibiotic	digitalis	mood-altering drug
antidepressant	disorientation	peristalsis
antihypertensive	diuretic	potassium loss
apathy	diuresis	rectum
bowel	enema	rehabilitation
cardiac stimulant	expectorant	sulfa drug
catheter	feces	suppositories
colon	hematuria	toxicity
colostomy	hypotension	tranquilizer
commode	laxative	vasodilator
dehydration		

SUGGESTED ACTIVITIES

1. Visit a long term care facility to see how the clients' activities of daily living are satisfied.

2. Examine care plans, noting the drugs that are commonly given.

3. Discuss with your instructor the purpose of commonly given drugs such as cardiac stimulants, diuretics, expectorants, antibiotics and mind-altering drugs.

4. Using a *Physician's Desk Reference (PDR)*, look up five commonly given drugs.

5. Assist during a recreation period at a care facility.

REVIEW

A. Brief Answer/Fill in the Blanks

1. List four activities of daily living (ADL) presented in this lesson.

   a. _____

   b. _____

   c. _____

   d. _____

2. Solid wastes are called _____.

3. Two aids to bowel elimination are _____ and _____.

4. Bowel elimination is encouraged by increased _____ and a diet that includes _____ and _____.

5. The resident's position must be changed every _____ to _____ hours.

6. Drugs that improve heart function are called _____.

7. Tranquilizers and sedatives are classified as _____ drugs.

8. _____ may occur if a resident is given drugs that increase urine output. These drugs are called _____.

9. Recreational and occupational activities help give residents a _____ to life and aid the rehabilitation process.

10. Two group recreational activities are _____ and _____.

B. True or False. Answer the following questions true (T) or false (F).

1. _____ Since it takes less time, the nursing assistant should carry out the ADL for the resident.

2. _____ Residents should recieve a complete bath every day.

3. _____ It is important to store dentures safely when not in use.

4. _____ Elderly people tolerate drug therapy less well than younger individuals.

5. _____ Rehabilitation means helping a person become fully independent in carrying out the ADL.

6. _____ Light-headedness and pulse change are signs of digitalis accumulation (toxicity) and should be reported.

7. _____ Sudden mood swings can be ignored, since these are not a significant change.

8. _____ The attitude of the nursing assistant can be important in motivating residents' participation in rehabilitation.

9. _____ Occupational activities are valuable only if they are financially profitable.

10. _____ A resident with a catheter connected to constant drainage needs to have both intake and output of fluids monitored.

CLINICAL SITUATION

John Rogers has a serious heart problem for which he is receiving a heart stimulant (digitalis) and a diuretic (Lasix) every day. What special observations would you make in regard to the care of this resident?

Answer: _____

_____

_____

_____

_____

LESSON 13 Nutritional Needs

OBJECTIVES

After studying this lesson, you should be able to:

- Name the six classes of nutrients and four food groups.
- State ways that the nursing assistant can promote good nutrition.
- List five diets commonly ordered in long term care facilities.
- Demonstrate feeding.
- Describe alternate ways that a resident might receive nutrition.
- Define and spell all vocabulary words and terms.

Eating to meet nutritional needs is one of the major ADL. Elderly people who live independent in the community are apt to prepare foods that satisfy their appetite without meeting the basic nutritional needs.

Appetite can be satisfied without meeting nutritional needs.

Proper nutrition provides us with the essential materials to:

- build and repair tissues
- carry out body functions
- provide energy for the work the body does

It takes energy to carry out specific activities such as walking or getting in and out of bed; but even when a person is quiet and inactive, energy is needed for the heart to beat and for the kidneys to produce urine. These are examples of vital body activities that sustain life.

The energy for body functions is supplied by the nutrients in the foods which we eat. When not enough nutrients are consumed, the body gradually uses up its storage supply and becomes depleted: illness follows close behind.

In order to better understand the nutritional needs of residents you need to learn about what nutrients do in the body and what sources are available for them. You also need to learn how to meet the special nutritional needs of residents.

NUTRIENTS

There are six classes of nutrients, but many foods contain more than one nutrient. The basic nutrients are:

Carbohydrates

Carbohydrates are the primary source of body energy. Many foods contain this nutrient. Fruits, vegetables, breads, cereal, and macaroni products are good sources. Carbohydrate foods supply the body with **fiber** in the form of cellulose. Fiber helps maintain **regularity** (bowel activity).

Fats

Fats provide energy and can be found in both plant and animal foods. Rich sources of fats include butter, pork, nuts, egg yolks, and vebetable oils.

Proteins

Proteins are essential for tissue building and repair. Foods rich in protein include meats, fish, poultry, eggs, beans, nuts, and lentils.

Vitamins and Minerals

Vitamins and **minerals** regulate body processes. The different kinds of vitamins are represented by letters. Vitamins A, D, K, and E are fat soluble and are found in fatty foods as well as in fruits and vegetables. Vitamins B and C are water soluble and are found in fruits, vegetables, and whole grain products. The minerals include sodium, potassium, calcium and iron.

Water

Water is essential to all life processes. Each person needs to take in about 2½ quarts (2½ liters or 2500 milliliters [ml]) of water in some form daily. (In certain circumstances, under a doctor's order water intake may be limited.) Water is consumed in drinks such as tap water, tea, coffee and other beverages and is also taken in with foods such as fruits and vegetables that have high water content, figure 13-1. In general, elderly persons do not take in enough water and must be reminded and encouraged to drink. This is especially true when they feel ill or have a fever, or when the weather is hot. You can help to ensure fluid balance in residents by:

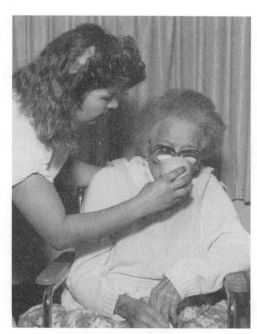

FIGURE 13-1. Residents need to be encouraged to take fluids often.

- making sure water is fresh and close at hand
- reminding the resident to drink
- keeping residents cool during hot weather
- increasing attention to fluid intake when the resident is ill or has a fever

Residents who are not getting adequate fluids may give warnings of *dehydration* such as:

- becoming confused
- showing less energy than usual
- becoming constipated
- complaining of thirst
- exhibiting dry skin
- producing less urine

Signs of Dehydration
• Dry skin
• Scanty urine
• Thirst
• Restlessness
• Elevated temperature
• Apathy

FIGURE 13–2. Signs of dehydration.

Be sure to report any signs of dehydration at once so that steps may be taken to correct the problem.

THE FOUR FOOD GROUPS

Foods can be classified into four basic groups, figure 13–3. Adequate selections from each group ensure proper nutrition. The four food groups are:

1. fruits and vegetables
2. milk group
3. grain group
4. meat group

Selections from the basic four food groups provide essential nutrients.

Fruits-Vegetables Group. The fruit and vegetable group provides **vitamins, minerals,** and **fiber.** Four or more servings of vegetables or fruits should be included in the daily diet. Fruits and vegetables can be made easier to chew by:

- cooking
- chopping
- dicing

Milk Group. The dairy product group is a good source of **proteins,** vitamins, and minerals. A minimum of two servings of milk are

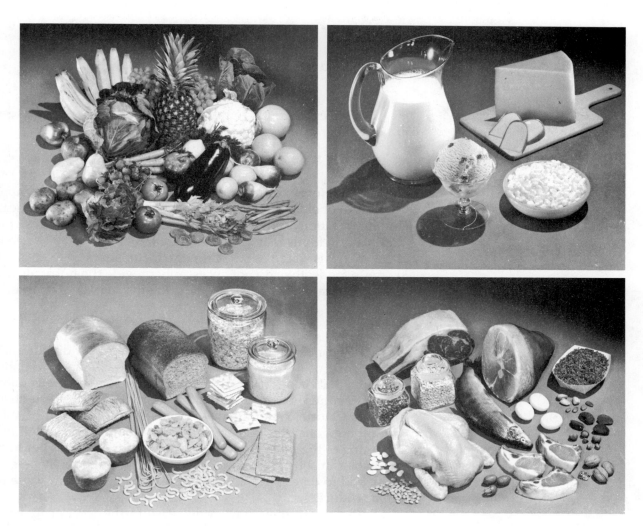

FIGURE 13–3. Four food groups.

recommended for adults. One serving of milk has about the same amount of calcium as one cup of yogurt, one and one-half slices of cheese, one cup of pudding, or two cups of cottage cheese. Milk substitutes include:

- cheese — 1½ slices
- cottage cheese — 2 cups
- puddings — 1 cup
- yogurt — 1 cup

Grain Group. The grain group provides **carbohydrates,** vitamins, minerals, and roughage. Four or more servings of this group should be served daily.

Meat Group. The meat group supplies protein and is also a good source of fats, vitamins, and minerals. Two or more servings should be taken each day. This group includes:

- meat
- fish
- eggs
- dried beans and peas
- nuts

The basic four food groups are used in planning diets for residents in long term care facilities.

NUTRITIONAL STATUS

Obesity (overweight) and dehydration are problems for more than 20 percent of older persons. Obesity is due to excessive caloric intake, and dehydration is often due to inadequate water intake. Easy-to-chew high-calorie foods may provide energy in excess of body needs; the extra energy is stored as fat. Although the person's appetite is satisfied by these foods, they do not necessarily provide the nutrients needed. Essential vitamins, minerals, and proteins may be deficient.

ASSURING PROPER NUTRITION

Meals for residents are carefully planned by a dietitian to meet special geriatric needs. The nursing assistant has a major responsibility in seeing that these meals are consumed. In general, the geriatric diet needs to continue to contain adequate levels of all nutrients except calories. Calorie content usually needs to be decreased because the elderly are generally less active. Coarse foods are avoided because the lining of the mouth of the elderly is thinner and easier to injure. Vegetables and fruits that are cooked and chopped may be easier to chew and to digest and are included for their nutrient value and as bulk producers.

Some elderly may have a decrease in the level of hydrochloric acid in the stomach juices, making the absorption of some minerals more difficult. Diminished production of the intestinal enzyme lactase and some drugs may limit the use of milk sugar (lactose). The general diet may be supplemented with vitamin and mineral capsules or tablets.

Remember, adequate fluids (water) are essential, and liquids should be included in meals and as planned nourishment three times each day — morning, afternoon and early evening. Additional fluids are offered whenever the opportunity arises.

Small servings are more appealing, especially when inactivity causes poor appetites, figure 13-4. Many facilities serve several (four or five) small meals instead of three larger meals. The evening meal is usually lighter to promote comfortable sleeping. In some individual cases, fluids may be limited in the evening hours so that the resident will not have to awaken to go to the bathroom so often.

TYPES OF DIETS

Some residents may need to have their diets modified because of health problems. Special diets are based on the four food groups, but consistency and method of preparation may be altered.

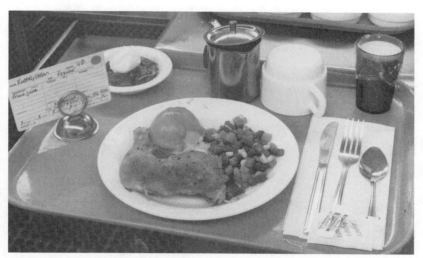

FIGURE 13–4. Well-balanced, smaller servings are more appealing to the elderly appetite.

Standard Diets

Both standard and specialized diets are available in long term care facilities.

Four standard diets are offered in long term care facilities. They are the:

1. Regular diet
2. Mechanical soft diet
3. Full liquid diet
4. Clear liquid diet

Regular Diet. The **regular diet** is prepared for most residents. It includes varied selections from the basic food groups.

Mechanical Soft Diet. The **mechanical soft diet** is based on the regular diet but includes liquids and semi-solid foods that are more easily chewed and digested, figure 13–5.

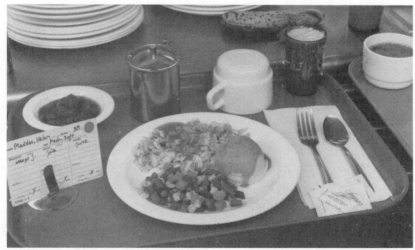

FIGURE 13–5. The mechanical soft diet is easy to chew and digest.

Full Liquid Diet. The **full liquid diet** meets nutritional needs with foods that can be put into liquid form at room temperature, figure 13–6.

It may be given to residents with diseases of the intestinal tract or those who are unable to chew because of infection or some other problem.

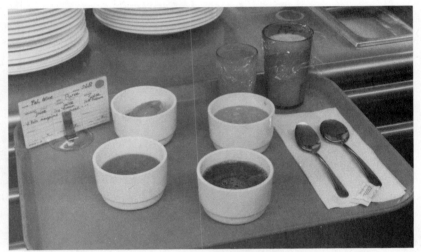

FIGURE 13–6. The pureed diet includes foods from each of the four food groups that have been placed through a blender.

Clear Liquid Diet. The **clear liquid diet** is usually prescribed when a resident is ill and needs to have fluids replaced. This diet is not given for prolonged periods because it does not provide adequate nutrition. Milk is not included in the clear liquid diet because the liquids must be clear (i.e., you can see through them), but broths and filtered fruit juices are permitted.

Special Diets

Special diets, also called therapeutic diets, are prepared for residents with individual health problems, figure 13–7. They include the:

1. Diabetic diet
2. Low sodim diet
3. Low fat diet
4. Calorie restricted diet
5. High protein diet

The **diabetic diet** is usually a carefully balanced diet for residents who have diabetes mellitus and who must restrict concentrated carbohydrates (e.g., candy or pastry) in their diet. They may eat nothing that is not on their diet, but it is equally important that they consume everything that is ordered for them.

The **low sodium diet** is prescribed for the resident with a heart condition or one who retains fluids. The **low fat diet** limits the amounts of fats in the diet and is served to residents with gallbladder or liver disease. The **calorie restricted diet** is given to residents in need of weight control. The **high protein diet** is provided for residents who are underweight and poorly nourished and when diseases such as cancer make unusual nutritional demands.

Diabetic	Amounts of carbohydrates, fats, and proteins are balanced and prescribed. Concentrated sweets are restricted.
Low Sodium (Sodium Restricted)	Amounts of sodium specifically prescribed such as 500 mg. sodium. Sodium rich foods such as milk and bacon or salted nuts are excluded.
Calorie Restricted	Limits the number of calories while ensuring an adequate intake of nutrients.
Low Fat	Foods with high fat content are restricted such as whole milk and eggs. Eliminates use of fats in preparation of food.
Antianemic	High in protein, iron and vitamins, served in six small meals per day. Hot, spicy foods excluded.
Low Residue	Roughage, fresh fruits and vegetables (except bananas and potatoes), nuts, and whole grains are limited.

FIGURE 13–7. Summary of special diets.

Remember, special diets are *therapeutic,* which means they are used as *treatments.* Always check to be sure that the resident receives the right tray.

NURSING ASSISTANT RESPONSIBILITIES ▪▪▪▪▪▪▪▪▪▪▪▪▪▪▪▪▪▪▪▪

Mealtime is a busy time in the long term care facility. The nursing assistant has a major responsibility to see that it goes smoothly and pleasantly. You will

Assistant duties include transporting, serving, feeding residents.

- assist residents to reach the dining room
- serve trays
- feed residents needing assistance

Eating may be one of the few generally pleasing activities left to the elderly. The meal should be sensually and socially satisfying as well as one that meets nutritional needs. Large dining areas permit residents to eat together and promote a social atmosphere.

Assisting with Feeding

If residents can go to the dining room, assist them to the toilet before mealtimes. Wash their hands and help them into the dining room. Wheelchairs and geri-chairs can be rolled into the dining room if residents are not ambulatory, figure 13–8. After washing your own hands, help serve the trays and assist as necessary (e.g., cutting meat, pouring liquids, buttering bread, unfolding and positioning napkins).

Feeding the Resident

Even when a resident is confined to bed, or when it is necessary to feed him or her (figure 13–9), you can make the experience more pleasurable if you:

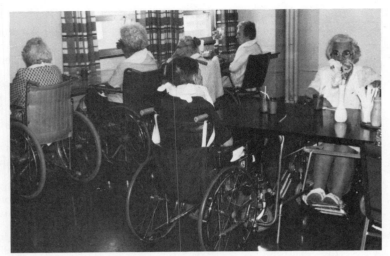

FIGURE 13–8. Residents are transported to communal eating areas.

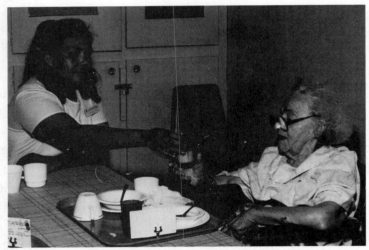

FIGURE 13–9. Nursing assistants help residents eat.

- never hurry the procedure
- position the resident comfortably
- remove all unpleasant things from sight
- allow the resident to help as much as possible
- identify the food offered
- follow the resident's preference, offering liquids frequently
- talk with the resident in an unhurried manner

If the resident has difficulty seeing, make sure there is as much light as possible. Describe the arrangement of the food on the plate, relating them to the face of a clock, figure 13–10. Explain placement of other items on the tray so the resident can feed himself or herself as much as possible.

Before delivering a food tray, wash your hands and check the tray for proper identification. Place the tray on the overbed table and position the resident in a sitting position, if permitted, or on the

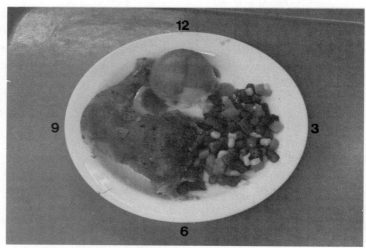

FIGURE 13–10. For residents who have difficulty seeing, describe the food as placed in relation to the face of a clock.

unaffected side if he or she has had a stroke. Prepare food as necessary, such as cutting it into small pieces, and feed small amounts slowly; avoid having the resident talk or laugh during feeding.

PROCEDURE: Feeding a Resident

1. Identify resident and explain what is to be done.
2. Offer bedpan or urinal, or assist resident to the bathroom.
3. Wash your hands and see that the resident washes also.
4. If permitted, elevate head of bed or assist resident to chair.
5. Clear overbed table and position in front of resident.
6. Remove unpleasant equipment from sight.
7. Check dietary name tag against resident's identification.
8. Place tray on overbed table and arrange food in a convenient manner.
9. Assist in food preparation as needed. Encourage the resident to do as much as possible for himself or herself.
10. Remove tray as soon as resident is finished. Make sure to note what he or she has and has

PROCEDURE: Assisting the Resident Who Can Feed Himself or Herself

1. Identify the resident.
2. Offer the bedpan or assist resident to the bathroom before feeding.
3. Wash your own hands.
4. Assist in the washing of the resident's hands and face, if needed.
5. Assist resident to sit in chair if permitted or possible.
6. If the resident is confined to bed, and if permitted, raise the head of the bed or adjust the resident through use of pillows.
7. Clear the overbed table.
8. Remove anything unpleasant from sight.
9. Obtain the resident's correct tray — *check identification.*
10. Identify foods and their placement on tray for resident, if necessary.
11. Assist by cutting up meat, pouring liquids, or buttering bread.
12. Allow the resident to do as much for himself or herself as possible.
13. Be pleasant and unhurried in your manner.

has not eaten. Record fluids on intake record, if required.

11. Push overbed table out of the way and assist the resident to return to bed or place in a comfortable position.

12. Make sure that call bell and water are within reach and that the room is tidy.

13. Wash hands.

PROCEDURE: Feeding the Helpless Resident

1. Wash hands.
2. Check the diet order. Add nothing to the tray unless it is on the diet order. Check the name card on the tray against the resident's identification.
3. Remove unnecessary articles from the overbed table.
4. Adjust the resident to a comfortable position.
5. Place napkin under resident's chin.
6. Butter bread and cut meat. Do not pour hot beverage until resident is ready for it.
7. Use drinking straw to give fluids.
8. Holding spoon at a right angle, give solid foods from point of spoon. Alternate liquids and solids. Describe or show resident what kind of food you are giving him or her. Test hot foods by dropping small amount on the inside of your wrist before feeding to the resident.
9. Allow resident to hold bread and assist to the extent that he or she is able.
10. Use napkin to wipe resident's mouth and hands as often as necessary.
11. Remove tray as soon as resident is finished. Make sure you note what the resident has or has not eaten.
12. Record fluids on intake record if necessary.
13. Wash hands.

Choking

There is always the danger of choking when feeding a helpless resident. Be on guard! A choking resident will be unable to speak, may cough or gag, or may grasp at his or her throat. Stop feeding at once.

If a resident becomes unconscious and food is visible in the mouth, grasp the lower jaw and tongue with one hand and lift. With the other hand, insert the index finger inside the cheek and into the throat at the base of the tongue and clear the mouth with a sweeping motion. Call out for help or use the intercom, figure 13–11.

A resident who is sitting and begins to choke can be helped in the same way. In addition, the Heimlich maneuver can be beneficial, figure 13–12. This requires practice but can be life-saving in an emergency. This method involves:

- Standing behind the resident.
- Placing your arms around the resident's waist.
- Clasping your hands together making a fist, with the thumb side against the resident's abdomen between the waist and the sternum.
- Giving six to ten upward and inward thrusts.

In many cases this may dislodge the food that is caught.

Remember, as you feed the resident, talk with him or her. Make the process an opportunity both for social exchange and close observation of the resident. Be sure to note how much food is taken in, which foods are enjoyed, and which foods are refused. If foods are refused, try to determine why the resident won't eat them. Report and record the information.

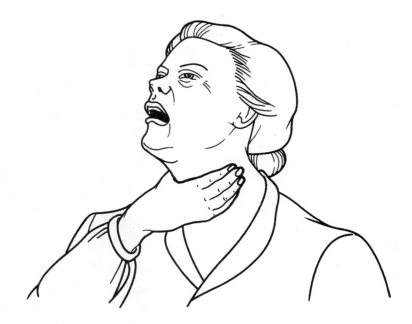

FIGURE 13–11. *The distress signal that the resident is choking.*

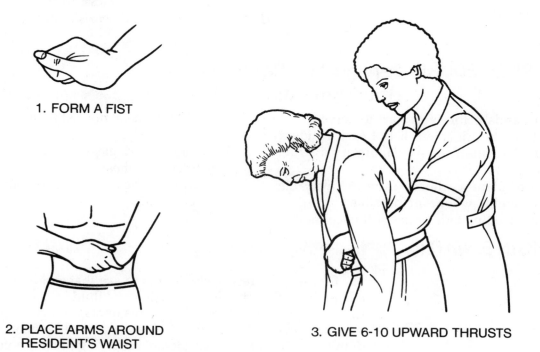

1. FORM A FIST

2. PLACE ARMS AROUND RESIDENT'S WAIST

3. GIVE 6-10 UPWARD THRUSTS

FIGURE 13–12. *Procedure for the Heimlich maneuver.*

SUPPLEMENTAL NOURISHMENT ■■■■■■■■■■■■■■■■■■■■■■■■■■■■

Follow nourishment
instructions carefully.

Serving between-meal nourishments is an important function of the nursing assistant. Milk, juice, custard, or other light nourishment is offered to the residents, figure 13–13. If this is your assignment, be sure to follow the dietary instructions carefully. Assist residents who need help and do not offer nourishment to those who are listed as "withholds." Use the nourishment list as a guide. Remember, instructions may change from day to day. All supplementary nourishments and meals must be recorded.

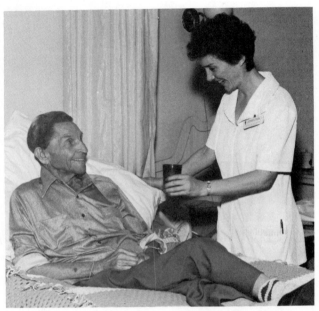

FIGURE 13–13. Between-meal nourishments help to meet nutritional needs.

■■■ PROCEDURE: Serving Supplementary Nourishments ■■■■■■■■■■■■■■■■■■■■■■■■

1. Wash hands before you start to serve.
2. Check the nourishment list of each resident for any limitations or special dietary instructions.
3. Allow resident to choose from the available nourishments whenever possible.
4. Provide feeding aids or assist those who are unable to take nourishment alone (figures 13–14 and 13–15).
5. Remove used glasses and dishes after the resident finishes.
6. Record on the intake and output (I&O) sheet if required.

CHANGING WATER ■■■■■■■■■■■■■■■■■■■■■■■■■■■■■■■■■■

One of your responsibilities is to see that residents always have adequate fresh water. Because adequate fluid intake is important for the older person, make sure that residents are drinking as they are supposed to do. If "forced fluids" are mandated, encourage the resident to take in more fluids. Before emptying pitcher note how much water is left. If the resident is on measured intake, the amount of fluid taken may be estimated by subtracting what is left from the originally

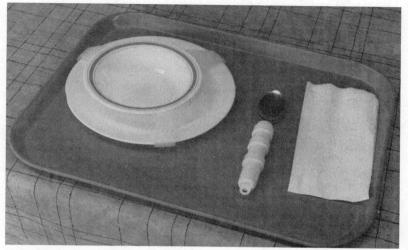

FIGURE 13–14. Note the fasteners that hold the bowl firmly in place and the firm grip spoon.

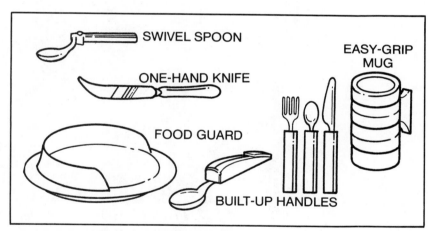

SWIVEL SPOON

ONE-HAND KNIFE

EASY-GRIP MUG

FOOD GUARD

BUILT-UP HANDLES

FIGURE 13–15. Other assistive devices.

full container. Since the procedure for changing water varies with each facility, be sure to check the procedure book. A sample procedure follows. Not all residents prefer or are allowed ice water, so check before you fill the water pitcher. Unless otherwise ordered, fresh water must always be kept within easy reach of every resident.

▪▪▪ PROCEDURE: Changing Water ▪▪▪▪▪▪▪▪▪▪▪▪▪▪▪▪▪▪▪▪▪▪▪▪▪▪

1. Wash your hands.
2. Check whether resident is allowed ice or tap water.
3. Wash, refill, and return pitcher to resident's bedside table.

4. Leave a clean glass beside the pitcher.
5. Leave a bendable straw beside the resident's glass.
6. Make sure that the water is close at hand.

ALTERNATE METHODS OF FEEDING ▪▪▪▪▪▪▪▪▪▪▪▪▪▪▪▪▪▪▪▪▪▪▪▪▪▪

Sometimes residents are too ill or weak to consume even a liquid diet. Then alternate methods of providing nutrition are needed. A **nasogastric tube** may be introduced through the nose and into the stomach (by a nurse or physician) so that liquid or pureed food may be directly introduced. This form of feeding is called *gavage* and requires special training to be sure the tube is in the proper place, figure 13–16. In some cases, a **gastrostomy** (an opening into the stomach through the abdominal wall) may be made and feedings are given through a gastrostomy tube. Gastrostomy feedings also require special skills and are performed by a nurse. You must inform the nurse if either of these tubes become dislodged.

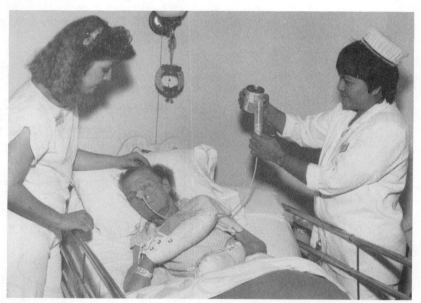

FIGURE 13–16. The nursing assistant offers support as the nurse gavages the resident.

Special fluids and nutrients are also administered directly into the blood stream by **intravenous (IV) feedings**, figure 13–17. The nurse will begin and end the **infusion** (introduction of IV fluid), but you must be alert to the level of fluid in the bag or bottle. Be sure to tell the nurse before the fluid completely runs out. The nurse will let you know how rapidly the fluid should drop (**flow rate**), and the position of the infusion site. Report any change in the flow rate or any swelling or discoloration at the infusion site.

Do not reposition the part of the arm receiving the IV infusion once the fluid has been started. A small board can sometimes give added support. Be sure that the tape or gauze holding the board is not too tight. Check it frequently and inform the nurse if the area is discolored or swollen.

Some infusions will be given with an infusion pump. If the infusion pump alarm goes off inform the nurse at once.

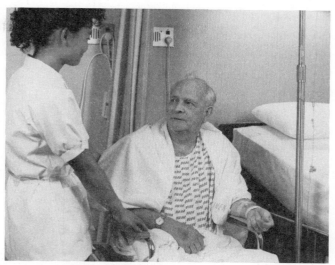

FIGURE 13–17. This resident is receiving an intravenous infusion of nutrients.

VOCABULARY

calorie restricted diet	high protein diet	minerals
carbohydrate	infusion	nasogastric tube
clear liquid diet	intravenous (IV) feeding	obesity
fats	lactose	protein
fiber	low fat diet	regularity
flow rate	low sodium diet	regular diet
full liquid diet	mechanical soft diet	vitamins
gastrostomy		

SUGGESTED ACTIVITIES

1. Practice feeding a classmate and then reverse the positions. Use samples of solids, liquids, and pureed foods.

2. List all the foods that you consume in a 24-hour period of time, placing them in the proper basic food groups.

3. Talk with a dietitian about the types of diets prepared for residents.

4. Practice the following procedures in the clinical setting:
   a. Serving trays
   b. Preparing residents for meals
   c. Assisting in the resident dining room
   d. Feeding the helpless resident
   e. Serving nourishments
   f. Providing fresh water

REVIEW

A. Brief Answer/Fill in the Blanks

1. Name the six basic nutrients.

   a. _____

   b. _____

    c. _____

    d. _____

    e. _____

    f. _____

2. The four food groups are:

    a. _____

    b. _____

    c. _____

    d. _____

3. The elderly diet needs to be _____ in calories and _____ in vitamins and minerals.

4. Regularity is promoted when _____ is included in the diet.

5. All life processes are dependent upon adequate_____.

6. Milk substitutes can be given to residents who cannot tolerate milk. These include:

    a. _____

    b. _____

    c. _____

7. Evening meals are usually lighter in content to promote more

    _____.

8. Three therapeutic diets frequently served in a long term care facility are:

    a. _____

    b. _____

    c. _____

9. Two alternate feeding methods are:

    a. _____

    b. _____

10. Meeting nutritional needs in the elderly may be difficult because chewing is _____ and digestion _____.

B. True or False. Answer the following questions true (T) or false (F).

1. _____ A dietitian plans the diet for the resident.

2. _____ Eating should be a social occasion.

3. _____ Elderly persons need approximately one quart of water daily.

4. _____ Three large meals are usually served to residents in long term care facilities.

5. _____ The source of nutrients is the food eaten.

6. _____ Dehydration is a major problem for the elderly.

7. _____ Concentrated sugars are included in the diabetic diet.

8. _____ Nursing assistants start intravenous infusions.

9. _____ Obesity is a nutritional problem associated with older people.

10. _____ Appetite may be satisfied and still not meet all the nutritional needs of the resident.

CLINICAL SITUATION

Mrs. Hartley is 92 and almost blind. Although she can make out light and dark, everything is blurred and as if in shadows. She has a cold and wants to rest in bed instead of going to the dining room to eat. You are serving trays. How might you improve the mealtime and insure proper nutrition?

Answer: _____

_____

_____

_____

_____

_____

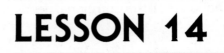

LESSON 14 Psychological, Spiritual, and Sociological Needs

OBJECTIVES

After studying this lesson, you should be able to:

- Identify Abraham Maslow and Erick Erickson and explain the contribution each has made to the understanding of human needs.
- Describe developmental tasks as they relate to the elderly.
- List the ways the elderly meet their psychological needs.
- Support the spiritual needs of the resident.
- Recognize sexual needs of older persons.
- Indicate the ways that the nursing assistant can assist in meeting psychological and spiritual needs.
- Define and spell all the vocabulary words and terms.

BASIC HUMAN NEEDS

Basic human needs are those activities required by all people to successfully and satisfactorily live their lives. The needs are the same for all people, at all ages — healthy or unwell.

Abraham Maslow and Erick Erickson, two leaders in the field of human behavior, have made valuable contributions to our understanding of the basic needs and how people go about satisfying them.

Maslow described the three groups of basic needs as:

- physical
- psychological
- sociological

He found that the physical needs must be satisfied first before the psychological or sociological needs can even be considered, figure 14–1.

The most basic human concerns are related to the physical functioning of our bodies and include nutrition, rest, oxygen, elimination, activity, and sexuality. Illness and age create stresses that make meeting these needs a challenge for both resident and care giver. For example, poorly fitting dentures and small appetites must be taken into consideration if nutrition is to be maintained at adequate levels. Once basic physical needs are met, attention can be given to the next level of needs — psychological (emotional) needs.

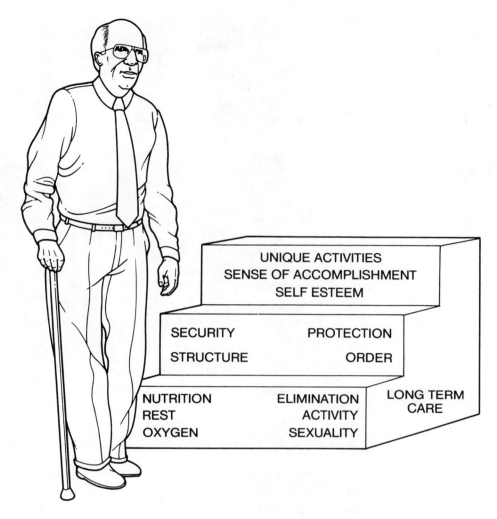

FIGURE 14–1. People meet needs in order of priority of importance. Physical needs must be satisfied first.

EMOTIONAL NEEDS

The basic emotional needs of the elderly are the same as those at any age. There is a need

- to love
- to be loved
- to be treated with respect and dignity

Emotional needs may not be as readily seen as physical needs.

When residents enter a long term care facility, they often feel depressed, threatened, frightened, and frustrated. They are in a new, strange environment and they fear that they will lose all privacy and control of their own lives. Residents need to feel protected and secure in the knowledge that those who care for them will not abuse them in any way. Care givers meet this need when they provide care promptly and gently, and when they treat residents as respected individuals capable of making choices and decisions, figure 14–2.

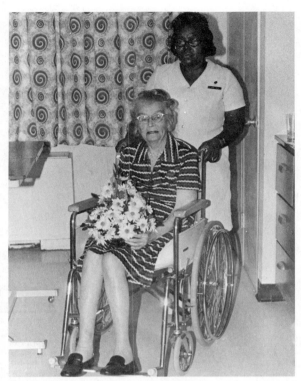

FIGURE 14–2. Newly admitted residents need much support as they adjust to their new home. (From Brooks, The Nurse Assistant, copyright 1978 by Delmar Publishers Inc.)

Elderly residents have fewer opportunities to satisfy their emotional needs. Most are aware that their bodies are failing, that they are separated from family and friends, and that others will be doing for them things they used to do for themselves. All of these facts are major stresses to emotional security.

Most residents — like most people in general — try to deal with emotional stress by relying on the strategies that have been successful for them in past years. Some may move backward in emotional responses, behaving as children might who are frightened and frustrated. Others may be so overwhelmed by stress that they become withdrawn, confused, and disoriented.

Personality_____

Each personality is unique — formed by life's experiences.

Exactly how each person goes about satisfying personal psychological needs depends on his or her **personality**. Personality is the sum of the ways we react to the events in our lives. Personality is gradually formed through experience.

Erickson suggests that as we mature from infancy to old age, we pass through several growing stages, and that during each stage a task has to be accomplished. He calls these the *tasks of personality development*, or **developmental tasks**. For example, the task of old age is to review the life's challenges and accomplishments and to find final contentment. The tasks of the various growth periods are summarized in figure 14–3.

TASKS OF PERSONALITY DEVELOPMENT	
Growing Stage	Task
Infancy	Learning to trust
Early childhood years	Recognizing identity as part of a family unit
School years	Skill development; constructive activities
Adolescent years	Developing identity as an individual
Young Adulthood	Forming intimate relationships; raising a family
Middle years	Carrying out one's chosen work
Old age	Integrating life's experiences

FIGURE 14–3. *Tasks of personality development as summarized by Erickson.*

MAJOR CHALLENGES TO ADJUSTMENTS ▪▪▪▪▪▪▪▪▪▪▪▪▪▪▪▪▪▪▪▪

Each phase of life brings with it adjustments to be made, stresses to be overcome, and challenges to be met. The challenges that develop personality often come as the result of a major life crisis. Three crises that present major challenges and adjustments to the older person are:

1. Loss of a mate
2. Living with illness and infirmities
3. Loss of independence

In the lives of many people, these three events occur in close succession and stress can be overwhelming, figure 14–4.

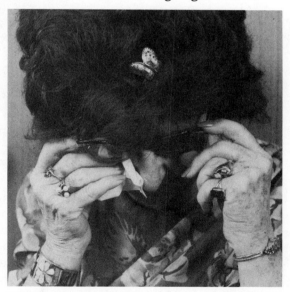

FIGURE 14–4. *People have reasons for feeling sad.*

Loss of Loved One__

A person who loses a spouse faces major psychological adjustments and a bereavement period that is a time of great uncertainty at any age. It is particularly traumatic when one is old, with failing health and limited resources. Many important decisions about the future must be made at a time when loneliness, confusion, and grief are at their height.

When her husband dies, a woman may sense a loss of her own identity. When his wife dies, a man loses much of his available social structure. If able, each will eventually adjust to his or her new life alone. Family and friends can be very helpful in the transition process, but it is the individual who must finally face and master the tasks of adjustment.

Sometimes a pet can become a loved member of the family to an elderly person. The loss experienced when the pet dies can also require major psychological adjustments similar to those experienced when a human family member is lost.

Major losses: a mate, health, independence.

Overcoming Grief

Having a **confidant** (someone to confide in) can help the elderly person work through the grief and adjustment period. The nursing assistant who has good **rapport** (interpersonal relationships) with the resident can be invaluable in fulfilling the role of confidant, figure 14–5. Giving the resident the opportunity to talk about lost loved ones helps to put feeling and memories into proper relationships. Working through feelings gives the resident an ultimate sense of strength and self-identity.

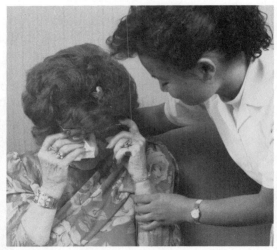

FIGURE 14–5. Be comforting. Recognize the resident's right to have such feelings.

Chronic Illness

Another major challenge faced by older folks is the adjustment that must be made to the frailty of age and infirmities as health is lost and illness becomes chronic. Although poor health is not necessarily part of the aging process, conditions such as diabetes mellitus, heart disease, arthritis, and emphysema are more common and put additional stress on changing body systems.

Many people try to deny the existence of the changes in stamina that are occurring and then become angry and frustrated as they come to realize they cannot control the changes going on in their bodies. However, most people gradually come to adjust to and accept their present condition and limitations. Eventually they come to realize that an individual's life does not go on forever and that death is inevitable. The process of moving toward this understanding and acceptance is called **disengagement**. It is a gradual process that is developmental in nature.

Loss of Total Independence_____

The third crisis involves the set of adjustments the elderly person makes in giving up independent living to become a resident in a long term care facility, figure 14–6. Prior to admission, many individuals undergo a series of emotional stresses. Making this decision is never easy for the family or for the person involved. Personal treasures may have to be given up, beloved pets put into new homes, and an entire life style changed. A person's sense of independence is threatened just by knowing that there is a need for facility care and support.

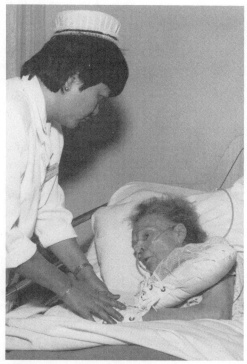

FIGURE 14–6. Loss of independence is a major adjustment for a person. The staff must be supportive as they provide total care.

After admission, the new surroundings and people can raise the levels of anxiety and stress to such a point that the new resident becomes confused and disoriented. Your calm consistency and patience are vital factors in helping the new resident to adjust successfully and to complete this developmental task.

COPING MECHANISMS

The success or failure in making positive psychological adjustments in later life depends to a large extent upon how well the developmental tasks of earlier life periods have been mastered, and how the personality has been formed. The ways of adjusting that a person has used successfully throughout his or her life become part of that person's **coping mechanism** or response pattern. As care givers, we must remember that residents will react to situations in the same ways that have worked for them in the past.

Each coping mechanism is a response to stress and is defensive, protecting the person's feelings of **self-esteem** (self-worth).

Common coping, or **defense mechanisms**, include:

- projection
- rationalization
- denial
- compensation

Projection is a way of blaming others for failures or problems. For example, a resident tells you her bed is wet because another assistant wouldn't bring the bedpan on time. The resident blames someone else for the problem rather than admit that she is incontinent (unable to hold back urine).

Rationalization can be defined as giving false but believable reasons for a situation. Rationalization is being used when a resident tells you that she could crochet just as well as someone else, but her "arthritis" makes it too difficult. You know that this resident plays the piano almost every day, moving her fingers across the keyboard quite easily.

Denial is arguing or pretending the problem does not exist. This defense mechanism is at work when a resident tells you this is one of the happiest times of his life, even though you know that the resident is having a very difficult time adjusting to the facility.

Compensation (making up for a situation in some other way) is being used when one resident cannot walk, for instance, but can draw people to him by telling amusing stories or jokes.

Examples of these defense mechanisms in operation can be seen in every long term care facility. In fact, they are the same coping mechanisms we all use at one time or another.

Coping mechanisms are used to overcome stress.

Stress Reactions

When coping mechanisms are inadequate, stress reactions develop and can take several forms. Chronic complaining, agitation, restlessness, poor sleeping patterns, periods of depression, and withdrawal are all signals that the coping ability of the individual is being excessively strained, figure 14–7. Residents may ignore their surroundings and become confused and generally uncooperative and demanding. Some may even become combative and abusive. Some residents may give up the struggle to assert themselves, becoming withdrawn and dependent.

MEETING RESIDENTS' EMOTIONAL NEEDS ▪▪▪▪▪▪▪▪▪▪▪▪▪▪▪▪▪▪

The nursing assistant who is in continuous contact with the resident has a tremendous opportunity to provide the emotional support so desperately needed by the residents. You can do this by:

Signs that coping mechanisms are failing:
- *chronic complaining*
- *agitation*
- *restlessness*
- *sleeplessness*
- *depression*
- *withdrawal*

- demonstrating that you and each member of the staff are aware of the resident's anxieties and really do care. You demonstrate your interest and caring by helping each resident continue his or her own life style as much as he or she is able.
- encouraging the resident to be as independent as possible.
- explaining the care that you give and providing the opportunity for choices whenever possible.

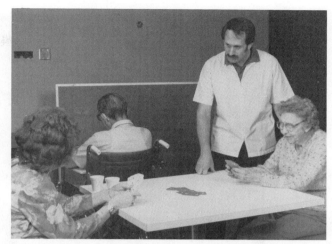

FIGURE 14–7. When stress is too great, coping mechanisms can fail and the resident withdraws.

- being a good listener and friend. This is especially important during periods of depression and loneliness.
- encouraging the resident to talk about fears and frustrations, as this will help reduce anxieties.
- not taking angry outbursts personally. Be able to recognize that such outbursts are the natural product of feelings of hopelessness.
- directing the resident's emotional energy in positive ways — for example, by encouraging the resident to take part in the facility's activities.
- being honest. Honest relationships have the best chance for success, and residents know if you are putting on an act.
- being patient and kind. This is the best kind of emotional support you can offer and will, in turn, help to build rapport and trust.
- recognizing the signs of stress reactions and being ready to offer encouragement and support.

SPIRITUAL NEEDS

A person's spiritual feelings play an important part in helping them through the crises and stress periods of their lives. Spiritual feelings are personal, are expressed in different ways, and may or may not be associated with a specific religious church or group, figure 14–8. You must be prepared to support a person's spiritual beliefs, whatever their source, in any way that you can.

Spiritual needs are as important to many people as any of the other basic human needs. Spiritual values form the guiding principles of what many consider to be right and wrong.

Residents may wish to talk to you about their beliefs or may need help in carrying out certain practices or rituals, figure 14–9. Be open to discussions with the resident. Listen, redirecting statements so that the resident has a chance to continue exploring his or her own thoughts. For example, if a resident asks you "Do you believe there

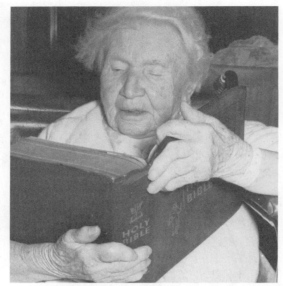

FIGURE 14–8. Spiritual feelings are very deep and must be respected.

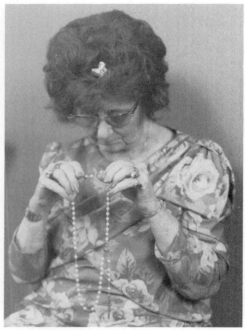

FIGURE 14–9. Some residents will be guided by a specific religion and its practices.

is a God?" your response could be, "You are thinking about God" or "What is your feeling about it?". These responses redirect the topic to the resident for further reflection.

There are several things that you can do to support the resident's spiritual needs. These include:

- being respectful of the resident's religious items — e.g., rosary, crucifix, Bible, Koran (figure 14–10).
- making sure that the resident knows about the availability of special services — e.g., vespers, communion, prayer meetings, masses, seders, Bible study meetings.
- helping residents prepare for and arrive on time for religious services.
- honoring requests for visits from the clergy. Make sure to report all such requests to the charge nurse. Help the resident get ready before the clergy arrives and provide privacy during the visit.
- reading aloud a resident's spiritual materials to him or her if requested.
- being aware of dietary restrictions practiced by the resident.
- discussing religious and spiritual beliefs without trying to make the resident's beliefs conform with your own.

If you find it difficult to care for the spiritual needs of a resident, talk the matter over with the charge nurse and together find someone who can be supportive.

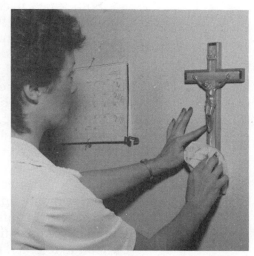

FIGURE 14–10. Treat personal religious objects respectfully.

SENSUAL FEELINGS AND SEXUAL EXPRESSION ■■■■■■■■■■■■■■

Sensual (pleasurable) feelings are just as important to the 70-year-old person as they are to the child or young adult, figure 14–11. And, sexual expression is both a basic psychological and physical need. Elderly people do not lose interest in their sexuality but their opportunities for expression are limited. Sexual behaviors are very sensual and give great pleasure and satisfaction. Some facilities recognize this basic need and make it possible for consenting adults to find privacy. Much depends upon the attitude of the staff, but elderly people should have choices and options for intimacy and sexual expression.

Sensual feelings come through:
- touch
- vision
- hearing
- taste
- smell

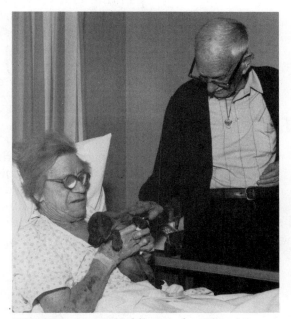

FIGURE 14–11. Holding and petting a puppy is a pleasant feeling.

Sometimes, in confusion, one resident may make sexual advances to another resident who is not interested. You must provide protection for the non-consenting resident. Often, you can simply divert the attention of the resident making sexual advances by suggesting another activity. Do not scold, but explain that the behavior is not appropriate.

Young staff members, especially, may feel that any sexually oriented behavior between older people is unacceptable. It is often difficult for young people to understand that sexual feelings continue throughout life. It takes a certain degree of maturity and understanding to accept the fact that human beings are sexual beings all their lives and that sexual expression takes many forms.

Other staff members may find that their own personal views of human sexuality limit their view of the resident's rights, or may find them in actual conflict with certain sexually oriented behaviors. For example, you may find the self-stimulating behavior of **masturbation** difficult to tolerate, but you must accept the fact that this may be the only sexual outlet available for some elderly residents. Make sure that residents who do masturbate have opportunity and privacy.

If a resident makes sexual advances to you, be firm but gentle in your rejection of these advances. Calmly let the resident know that the behavior is not appropriate or acceptable. Even if you are irritated, do not show anger.

SOCIOLOGICAL NEEDS

When the more primary physical and psychological needs are met, the resident is free to pursue activities that are unique to them as individuals. These activites make the resident feel good about himself or herself and about his or her situation, promoting a sense of accomplishment, figure 14–12. Sociological needs are met by interactions with others and opportunities to express oneself. Handicrafts, painting and drawing, dancing, music (group singing, playing an instrument), card and other games, and study groups are a few examples of activities that elderly people can take part in to meet sociological needs.

Care givers can promote this process by assisting residents to activity areas and by encouraging each resident to engage in those activities which he or she selects and finds most satisfying.

EMPLOYEE STRESS

As you can see, working in a long term care facility requires much personal giving. Helping residents work through their stresses is not easy. The emotional drain is great and you must find ways to reduce your own stress without involving the residents.

Unresolved stress can be troublesome for you.

You can help protect your own mental health by:

- developing healthy balancing relationships in your own personal life
- learning to use personal relaxation techniques
- identifying the problems in your work that are causing stress
- clarifying your own feelings about the problems causing stress
- evaluating possible solutions
- choosing the correct response

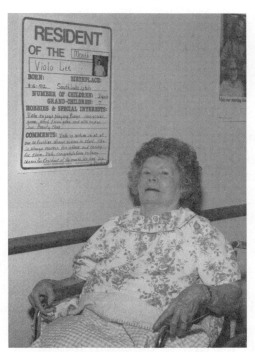

FIGURE 14–12. Highlighting the resident of the month is a way of promoting self-esteem and helping residents learn more about one another.

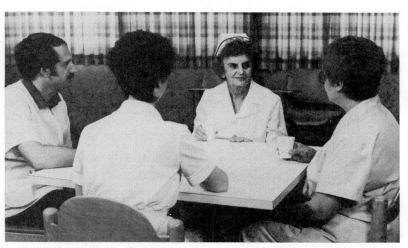

FIGURE 14–13. Staff conferences are a good way to find solutions to the stresses associated with the job.

A staff conference is often the best way to cope with resident behavioral problems, figure 14–13. In such a conference, the staff has the opportunity to share experiences and feelings and to suggest possible solutions. For example, if a resident is behaving in a way that is annoying to members of the staff — perhaps trying to manipulate staff members — the problem can be discussed in the conference period. Feelings can be aired and a common approach toward dealing with the problem resident can be reached.

Staff conferences also can be used to solve, or help to solve, inter-staff conflicts. Staff harmony is an important factor in creating the optimum environment for resident care. No hint of personal conflict should ever reach the residents. Staff disharmony only adds to a resident's confusion and stress.

VOCABULARY

compensation	developmental tasks	rationalization
confidant	disengagement	rapport
coping mechanism	masturbation	self-esteem
defense mechanism	personality	sensual
denial	projection	

SUGGESTED ACTIVITIES

1. Discuss with classmates the developmental tasks associated with your age group, such as:
   a. training to become gainfully employed

b. establishing personal relationships

c. supporting a family

d. becoming independent from your childhood family structure

2. Describe ways you have seen older people in your family or acquaintances handle stress. Try to identify factors which were helpful to the adjustment.

3. Role-play the following situations:
a. a resident who seems depressed
b. a resident who is angry and abusive

4. Try to think through your own feelings about your own sexuality and the sexual behavior of others. Does age make a difference in the standards that you accept?

REVIEW

A. Brief Answer/Fill in the Blanks

1. People solve problems as they get older in ways they have found _____ in the past.

2. Basic emotional needs of the elderly include the need to _____ and to _____, to interact _____ with others, and to be treated with _____ and _____.

3. Three developmental challenges to be mastered by the elderly include loss of _____, adjustment to _____ and _____, and loss of _____.

4. Changes which the elderly undergo threaten their sense of _____ or self-esteem.

5. _____ occurs when coping mechanisms fail.

6. Name three stress reactions commonly seen in residents:

a. _____

b. _____

c. _____

7. Spiritual expression is very personal and can help the resident who desires it to _____ with stressful events.

8. Relationships that are _____ have the best chance for success.

9. Two leaders in the field of human behavior described in this lesson are _____ and _____.

10. Personal views regarding sexuality limit the expression of _____.

B. Matching. Match the correct defense mechanism at right with the example in the left-hand column.

1. _____ Mr. Brooks spills a glass of water and explains that it happened because the glass was too close to the edge of the overbed table.

2. _____ Miss Alcott wants to stay in her room because, she says, the other residents don't like her.

a. projection
b. denial
c. compensation
d. rationalization

3. _____ Mrs. Jones spends most of her time out of bed helping other residents, even when they do not want or need help.

4. _____ When the nursing assistant tries to talk to Miss Anderson about her incontinence (she had wet the bed the night before), Miss Anderson says, in a tone of injured innocence, "Why, I don't know what on earth you are talking about!"

5. _____ Mr. Ramirez tells everyone how much his family loves him and that they would visit him more often if they only lived closer. You know that his family lives in the same town as the facility.

CLINICAL SITUATION

Mr. Warner, age 87, has been a resident in your facility for four years. During that time you have come to know him well. He is in a wheelchair but his mind is still very clear. He confides to you one morning that he really misses "having a woman" and wishes that there were a way he could relieve his sexual tension. What is your response?

Answer: _____

_____

_____

_____

SECTION III Achievement Review

A. **Multiple Choice.** Select the one best answer and circle the correct letter.

1. Senile lentigines are associated with the elderly person's
   a. teeth
   b. skin
   c. hair
   d. feet
   e. back bone

2. The basic nutrients include
   a. minerals and vitamins
   b. fats
   c. carbohydrates
   d. proteins
   e. all of the above

3. Each person should take in approximately how much water daily?
   a. 1 pint
   b. 1½ pints
   c. 1 quart
   d. 2 quarts
   e. 2½ quarts

4. Which of the following would not be part of the fruit and vegetable group?
   a. oranges
   b. chicken
   c. melon
   d. strawberries
   e. squash

5. Your resident doesn't like milk. You might substitute
   a. potatoes
   b. nuts
   c. pudding
   d. peaches
   e. eggs

6. Your resident has difficulty chewing fresh vegetables. You could solve this problem by
   a. substituting whole wheat bread
   b. cooking or dicing the vegetables
   c. making sure the resident drinks 6-8 glasses of water daily
   d. substituting eggnog
   e. including dried beans in the diet

7. Residents should take in how many servings of fruits and vegetables each day?
   a. 1 serving
   b. 2 servings
   c. 3 servings
   d. 4 servings
   e. 5 servings

8. Your resident is on a full liquid diet. You could give him/her
   a. ground meat
   b. grapes
   c. cooked peas
   d. junket
   e. fresh carrots

9. When helping to feed someone who is blind, you should
   a. do all the feeding yourself
   b. describe the food placement related to a clock
   c. always put the proteins in the same place
   d. let the resident figure out the position of food on the tray independently
   e. always put hot liquids close to the resident

10. Rigid ideas about groups of people are called
    a. myths
    b. stereotypes
    c. conclusions
    d. thoughts
    e. opinions

B. **Matching.** Match the correct words on the right with the statements on the left.

1. _____ low blood pressure

2. _____ mood elevating drug

3. _____ chemicals which regulate body functions

4. _____ solid waste

5. _____ means to bend

6. _____ bowel aids

7. _____ bedside toilet

8. _____ source of nourishment

9. _____ weakening

10. _____ inadequate water

a. debilitating
b. dehydration
c. commode
d. feces
e. antidepressants
f. nutrients
g. flex
h. laxatives
i. hormones
j. sedatives
k. hypotension

C. **True or False.** Indicate which of the following statements are true (T) about the elderly, and which are myths (F).

1. _____ cannot care for themselves

2. _____ have sensory losses

3. _____ have slower sexual response

4. _____ have no interest in sex

5. _____ are unable to learn

6. _____ have no interest in life

7. _____ are all living in poverty

8. _____ undergo postural changes

9. _____ no longer contribute in a positive way to society

10. _____ experience memory changes

D. **Describe/demonstrate the following for your instructor.**

1. Physical changes associated with aging.

2. Why messages may be misinterpreted by the elderly.

3. Ways that you can help fulfill residents' spiritual needs.

4. Ways that a person shows that he or she is under stress.

5. How you would handle conflict between two residents.

6. Examples of the defense mechanisms of *projection, rationalization, denial,* and *compensation.*

E. **Spell the words correctly that mean the following:**

1. normal aging changes _____

2. that the knees are slightly bent _____

3. emotional and social adjustments _____

4. a person's deepest beliefs _____

F. **Word Search.** Find the correct word for each definition listed. (Identify by line or column.)

1. _____ being older than 85 years of age

2. _____ getting up at night to urinate

3. _____ sense of balance

4. _____ being over 20 percent overweight

5. _____ nutrient used as stored energy

6. _____ nutrient needed for building and repair

7. _____ defense mechanism in which the person refuses to admit there is a problem

8. _____ sexual self-satisfaction

9. _____ feeding tube that is passed from the nose into the stomach

	A	B	C	D	E	F	G	H	I	J	K	L	M	N	O
1	N	A	S	O	G	A	S	T	R	I	C	B	N	C	U
2	P	R	O	P	R	I	O	C	E	P	T	I	O	N	B
3	M	A	S	T	U	R	B	A	T	I	O	N	C	Q	X
4	L	D	R	O	A	V	E	B	M	L	E	P	T	I	W
5	A	W	P	M	X	B	S	Q	D	W	N	R	U	C	A
6	S	F	R	A	I	L	I	S	E	N	I	O	R	X	F
7	B	A	F	D	N	O	T	C	N	U	Z	T	I	S	U
8	G	T	P	B	W	X	Y	Z	I	T	O	E	A	R	E
9	U	S	F	O	Q	B	D	O	A	H	L	I	U	Y	O
10	A	V	O	T	D	I	C	Y	L	B	I	P	Q	N	C

SECTION IV   BASIC SCIENCE CONCEPTS

LESSON 15   Understanding the Body

OBJECTIVES

After studying this lesson, you should be able to:

- Explain the organization of the body into cells, tissues, organs, and systems.
- Locate body parts and organs, using proper anatomic relationships.
- Describe observations using proper technology.
- Define and spell correctly all the vocabulary words and terms.

There are sound reasons for the care given to the residents. The type of care given is based on an understanding of how the body is structured and functions normally and of the changes brought about by age and disease.

These reasons, or principles, are derived from four sciences:

There is scientific foundation for the care that is given.

- **Anatomy:** The study of structure
- **Physiology:** The study of function
- **Gerontology:** The study of aging
- **Pathology:** The study of disease

In this lesson and Lesson 16, you will have the opportunity to learn more about these important sciences and how they relate to the care that you give.

ANATOMIC TERMS

Special terms are used to describe the location and relationship of body parts and organs. Knowing these terms will help you to study and learn more easily and will help you to communicate more accurately as you report and record your observations, figure 15–1.

The Anatomic Position

Descriptive terms give everyone a common frame of reference. Before applying the terms, we must place the resident in our minds

190

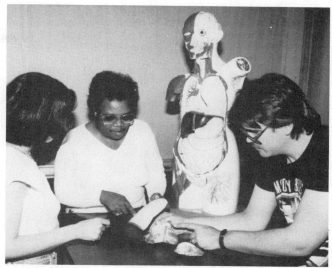

FIGURE 15–1. An understanding of the structure of the body helps you to understand the related nursing care.

as if he or she were standing in the **anatomic position**. When the resident is in the anatomic position he or she

- is standing
- is facing the observer
- has hands at the sides
- has palms forward (figure 15–2)

This means that the heels will always be towards the back (described as *dorsal* or *posterior*) even if the resident is resting on the abdomen or lying on the side. The breasts will always be described as facing front (*ventral* or *anterior*) even if she is sitting in a wheelchair or walking away from you. Notice also that the resident's left hand will be on the same side as your right hand. It is the same as looking at a mirror image.

Descriptive Terms

Planes are imaginary lines that section the body.

Planes are imaginary lines drawn through the body, figure 15–3.

The Midplane. The **midplane**, or midline, is drawn down the center of the body from head to floor. This plane divides the body into two equal sides. **Medial** parts are close to the midline; **lateral** parts are farthest away from the midline. For example, in anatomic position, the thumbs are more lateral and the little fingers are more medial.

The Transverse Plane. The **transverse plane** is a line drawn parallel to the floor that divides the body into two parts — upper and lower. **Superior** is the term meaning above this line; **inferior** is the term applied to areas below the line. For example, if a transverse plane is drawn between the knees and ankles, the knees would be described as superior to ankles which are inferior.

Points of Attachment

The head and body are referred to as the *torso*. The arms and hands are referred to as the **upper extremities**; the **lower extremities** are the legs and feet.

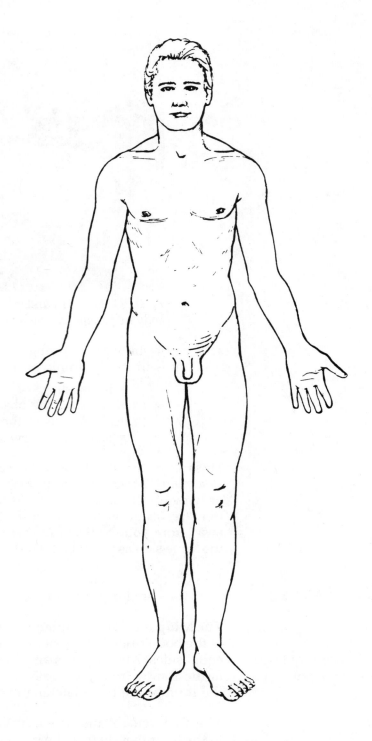

FIGURE 15–2. The anatomic position.

The **point of attachment** of the arms and torso is at the shoulder; the point of attachment of the leg and torso is at the hip. Since the upper arm is closest to the shoulder, where it is attached, this part is described as **proximal** when compared to the fingers, which are farthest away. The fingers are **distal**, or farthest away from the point of attachment of the upper extremity.

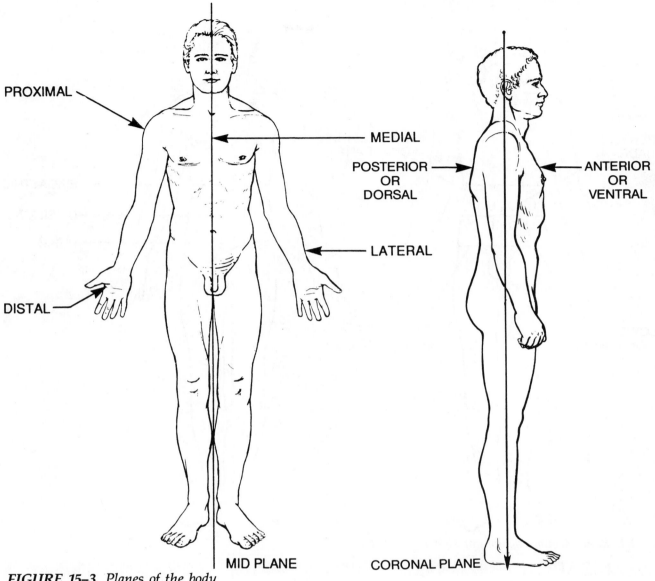

FIGURE 15–3. Planes of the body.

- **Anterior** or **ventral** refers to the front
- **Posterior** or **dorsal** refers to the back
- **Lateral** refers to the side (away from the midline)
- **Medial** refers to the center of the body (midline)
- **Proximal** means closest to the point of attachment
- **Distal** refers to the point farthest away from the point of attachment

FIGURE 15–4. Summary of points of attachment.

Abdominal Quadrants

If a resident places his or her hand on the anterior abdominal wall, complaining of pain, you must be able to describe the area in proper terms. For reference, the anterior wall of the abdomen is divided into four parts or quadrants, figure 15–5. The center of this area is the **umbilicus**.

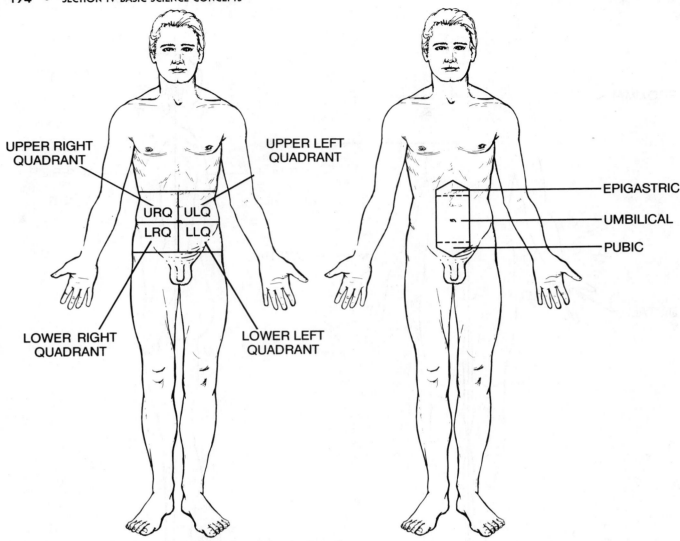

FIGURE 15–5. Regions of the anterior abdominal wall.

ORGANIZATION ■■■■■■■■■■■■■■■■■■■■■■■■■■■■■■■■■■■■■■■

Cells
Tissues
Organs
Systems

The body is organized in such a way that all parts are interdependent. The basic unit of the body is the **cell**. Groups of similar cells are organized into **tissues**, and different tissues form **organs**. The organs are organized into **systems** that carry out the body functions.

CELLS ■■

Each cell carries on the functions that the body performs, but on a smaller scale, figure 15–6. These functions include breathing (respiration), reproduction, nutrition, excretion (eliminating wastes), and work of some kind. Different cells perform different kinds of work necessary for the body as a whole to function. Some of the various specialized types of cells are:

- epithelial cells
- nerve cells
- muscle cells
- connective tissue cells

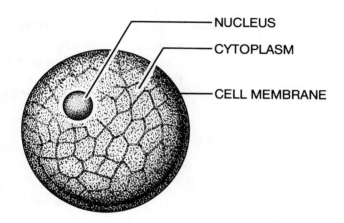

NUCLEUS
CYTOPLASM
CELL MEMBRANE

FIGURE 15–6. Cell structure.

Epithelial cells, which are very close together, form protective coverings and sometimes produce body fluids like **mucus**.

Nerve cells carry messages to and from the different parts of the body, coordinating activities and making us aware of changes in the environment.

Muscle cells can **contract** (shorten) or **relax** (lengthen), changing their shape and the position of parts to which they are attached. They also surround body openings such as the mouth.

There are many kinds of **connective tissue cells**. They hold all the parts together, supporting and connecting them.

TISSUES

Tissue types:
- epithelial
- nervous
- connective
- muscle

Groups of similar cells are organized into tissues. The basic tissue types are:

- epithelial tissue
- connective tissue
- nervous tissue
- muscle tissue

Epithelial tissue is specialized in its ability to absorb, *secrete* (produce) fluids, *excrete* (eliminate) waste products and protect.

Bone, blood, fibrous and elastic tissues are examples of **connective tissues**. There is a great variety of connective cells and tissues which they form.

Nervous tissue forms the brain and spinal cord and the nerves of the body. This tissue is also found in the special sense organs such as the eyes, ears, and tastebuds. The activities of all the rest of the body are directed and coordinated through the nervous tissues.

There are three kinds of **muscle tissue**: **cardiac muscle** tissue, which makes up the walls of the heart; **visceral** or **smooth muscle** tissue, which forms the walls of body organs such as the stomach and intestines; and **skeletal muscle** tissue which is attached to bones for movement.

ORGANS

Each organ, which is made up of more than one kind of tissue, carries on special functions that contribute to the function of the body systems. Some organs, like the **kidneys**, are found in pairs. Some single organs can contribute to more than one system. For example, the **pancreas** contributes secretions to both the endocrine and the digestive systems. Study figure 15–7 to learn the names and location of the organs.

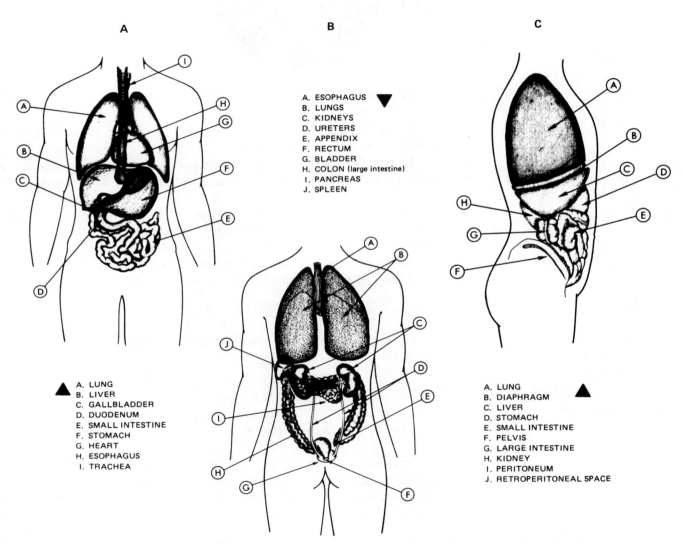

FIGURE 15–7. *The major organs of the body: A, anterior view; B, posterior view; C, lateral view.*

SYSTEMS

Organs may contribute to more than one system.

There are nine major body systems. Figure 15–8 shows the organs that contribute to the function of each system. Notice that some organs are included with more than one system. For example, the ovaries contribute to the endocrine system and to the reproductive system.

SYSTEM	ORGANS	FUNCTIONS
Circulatory	Heart, arteries, veins, capillaries, spleen, lymph nodes, lymphatic vessels	Carries materials needed for body function from where they are produced to where they are needed or excreted.
Endocrine	Parathyroid, pituitary gland, thyroid gland, pineal body, ovaries, adrenal gland, thymus, testes, islands of Langerhans	Produces hormones (chemicals that regulate body functions).
Gastrointestinal	Mouth, esophagus, intestines, gallbladder, pharynx, stomach, appendix, liver, pancreas, teeth, tongue, salivary glands	Digests, transports, and absorbs nutrients; eliminates solid wastes.
Integumentary	Skin, hair, nails, sweat and oil glands	Protects the body; helps control temperature.
Musculoskeletal	Bones, joints, muscles, tendons, ligaments	Protects vital organs and moves the body.
Nervous	Brain, spinal cord, nerves, ganglia	Coordinates activities through-out the body by nervous stimuli.
Reproductive	Male: Testes, epididymis, urethra, seminal vesicles and ducts, ejaculatory ducts, prostate gland, bulbourethral glands, penis, spermatic cord Female: Breasts, ovaries, oviducts, uterus, vagina, Bartholin glands, vulva	Controls reproduction and sexual activity.
Respiratory	Nose, pharynx, larynx, trachea, bronchi, lungs, sinuses	Brings gases (oxygen and carbon dioxide) into and out of the body.
Urinary	Kidneys, ureters, urethra, urinary bladder	Eliminates liquid wastes from the body; balances water and chemicals.

FIGURE 15–8. Summary of the body systems.

MEMBRANES

Membranes are sheets of epithelial and connective tissues that cover the body, line body cavities, and produce some body fluids. Important membranes include:

Mucous Membranes. These produce a fluid called *mucus,* line those body cavities that open to the outside. Since the respiratory system, the digestive system, and the genitourinary system all open to the outside they are lined with mucous membranes.

Synovial Membranes. These form *synovial fluid* and line joint cavities. The synovial fluid is a clear fluid resembling the white of an egg. It helps to cut down the friction between the bones of active joints and the tendons.

Membranes:
- protect
- secrete
- cover
- produce body fluids

Serous Membranes (*serous:* resembling). These cover the internal organs and line the closed cavities of the body. They produce a *serous fluid* that helps cut down on friction as the organs work and move. Important serous membranes are the:

- *pericardium,* which surrounds the heart
- *pleura,* which surrounds the lungs and lines the thoracic cavity
- *meninges,* which cover the brain and spinal cord and line the dorsal cavity
- *peritoneum,* which covers the digestive organs and lines the abdominal cavity

Cutaneous Membrane. This is another name for the *skin*, which covers the entire body. Special epithelial cells in this membrane, called glands, secrete perspiration and oils.

CAVITIES

The body seems like a solid structure, but actually, there are spaces (**cavities**) within it that contain the organs, figures 15–9 and 15–10. There are two main cavities:

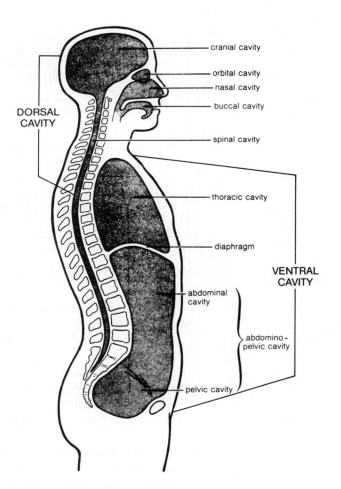

FIGURE 15—9. Side view of body cavities.

• the dorsal cavity
• the ventral cavity

Each is further subdivided by membranes.

Dorsal Cavity_____

The **dorsal cavity** houses the brain and spinal cord. It is found within the skull and vertebral column and is lined by the meninges.

Ventral Cavity_____

The **ventral cavity** contains major organs including the heart, the lungs, and the organs of digestion and reproduction. The ventral cavity is divided by the muscular **diaphragm** into an upper (superior) **thoracic cavity** and a lower (inferior) **abdominopelvic cavity**. Each of these cavities are further divided by membranes.

Body cavities contain organs.

Thoracic Cavity.

This cavity is divided into two *lateral pleural cavities*, that house the lungs. The **pericardial cavity** is found between the pleural cavities and houses the heart.

The **mediastinum** is the space between the pleural cavities, posterior to the pericardial cavity. The **esophagus** and **trachea** are found in the mediastinum.

Abdominopelvic Cavity.

Below the diaphragm, the membraneous peritoneum separates the abdominopelvic cavity into the:

• **peritoneal cavity**, which contains the liver, gallbladder, stomach, pancreas, most of the small and large intestines, and the spleen
• **pelvic cavity**, which contains most of the reproductive organs and the urinary bladder
• **retroperitoneal space**, (*behind* the peritoneum), which contains the kidney, adrenal glands, and ureters

CAVITY	ORGANS
Dorsal	Brain, pineal body, pituitary gland, nerves, spinal cord
Thoracic	Lungs, heart, great blood vessels, thymus gland
Abdominal	
Peritoneal	Stomach, small intestine, most of large intestine, liver, gallbldder, pancreas, spleen
Pelvic	Male: Seminal vesicles, prostate gland, ejaculatory ducts, urinary bladder, urethra, rectum
	Female: Uterus, oviducts, ovaries, urinary bladder, urethra, rectum
Retroperitoneal space	Kidneys, adrenal glands, ureters

FIGURE 15–10. Organ placement in body cavities.

■■■

VOCABULARY

abdominal	mediastinum	posterior
abdominopelvic cavity	membrane	proximal
anatomic position	meninges	quadrant
anatomy	midplane	relax
anterior	mucous membrane	retroperitoneal space
cardiac muscle	mucus	serous membrane
cavity	muscle cell	skeletal muscle
cell	muscle tissue	skin
connective tissue	nerve cell	smooth muscle
contract	nervous tissue	superior
cutaneous	organ	synovial membrane
diaphragm	pancreas	system
distal	pathology	thoracic cavity
dorsal cavity	pelvic cavity	tissue
epithelial	pericardial cavity	torso
esophagus	pericardium	trachea
gerontology	peritoneal cavity	transverse plane
inferior	peritoneum	umbilicus
kidneys	physiology	upper extremities
lateral	plane	ventral cavity
lower extremities	pleura	visceral muscle
medial	point of attachment	

SUGGESTED ACTIVITIES

1. Practice identifying the descriptive terms when people are in the anatomic position and in other positions.
2. Study a model or your own body to find the general location of body parts and organs.
3. Study a model or charts to locate body parts and organs.

REVIEW

A. Brief Answer/Fill in the Blanks

1. The basic unit of the body is the _____.
2. The body is organized into _____, which is organized into _____, and then into _____ and _____.
3. Name four tissue types.
   a. _____
   b. _____
   c. _____
   d. _____
4. The brain and spinal cord are made of _____ tissue.
5. Name three organs of the urinary system.
   a. _____
   b. _____
   c. _____

6. The palms are located on the _____ or _____ surface of the hands.

7. Another term for dorsal is _____.

8. The horizontal plane divides the body into _____ and _____ parts.

9. The ovaries contribute to the _____ and the _____ systems.

10. Name five organs in the abdominal cavity.

a. _____

b. _____

c. _____

d. _____

e. _____

B. Matching. Match the term in the right column with its description in the left.

1. _____ Elimination of wastes

2. _____ Farthest from point of attachment

3. _____ Close to midline

4. _____ Disease

5. _____ Study of aging

6. _____ Fluid produced by mucous membranes

7. _____ Around the heart

8. _____ Study of function

9. _____ Closest to point of attachment

10. _____ Study of structure

a. proximal
b. gerontology
c. anatomy
d. physiology
e. pericardial
f. pathology
g. mucus
h. excretion
i. distal
j. serous fluid
k. medial
l. lateral

C. Identification.

1. Name the areas indicated in the diagram.

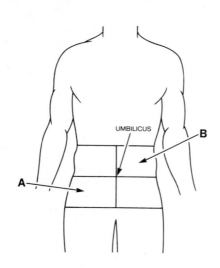

UMBILICUS

A

B

2. Name the organs indicated.

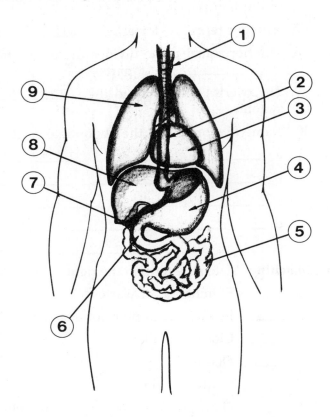

CLINICAL SITUATION

Mrs. Driscoll has had a stroke and she cannot move her left arm and leg. The left side of her face is also paralyzed so that her left eyelid droops. She fell when she became ill and broke the distal bone in her right thumb. She has a bruise on the medial superior portion of her right breast. On the photo below, indicate the areas of disability and injury.

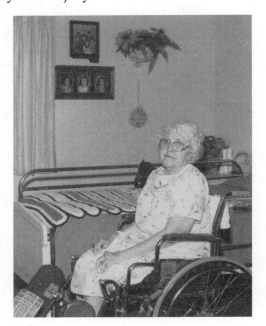

LESSON 16 The Effects of Aging and Disease

OBJECTIVES

After studying this lesson, you should be able to:

- Explain current theories of aging.
- Describe the general effect of diseases on the aging process.
- Name and describe two diseases that can affect any body system.
- Recognize at least five signs of approaching death.
- Demonstrate post mortem care.
- Define and spell all the vocabulary words and terms.

Residents suffer from many different disabilities and diseases that make self care difficult. Some of the changes are due to the aging process, others to actual disease. In this lesson, specific conditions are discussed with the individual systems that are primarily affected. Two conditions that affect the elderly can affect body systems: they are *cancer* and *infections*.

THEORY OF AGING

Aging is an ongoing process.

Aging is a progressive process that begins even before birth and continues until death. It goes on at different rates in different people. No one fully understands the complex series of changes that constitute aging and that occur in all living beings, but several ideas have been advanced. Some people believe that:

- The rate of aging is an inherited factor that is "built into" our personal genetic code.
- The body undergoes wear and stress during life that eventually results in less and less functional ability.
- During aging, increasingly smaller amounts of the chemicals which control body activities, including immune processes, are produced, so that fewer protective substances are available and there is greater susceptibility to disease.

SENESCENCE AND DISEASE

Disease speeds the aging process.

Senescent (aging) changes take place in every body system, but not at any specific time or at any specific rate, figure 16-1. Disease increases the natural aging process, altering its rate, and the process of aging intensifies the effect of disease.

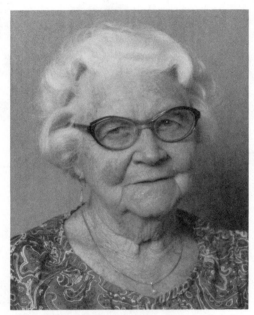

FIGURE 16–1. Note the signs of aging in this resident.

The effects of aging and disease bring about changes in the structure and function of the body. These changes are evidenced as:

- signs
- symptoms

Signs are changes that *you can see* — e.g., the way the resident looks or reacts. For example, an elevated blood pressure, a skin rash, and a rapid pulse rate are signs.

Symptoms are feelings *experienced by the resident*. Nausea, dizziness, light-headedness, and pain are all examples of symptoms that may be described to you by the person experiencing them.

Disease (*pathology*) sometimes follows a predictable course or progression. This probable outcome is called a **prognosis**. The prognosis may be described as:

- unfavorable — if the condition is expected to worsen
- favorable — if the condition is expected to improve
- guarded — if the outcome is uncertain

Disease does not always affect the body in the same way.

In some conditions, signs and symptoms may appear and then disappear. These conditions are described as being in **exacerbation**, when there are signs. When the signs and symptoms temporarily go away, the condition is referred to as being in **remission**. Arthritis is an example of a condition in which there are periods of exacerbation and remission.

Disease conditions may be:

- acute
- chronic

Acute conditions are those that have a sudden or abrupt onset. They last a relatively short period. An abscess and a broken leg are examples of acute conditions.

Chronic conditions last a long time. Diabetes, emphysema, and arthritis are common chronic conditions affecting the elderly.

Sometimes disease brings about visible changes in the structure of tissues. Such a change is called a **lesion**. Sometimes the lesion is small and at other times large. A bedsore (*decubitus ulcer*) is a lesion that results from pressure and inadequate blood flow to the area.

INFFCTIONS

Infections are caused when **pathogenic** (disease-producing) microorganisms gain entrance into the body, begin to multiply, and then damage the body tissues. Infections can be:

- local (confined to one area) — such as a *boil* or skin *abscess*
- generalized — such as pneumonia, which involves the lungs
- septicemic — such as infection in the blood stream

Body Response

Infection and cancer are major disease states in the elderly.

The body responds to an acute infection by a special process called **inflammation**, figure 16–2. The signs of inflammation include:

- redness
- heat
- pain
- swelling
- loss of function in the affected area

If you note any of these signs and symptoms, be sure to report them.

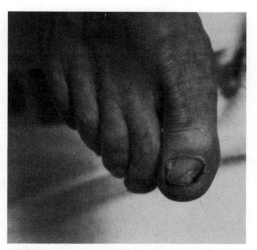

FIGURE 16–2. This improperly cut toenail has become infected. Note the reddened, swollen tissue around the nail bed.

Many times infections are associated with the production of pus, which may drain. Report the character, color, odor, and amount of any drainage. The drainage contains many infectious organisms and must be carefully handled so that the infection will not be transmitted to others. Information about how to prevent the spread of infection is detailed in Lesson 7.

CANCER

Remember, cancer can affect any body system and, if uncontrolled, can cause death. Throughout life, cells in the body undergo reproduction to meet body needs. For example, if a resident injures a finger with a paper cut, new cells will fill in the injury so that healing repairs the area. Growth is also dependent on the formation of new cells. The process of new cell production (**mitosis**) is controlled, and normally when the need is met, the production of cells stops. In cancer, the cells keep reproducing, eventually taking over the spaces normally filled by healthy cells. The normal cells are crowded out and die. Eventually, the person's life is threatened as the unhealthy cells spread (**metastasize**) throughout the body. Cancers (**malignancies**) are called **neoplasms** or **tumors** and can involve any body organ or tissue. Older people are especially prone to the development of certain cancers such as cancer of the lungs, digestive organs, and reproductive tract.

Unless treated with surgery, radiation, or drugs, most cancers will usually cause death. Sometimes the treatment saves a person's life but causes serious side effects and disability. The earlier cancer is detected, the sooner it can be treated and the more favorable the prognosis. Early signs and symptoms that indicate a developing cancer are listed in figure 16–3. Review them carefully. Late signs are listed in figure 16–4. The most striking of these is **cachexia**, which is a general wasting due to competitive struggle between malignant and normal cells for available nutrients.

Cancer is uncontrolled cell division that can spread.

- Any unusual bleeding or discharge
- A lump or thickening in the breast or elsewhere
- Any sore that does not heal
- Persistent change in normal bladder or bowel habits
- Any change in a wart or mole

FIGURE 16–3. Early warning signs of cancer.

The Effects of Therapy

Radiation

Radiation treatments are performed in an acute care hospital. You will see some of its effects when the resident returns to you for care. The radiation is either delivered by a machine from outside the body or from radioactive materials placed in the tumor area. The radiation rays will damage the unhealthy (malignant) cancer cells as well as causing some damage to surrounding normal cells.

Some residents will receive outpatient therapy and make daily or weekly trips out of the LTCF for treatment.

Radiation can cause serious side effects, including:

- Cachexia
- Fever, perhaps due to the abnormal metabolic process or in response to the presence of abnormal cells
- Loss of weight and anemia
- Pain due to pressure, obstruction, and ischemia (loss of blood flow)
- Inflammations of the skin
- Thrombophlebitis (inflamed veins and blood clots)
- Hormonal irregularities
- Lesions in the nervous system

FIGURE 16–4. Late signs of cancer.

- nausea
- vomiting
- loss of appetite (**anorexia**)
- anemia, from too few red blood cells
- bone marrow depression

Bone marrow depression causes a lowered ability to produce blood cells, so that the body is unable to fight infection because of decreased white blood cells. The resident may bleed more readily because of too few **thrombocytes** (blood platelets). Residents experience a loss of stamina, tire easily and may lose hair on their heads (**alopecia**), which can be particularly distressing to them.

Cancer therapy:
- radiation
- surgery
- chemotherapy
- supportive care

Drug Therapy

Many different drugs are employed in cancer treatment today. Often a combination of drugs (**chemotherapy**) is given. The drugs can be given directly into the body through a vein or injected into a muscle or be taken by mouth (**orally**). Side effects that can accompany chemotherapy are similar to those seen when residents receive radiation. In addition, skin rashes and irritations and mouth lesions may occur.

Surgery

Surgical procedures remove the cancer but sometimes leave the resident with permanent disabilities. For example, part of a limb may be **amputated** or part of the intestinal tract may be removed and a new opening (**ostomy**) made into the abdominal wall. Surgical procedures carry with them the risk of poor reactions to the anesthesia. Some people, particularly the elderly, do not respond well to anesthetic drugs.

Nursing Assistant Responsibilities___

Residents with a diagnosis of cancer need a great deal of emotional support. The diagnosis alone is frightening, so that even if the prognosis is favorable, there is uncertainty and stress. Some of the drugs used in chemotherapy may cause feelings of depression, and the side effects of therapy may require major adjustments. You can best help the resident by:

- being positive but realistic in your approach.
- helping the resident look and feel as attractive as possible (figure 16–5).
- not offering false hope.
- being aware of changes in behavior or physical appearance.
- being ready to listen to concerns (figure 16–6).
- being understanding when frustration and fear are expressed in anger or unreasonableness.
- watching for and reporting evidence of the side effects so that steps may be taken to control them and reduce discomfort.
- reporting pain, bleeding, or anything unusual right away.
- planning care so that fatigue is lessened, using frequent rest periods.
- encouraging adequate intake of fluids and nourishment (figure 16–7).
- giving careful, frequent attention to skin and mouth hygiene. This can help reduce some of the discomfort associated with therapy.

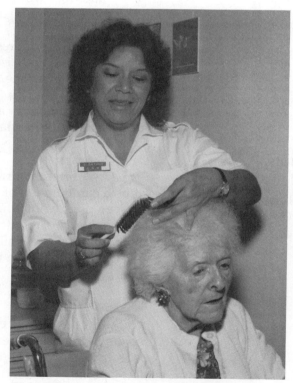

FIGURE 16–5. Help the resident feel as attractive as possible.

Small meals, attractively served, are one way to encourage intake. High calorie and protein supplements should be given. Staying with the resident as he or she eats can be very supportive. Remember, appetite is usually greatly diminished so plan to offer fluids in between meals.

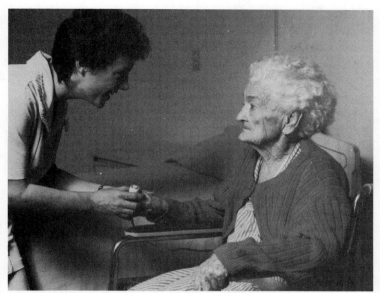

FIGURE 16–6. Be encouraging but do not offer false hope.

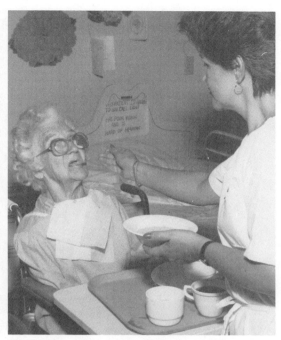

FIGURE 16–7. Offer small portions of high calorie foods and protein supplements.

The resident will be your prime focus, but often family members will need emotional support as well. This is especially true when the prognosis is unfavorable. You will need to offer support throughout the entire treatment period and long after.

When cancer has extended beyond the control of therapy, a **terminal diagnosis** is made. The resident may or may not be informed when curative treatment is no longer feasible or possible. The treatment which is continued is designed only to keep the resident comfortable. This type of therapy is known as supportive or **palliative**. Sooner or later, each resident with a terminal diagnosis becomes aware that the therapy is not going to bring about a cure.

TERMINAL DIAGNOSIS

Malignancies can lead to a terminal diagnosis, but other chronic conditions and age itself can eventually come to a terminal point. Dying and death are part of the natural progression of the life cycle. Everyone eventually faces a termination of his or her life on earth. Each person will react to his or her approaching death in a unique way.

Your response should be guided by the personal preference of the resident. Some will wish to talk and share their feelings, figure 16–8. Others may keep more of their feelings to themselves. All staff members should know what the resident has been told about his or her condition and whether or not a code is to be called when the resident is in danger of dying. The extent of the explanation is a medical decision and all staff members must abide by it.

Code Blue Order. Unless otherwise ordered, every effort must be made to keep the resident alive. Be prepared to assist with CPR.

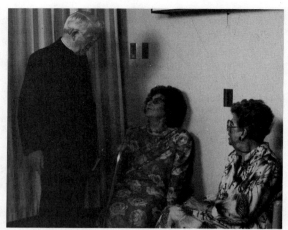

FIGURE 16–8. Visits from the resident's friends and clergy can be very supportive.

In some facilities, nursing assistants who have been certified are permitted to initiate this technique. Usually, when a resident is in danger of dying, a **code blue** order is called. Personnel rush to the scene and attempt to revive the resident by resuscitation. This is a very hectic time, so unless you have specific responsibilities:

- stay out of the way.
- be prepared to assist, if asked.
- help keep other residents calm.

No Code Order. Sometimes a resident whose illness is terminal will have a **no code** order. This means that if the resident ceases breathing, resuscitation will not be performed. The resident will be allowed to end his or her life with dignity. All personnel should be aware when a no code order is written. It is often difficult to carry out a no code order when you have come to know and love the resident. Try to remember that life needs both quantity and quality, and that the quality of life, when on support systems, is very limited. The no code order is a medical decision, often it is written at the expressed desire of a particular resident. All staff members should know as soon as the order is written.

Stages of Grieving

Grieving is a process which takes time.

After a terminal diagnosis is made and the resident and his or her family become aware of the situation, most residents and their families will pass through a series of steps known as the *stages of grieving**. These are:

- denial (figure 16–9)
- anger
- bargaining
- grieving
- final acceptance

*Elizabeth Kubler-Ross has done much of the pioneer work in the understanding of the grieving process. See her book *On Death and Dying*, published by Macmillan.

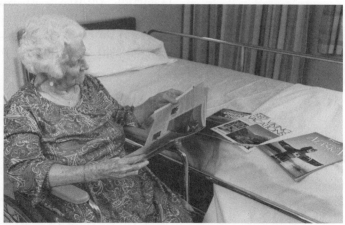

FIGURE 16–9. This resident with a terminal diagnosis is in the process of denial as she plans an extended trip.

As the resident and his or her loved ones move toward final acceptance of the resident's dying, they go through a similar process. (Some people, of course, never do progress through these stages to the point of accepting death as an inevitable part of the life experience.) The stages in the grieving process are not necessarily followed in sequence, and often people will move back and forth between stages, before moving forward.

As an example of the grieving process, Mrs. Bloomberg has been told of her terminal diagnosis. In the beginning she refuses to accept the facts. She acts cheerful and says, "I know that there are other therapies that could help. I'm too young to die. I still have much to accomplish on this earth." She may even tell you about her future plans. She is obviously in the stage of *denial*.

As time passes and she gets no better, she becomes *angry* and says, "It's all so unfair. I don't deserve this!" Mrs. Bloomberg strikes out verbally at you and her family. Then, the anger gives way to *bargaining*. She spends time in prayer, reading her Bible, and visiting the chapel. You hear her say, "If only God (nature or the doctors) can do something, I will make novenas, give cash, and be a better person from now on."

When the bargaining fails, the grieving process continues to the next stage. Mrs. Bloomberg speaks of past errors and says how sorry she is that there wasn't time to do or say certain things. She reviews her life and mourns the losses.

Hopefully, she finally reaches a point of *acceptance*. She seems calmer and more in control. She takes steps to write a will or give away some of her things.

Not all residents will achieve complete mastery of the stages, but at each level they will need the emotional support of a caring, understanding staff.

Anointing of the Sick. If a Catholic resident appears in danger of dying, a Catholic priest must be called, so that there is an opportunity for this special religious sacrament to be offered. It is known as the

last rites, figure 16–10. Families may wish to be together with the resident during this time, although they will leave during the period of personal confession. Even it they recover, Catholics consider it a privilege to have this opportunity.

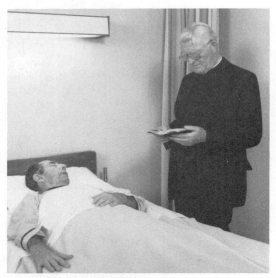

FIGURE 16–10. Catholic residents consider it a priviledge to receive the sacraments of the sick, or the "last rites," when they are seriously ill.

Non-Catholics may desire the spiritual support of the clergy of their own faith, or perhaps spiritual readings may provide some comfort. Be open to their needs and requests.

Nursing Assistant Responsibilities

You have a very special opportunity to be of service to the resident with a terminal diagnosis and to his or her family. Because of your day-to-day contact, you are in a position to provide the emotional and physical support needed. You can help the resident by:

- making frequent contact with the resident.
- increasing contact as death approaches.
- keeping the resident comfortable and clean.
- continuing to meet basic physical needs.
- continuing to monitor vital signs carefully.
- keeping the room quiet but well-lighted.

Blankets can be added to provide warmth during the final hours. Change soiled linen as you would for any other resident. Give oral care frequently, especially if the resident is mouth-breathing, since this is very drying to the mucous membranes. Mouth care is an important comfort measure.

SIGNS OF APPROACHING DEATH

Approaching death is signaled by a slowing of body functions and a loss of control including the following signs and symptoms:

All body processes slow down during the dying process.

- The body seems to relax and the jaw drops.
- Breathing becomes labored.
- Control of bowels or bladder may be lost (incontinency).
- Circulation slows.
- Blood pressure drops.
- Extremities become colder.
- Profuse perspiration is common.
- Respirations become labored (**dyspnea**) or temporarily cease (**apnea**).
- Periods of dyspnea followed by apnea, known as *Cheyne-Stokes* respirations, may occur.
- The pulse becomes more rapid and weaker.
- The skin pales and may become **mottled** (discolored).
- The eyes do not respond to light.
- Hearing is lost.

Hearing is the last sense to be lost and may still be present even though the resident doesn't seem responsive. Be careful of what you say. Continue to talk to the resident in a normal tone even if the resident is **comatose** (unconscious).

Gradually, breathing becomes more labored and then ceases. If the nurse is away from the bedside, note the time that breathing ceases and inform the charge nurse when the vital signs are lost. If the resident's family is with him or her at the time of death, they will be asked to step outside while the nurse examines the resident and then calls the physician.

Provide a comfortable, private area for the family and stay with them unless they prefer to be alone. This is not an easy time for the family or for you. Residents often become like close acquaintances and you will most likely experience grief and a sense of loss. It is all right to let the family know how much the resident meant to you, so do not be embarrassed if you feel like crying. Do, however, try to control your emotions, since the family members will need your support.

POST MORTEM CARE

The care given immediately after death is called **post mortem** care. Make sure the resident is positioned naturally, with limbs straightened. Return dentures to the mouth if they were normally worn. Make sure the linen is clean. Family members may want to spend a little time with the body. Stay with them, if requested, but provide privacy otherwise, figures 16–11 and 16–12.

After the family leaves, the body may be bathed and dressings, tubings, and equipment removed. You should also:

- cover the body with a clean sheet.
- gather, identify, and tag belongings.
- close the door and leave the curtains drawn.

Although the exact procedure varies, the body may be moved to a holding area if available. Continued preparations of the body for internment are usually carried out by the mortuary staff when they

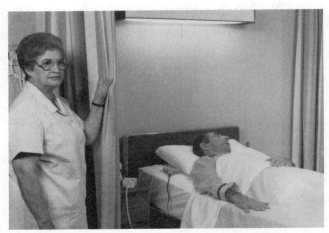

FIGURE 16–11. *Provide privacy after the resident dies for the family who wish to spend a few moments alone.*

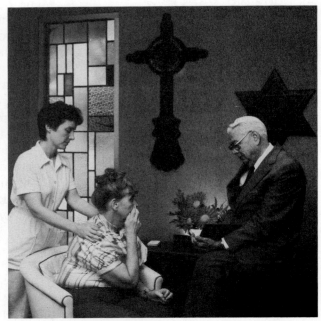

FIGURE 16–12. *After the resident dies, the family will need support.*

arrive. If a morgue is available and the mortuary people will be delayed, you may need to complete the procedure of post mortem care. A sample guide is included here.

Following the death of a resident, your behavior should be dignified and restrained. You will need to be supportive of the other residents who will want information. Be frank and direct without giving excessive details. A simple "yes" when asked if the resident died may be sufficient. At times, residents may want to recall their relationship to the recently expired person. Be supportive as they express their feelings of grief, figure 16–13.

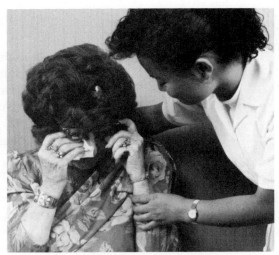

FIGURE 16–13. *Remember that residents become very close, and when one dies you must be prepared to offer comfort to those who are left.*

▓▓▓ PROCEDURE: Post Mortem Care ▀▀▀▀▀▀▀▀▀▀▀▀▀▀▀▀▀▀▀▀▀▀

1. Wash hands and assemble the following equipment:
   a. shroud or clean sheet
   b. basin with warm water
   c. washcloth
   d. towels
   e. identification cards (3)
   f. cotton
   g. bandages, as needed
   h. pads, as needed
2. Close door, or screen off unit.
3. Remove all equipment and used articles.
4. Work quickly and quietly; maintain an attitude of respect.
5. Place the body on the back, head and shoulders elevated. Close eyes by grasping eyelashes. Replace dentures. Secure jaw if needed.
6. Bath as necessary. Remove any soiled dressings and replace with clean ones.
7. Pad the areas between the ankles and knees with cotton. Tie lightly.
8. Pad the anal area in case of drainage.
9. Put the shroud on the body.
10. Collect all belongings. Wrap and label them.
11. Fill out the three identification cards and fasten one on the body and one on the resident's clothing and valuables (securely wrapped).
12. Empty corridor of residents and visitors. With assistance, place body on gurney. Cover with sheet and take to the morgue. Place third identification card on morgue compartment.

VOCABULARY

acute	exacerbation	ostomy
alopecia	inflammation	palliative therapy
amputated	last rites	pathogenic
anorexia	lesion	post mortem
apnea	malignancy	prognosis
cachexia	metastasize	remission
cancer	mitosis	septicemic
chemotherapy	moribund	sign
Cheyne-Stokes respiration	mottling	symptom
chronic	neoplasm	terminal
code blue order	no code order	thrombocyte
comatose	orally	tumor
dyspnea		

SUGGESTED ACTIVITIES

1. Under supervision, give care to terminal residents.

2. Invite clergy of different faiths to discuss their experiences with terminally ill people.

3. Write a brief statement beginning with "I feel that death is . . ."

4. Discuss the theories of aging with either the instructor or classmates.

5. Read *On Death and Dying* by Elizabeth Kubler-Ross and discuss your feelings about a no code order.

6. Discuss stages of grieving and nursing assistant actions that can support the resident.

REVIEW

Brief Answer/Fill in the Blanks

1. Aging is a progressive process beginning _____.

2. Disease _____ the aging process.

3. A condition in which signs and symptoms temporarily go away is said to be in _____.

4. Changes in the normal structure of tissues, due to disease, are called _____.

5. Two disease processes that can affect any body system are _____ and _____.

6. A disease that has an abrupt onset and short course is called _____.

7. Name three treatments used to treat cancer.

   a. _____

   b. _____

   c. _____

8. List five side effects of cancer therapy that need to be noted and reported.

   a. _____

   b. _____

   c. _____

   d. _____

   e. _____

9. Attitude is important in cancer therapy. The staff should be positive but _____.

10. _____ therapy keeps the resident with an incurable malignancy comfortable.

11. List five signs of approaching death.

   a. _____

   b. _____

   c. _____

   d. _____

   e. _____

12. List the five stages of grieving (or dying).

   a. _____

   b. _____

   c. _____

   d. _____

   e. _____

CLINICAL SITUATION

Ms. Mitterand has a diagnosis of terminal cancer of the uterus. Although she has had surgery, followed by a course of radiation, the prognosis is poor. She has been a resident of your facility both before and after surgery. You have cared for her frequently and she has always been pleasant, but now she is angry most of the time and lashes out verbally at everyone. How should you respond?

Answer: _____

_____

_____

SECTION IV Achievement Review

A. **Multiple Choice.** Select the one best answer and circle the letter of the correct answer.

1. A group of similar cells that carry out a specific body function is called a
   a. cell type
   b. tissue
   c. organ
   d. system
   e. structure

2. The membrane that lines body cavities that open to the outside, such as the nose and mouth, is called
   a. serous
   b. protective
   c. mucous
   d. synovial
   e. cutaneous

3. Nervous tissue forms the
   a. stomach and spleen
   b. muscles and bones
   c. brain and spinal cord
   d. uterus and colon
   e. urethra and bladder

4. The kidneys contribute to which system?
   a. urinary
   b. reproductive
   c. digestive
   d. nervous
   e. respiratory

5. Another way to refer to the *front* of the body is to say
   a. posterior
   b. dorsal
   c. proximal
   d. distal
   e. anterior

6. The fingers are best described in their relationship to the wrist as being
   a. anterior
   b. distal
   c. proximal
   d. posterior
   e. dorsal

7. A resident places his hand over the area you know is the location of the appendix. You should chart this location as the
   a. lower right quadrant
   b. upper right quadrant
   c. umbilical area
   d. upper left quadrant
   e. lower left quadrant

8. The large muscle that separates the anterior body cavity into an upper and lower part is the
   a. intercostal muscle
   b. diaphragm
   c. rectus abdominis
   d. latissimus dorsi
   e. pectoralis major

9. The upper cavity formed by the muscle named in question 8 is called the
   a. pelvic
   b. abdominal
   c. thoracic
   d. cranial
   e. vertebral

10. The serous membrane that covers the lungs is the
   a. pleura
   b. meninges
   c. pericardium
   d. peritoneum
   e. omentum

B. **True or False.** Answer the following statements true (T) or false (F).

1. _____ Aging is a process that begins even before birth.

2. _____ Senescent changes take place at the same rate in every body system.

3. _____ The effects of aging bring about changes in both structure and function.

4. _____ Light-headedness is a symptom that you should report.

5. _____ Cancer and infections can affect any body system.

6. _____ A boil is an example of a systemic infection.

7. _____ Cancers are often called tumors or malignancies.

8. _____ Radiation treatments for cancer are usually performed outside the LTCF.

9. _____ Side effects of chemotherapy and radiation include nausea, vomiting, diarrhea, and lowered blood cell production.

10. _____ When caring for a resident with cancer, you should plan the care to minimize fatigue.

C. **Identification.**

1. Locate the body organs listed (a — e) and label them in the diagram.

   a. Heart
   b. Liver
   c. Lungs
   d. Small intestine
   e. Stomach

2. Identify the systems to which each of the following organs belong.

a. brain _____

b. heart _____

c. lungs _____

d. kidneys _____

e. ovaries _____

D. **Matching.** Match the correct terms or words on the right with the statements or phrases on the left.

1. _____ a condition that comes and goes rather quickly

2. _____ a cancerous growth

3. _____ a condition that ends in death

4. _____ supportive treatment that makes the person comfortable but doesn't cure the condition

5. _____ special service for ill and dying Catholic residents

6. _____ new cell production

7. _____ the study of structure

8. _____ the study of aging

9. _____ the study of disease

10. _____ a condition in which signs and symptoms seem to go away even though the condition is still present

a. remission
b. malignant
c. anatomy
d. mitosis
e. gerontology
f. last rites
g. acute
h. pathology
i. terminal
j. palliative
k. chronic

E. **Write and spell correctly the term(s) that mean**

1. aging changes _____

2. probable outcome _____

3. infection in the blood_____

4. spread of cancer cells_____

5. treatment with drugs _____

F. **Write a brief statement about the grieving process indicating the stages and how you might recognize and help a resident or the family at each stage.**

Stage	Signals	Nursing Assistant Action

SECTION V PROCEDURAL SKILLS

LESSON 17 Basic Nursing Care Skills

OBJECTIVES

After studying this lesson, you should be able to:

- Demonstrate procedures related to admission, discharge, and transfer of a resident.
- Recognize the emotional impact of these procedures on residents and their families.
- Record and report initial observations.
- Take and record vital signs accurately.
- Define and spell the vocabulary words and terms.

ADMITTING THE NEW RESIDENT

The decision to admit someone to a long term care facility is never an easy one. It is often filled with anxiety, guilt, fear, and depression for the resident and the family.

The new resident probably has experienced many losses already, and admission means a further loss — that of independence. He or she may have lost a spouse and now, along with failing strength and health, the comfort and security of familiar surroundings is about to be lost. Families often feel guilty because the family member cannot be provided for at home. There may be financial burdens also that are intensified by the financial costs of admission. Some residents may feel embarrassed at having to accept public help in financing their care.

Admission requires a major adjustment.

Stress makes it more difficult to hear and understand.

Both the family and the new resident will feel uncertain about and somewhat fearful of the new environment and will need support and encouragement. Their anxiety may make it difficult for them to remember things that you explain to them. Be prepared to repeat statements. Reassure them that their feelings are natural and help them express these feelings. Their first impression of you and the facility will be a lasting one, so make it positive, figure 17–1. Smile and be calm and patient. Include the family as much as you can in the admission process and orientation tour.

222

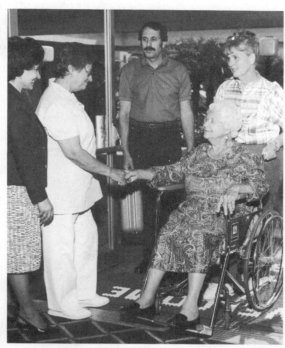

FIGURE 17–1. Remember, the first impression during admission is a lasting one. Make it positive.

NURSING ASSISTANT RESPONSIBILITIES ▪▪▪▪▪▪▪▪▪▪▪▪▪▪▪▪▪▪▪▪▪▪▪

Arrangements are made through the office for the new admission, and financial matters are handled by the office staff. You, however, have a major responsibility in making the transition as comfortable and as easy as possible for both family and resident. The manner in which you carry out the admission procedure should demonstrate caring and efficiency. You can help ease the transition process for the resident and their family by:

- being calm and patient.
- making explanations short and clear.
- making the resident feel welcome.
- helping the resident get settled.
- introducing the resident to others.
- orienting the resident and family to the facility and services.

Before the Admission_____

Prepare for the resident before he or she arrives. Find out all you can before meeting the person. For example:

1. Determine the person's name.
2. Find out how he or she is being transported.
3. Learn whether special equipment will be needed such as an overbed bar (**trapeze**).
4. Ask about orders and if special help will be needed to safely make the transfer.
5. Check the room for tidiness and readiness, making it as open and as inviting as possible.

6. If others share the resident's room, let them know about the new admission.

Meeting the New Resident_____

Your positive attitude can ease the transition.

Greet the new resident by name and introduce yourself. Escort the resident and visitor(s) to the resident's unit. Introduce everyone in the room, figure 17–2. Let the new resident know where her or his personal space will be. Assure the resident that even though there are roommates, her or his privacy will be protected.

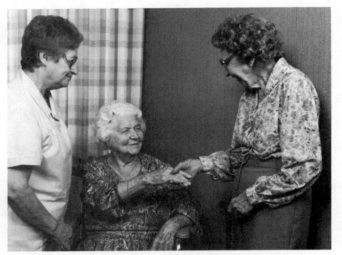

FIGURE 17–2. Introduce the new resident to her roommate and other residents.

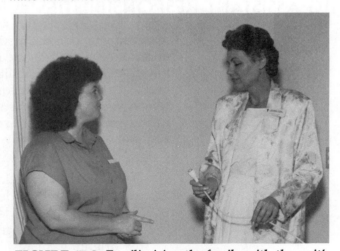

FIGURE 17–3. Familiarizing the family with the unit's equipment.

Encourage the new resident to assist in making decisions about placement of personal items. Those who will be making the facility their home are encouraged to bring personal items from home. These items include furniture, pictures, keepsakes, and religious articles. The resident feels that you appreciate the value of these items when you make positive comments about them and treat the things with respect.

Both the resident and the family should know how to operate equipment in the unit, figure 17–3. Orient the visitors and residents first to the immediate area and then to the rest of the facility. Be sure to include any facility rules, such as limitation of smoking areas, visiting periods, and the availability of services and activities. Knowing about such routines as mealtimes and activity periods and the availability of religious services and barber services can help the resident to adjust more easily and aids the family in their planning.

As you make a personal inventory of the resident's belongings, be sure the family signs for and takes home valuables for safety's sake. Be very specific about valuables as you list them. Do not make judgments about value. For example, don't write "gold ring." Write "yellow-colored band." Describe ring stones by color, such as white stone, rather than as a gem, such as diamond.

Personal belongings of value that remain with the resident should be placed in the safe for storage. Make sure that they are properly labeled, described, and signed for by two people. Articles remaining in the unit of a personal nature, such as a cane or eyeglasses or hearing aid, must be marked according to facility policy.

Demonstrate to the resident the way in which the position of the bed can be controlled and the way in which help can be quickly summoned using the call bell or intercom. Orient the new resident to the location of call bells in the lavatory (bathroom) and shower. Make sure the resident knows the location of bathroom facilities and dining room.

MAKING INITIAL OBSERVATIONS ■■■■■■■■■■■■■■■■■■■■■■■■■■■

Remember that there are nine body systems, figure 17–4. As you assist your resident in the admission process, keep these systems in mind. Look and listen carefully as you work. Make notations of your observations, as they will serve as important sources of comparison later on.

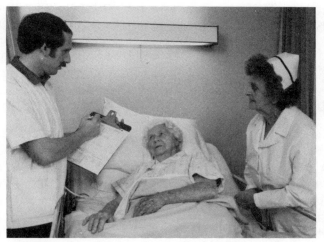

FIGURE 17–4. Think of each body system as you make your assessment.

More complete but similar base-line assessments will be made by the nurse and used to develop the nursing care plan, but since you will be reporting changes you observe, your initial observations will give you a basis for making comparisons. For example, you might note that the resident's skin is dry and scaly on admission. However, as the resident is encouraged to gradually take more fluid, you might later note that the skin seems less dry. Without accurate initial observations, you could not make this comparison or comment.

Use a systems approach as you make observations.

Here are some things you might want to consider in relation to the body systems as you make your observations:

- *Integumentary System* — color, flexibility, dryness; areas of redness or breakdown; any sores or bruises, swellings, or scars.
- *Musculoskeletal System* — deformities, amputations; ability to walk, sit, or move; any pain associated with movement, posture.
- *Circulatory System* — heart rate, pulse, blood pressure.
- *Respiratory System* — any difficulty in breathing; cough, blueness of skin (cyanosis), short of breath (SOB) on exertion.
- *Nervous System* — response to questions (articulation and words); paralysis, orientation as to time or place; condition of eyes and ears.
- *Urinary System* — frequency of urination; inability to hold urine; catheter drainage if present.
- *Digestive System* — intolerance to foods or types of foods; elimination problems (incontinent), ethnic food preferences.

Residents with deeper pigment in their skin present a special problem when assessing the skin. For example, cyanosis is not as easily recognized in dark-skinned persons and jaundice is less obvious in yellow-skinned persons. Therefore, also look for color changes in the whites of the eyes, the palms of the hands, soles of the feet and the mucous membranes of the mouth.

Take vital signs:
- **temperature**
- **pulse**
- **respiration**
- **blood pressure**

Skin breakdown may be signalled by impending drying, color change such as darkening and heat.

These systems, as well as the reproductive and endocrine systems, will be completely reviewed as the nurse makes a nursing assessment and develops a nursing diagnosis.

▪▪▪ PROCEDURE: Admitting a Resident ▪▪▪▪▪▪▪▪▪▪▪▪▪▪▪▪▪▪▪▪▪▪▪▪▪▪▪▪▪▪▪▪

1. Wash hands and assemble the following equipment:
   a. pad and pencil
   b. resident's record
   c. stethoscope
   d. blood pressure cuff
   e. equipment for taking temperature
   f. watch with second hand
   g. equipment for urine specimen
2. Prepare the unit for the resident by making sure that all necessary equipment and furniture are in their proper places. Check for adequate lighting and provide ventilation.
3. Identify the new resident by asking his or her name and by checking the identification.
4. Introduce yourself and take the resident and family to the unit. Behave in a courteous manner.
5. Screens unit. Ask the new resident to be seated, or if ordered, after helping resident to

undress, assist him or her into bed from stretcher or wheelchair; adjusts side rails. Ask the family to wait in the lounge or lobby while you carry out the admission procedure.

6. Introduce the resident to others in the room.
7. Explain the signal system (e.g., call bell) and the standard regulations.
8. Insofar as it is permitted, explain what will happen in the next hour. Has family return to unit.
9. Screen the unit.
10. Care for clothing and personal articles according to facility policy.
11. List valuables or jewelry that have not been left at the office. Ask the resident to sign the list, if possible.
12. Have relatives also sign the list and take the valuables home or place them in the facility's safe.
13. Check the resident's weight and height.
14. Take temperature, pulse, respiration, and blood pressure.
15. Clean and replace equipment according to facility policy.
16. Leave fresh water if permitted.
17. Leave call bell close at hand.
18. Record information, according to facility policy, on the resident's chart.

DETERMINING VITAL SIGNS

You will be carrying out several different procedures as you admit residents. To perform them accurately, you need to understand why the procedures are done, what equipment is needed and the correct way to proceed.

All residents will have the **vital signs** (*vital* means living) taken and recorded on admission and frequently throughout the resident's stay. The vital signs are:

- temperature
- pulse rate
- respiratory rate
- blood pressure
- weight and height

Although weight and height determinations are not vital signs, they are important factors to be considered in overall health and the administration of drugs. The vital signs give a great deal of information about the general health of the individual and changes in the health status. It is essential that you be accurate in making these determinations and recording them.

Equipment Needed_____

Clinical **thermometers** are used to determine temperature. A watch with a second hand is needed to count the pulse and respiratory rate. Both a **stethoscope** and **sphygmomanometer** (blood pressure cuff) are needed to measure the blood pressure. Weight may be determined with a scale and height with the ruler attached to an upright scale or a tape measure. Each vital sign and height and weight determinants will be discussed separately, although they are usually carried out as combined activities.

TEMPERATURE

Temperature is the measurement of body heat. One of two temperature scales may be used. A formula can be used to convert from one scale to another. Normal body temperature is about 98.6° Fahrenheit (37° Celsius).

Temperatures are usually taken orally, but if the resident is unable to keep the mouth closed, has respiratory difficulty, is receiving oxygen, or is uncooperative or confused, the temperature can be taken with a thermometer placed and held in the rectum (rectal temperature) or, as a last alternative, in the armpit (axillary temperature). The rectal temperature registers one degree higher and the axillary temperature registers one degree lower than an oral temperature.

Temperature can be increased by:

- infection
- dehydration
- physical exercise
- hot water

It can be decreased by:

- shock
- cold weather
- alcohol sponge bath
- medications

Clinical Thermometers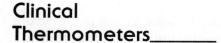

Three types of glass clinical thermometers are in general use: oral, security, and rectal thermometers, figure 17–5. These thermometers differ mainly in the size and shape of the bulb (the end which is inserted into the resident). When only security or stubby type, thermometers are in use, the rectal thermometers are marked with a red dot at the end of the stem.

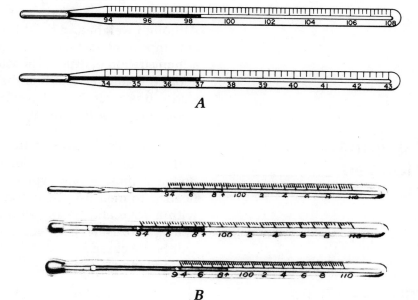

FIGURE 17–5. A, Fahrenheit and celsius thermometer scales; B, clinical thermometers. From top to bottom: oral, security, and rectal.

Reading the Glass Thermometer. Mercury (a heat-sensitive element which appears as a solid color line) in the bulb of the thermometer rises in the hollow center of the stem. To read the thermometer, hold it at eye level and find the solid column of mercury, figure 17–6. Look along the sharper edge between the numbers and lines. Starting with 94°F (34°C), each long line indicates a 1-degree elevation in temperature. Only every other degree is marked with a number. In between each long line are four shorter lines. Each shorter line equals two tenths (2/10 or .2) of 1 degree. The thermometer is "read" at the point at which the mercury ends (stops rising). If it stops between two lines, read it to the closer line.

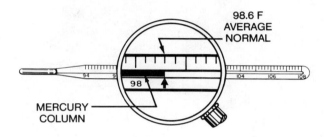

FIGURE 17–6. Reading a thermometer. This thermometer reads 98.6°F.

General Thermometer Safety Precautions_____

- Check glass thermometers for chips.
- Shake mercury down before use, *away* from resident or hard objects.
- Do not leave resident alone with thermometer in place.
- Allow to register for 3 minutes orally or 2 minutes rectally.
- Hold rectal and axillary thermometers in place.
- Lubricate before inserting in rectum.
- Wipe thermometer from end to tip before reading.

Contraindications — Oral Temperatures: Patient is

- uncooperative
- restless
- unconscious
- chilled
- confused
- coughing
- unable to breath through the nose

Contraindications — Rectal Temperatures: Patient

- has diarrhea
- has fecal impaction
- is combative
- has rectal bleeding
- has hemorrhoids
- has colostomy

Electronic Thermometers_____

Some facilities use a battery-operated electronic thermometer to take temperatures, figure 17-7. The temperature is registered in large numbers on the viewer. The probe is the portion that is placed into the resident. The probes are colored blue for oral use and red for rectal use. The probe is covered with a disposable sheath which stays on during use and is then discarded.

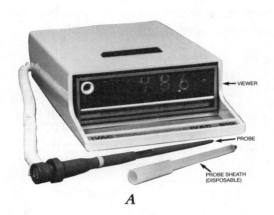

A

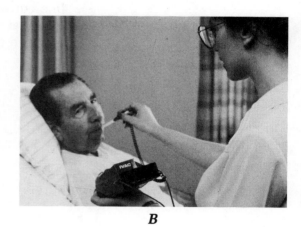

B

FIGURE 17-7. An electronic thermometer. A, The temperature is registered in large, easy-to-read numerals. The disposable, protective sheath is placed over the thermometer tip. The tip is then inserted into the resident's mouth in the usual manner. (Courtesy of Ivac Corporation); B, Place the probe under the resident's tongue.

PROCEDURE: Measuring Oral Temperature

1. Wash hands and assemble the following equipment on a tray:
   a. pad and pencil
   b. container with tissues
   c. container for soiled tissues
   d. watch with second hand
   e. container with clean thermometers
   f. container for used thermometer
2. Identify resident and explain what you plan to do.
3. Have resident rest in comfortable position in bed or chair.
4. Remove thermometer from container by holding stem end.
5. Wipe with tissue and check to be sure the thermometer is intact.
6. Read mercury column. If necessary, shake down to below 96°F.
7. Insert bulb end of thermometer under resident's tongue, toward side of mouth. Tell resident to hold thermometer gently with lips closed for 3 minutes.
8. Remove thermometer, holding by stem.
9. Wipe from stem toward bulb end.
10. Discard tissue in proper container.
11. Read thermometer and record on pad.
12. Place thermometer in container for used thermometers. If thermometer is to be reused for this resident, wash it in cold water and soap and dry it. Return to the individual disinfectant-filled holder.
13. Clean and replace equipment according to facility policy.
14. Record the temperature on the resident's chart. Report any unusual variation in reading immediately to supervising nurse.

▮▮▮ PROCEDURE: Measuring Rectal Temperature (Glass Thermometer) ▮▮▮▮▮▮▮▮▮▮▮▮▮▮▮▮▮

1. Wash hands and assemble equipment as for oral temperature. Add lubricant to equipment. Use rectal thermometer with rounded bulb.
2. Identify resident and explain what you plan to do.
3. Screen unit.
4. Lower back rest of bed. Ask resident to turn on side. Assist, if necessary.
5. Place small amount of lubricant on tissue.
6. Remove thermometer from container by holding stem end and read mercury column. Check to be sure it registers below 96°F. Check condition of thermometer.
7. Apply small amount of lubricant to bulb with tissue.
8. Fold the top bedclothes back to expose anal area.
9. Separate buttocks with one hand. Insert the thermometer gently 1½ inches into rectum.
10. Hold in place for 2 minutes. Replace bedclothes as soon as thermometer is inserted.
11. Complete procedure as for oral temperature, steps 8–14.
12. Record an "R" (for rectal) beside temperature reading.

▮▮▮ PROCEDURE: Measuring Axillary or Groin Temperature (Glass Thermometer) ▮▮▮▮▮▮▮▮▮▮▮▮▮▮▮▮▮

1. Wash hands and assemble equipment as for oral temperature.
2. Identify resident and explain what you plan to do.
3. Wipe the axillary or groin area dry and place the thermometer. The resident should hold arm close to body if axillary site is used. Thermometer must be in the fold against the body if groin site is used. Leave thermometer in place for 10 minutes.
4. Complete procedure as for oral temperatures, steps 8–14.
5. In recording, place "AX" after axillary temperature (for example, 98°F AX). For groin temperature, use the abbreviation "GR" (98°F GR).

▮▮▮ PROCEDURE: Measuring Oral Temperature Using Electronic Thermometer ▮▮▮▮▮▮▮▮▮▮▮▮▮▮▮▮▮

1. Wash hands and assemble the following equipment:
   a. electronic thermometer
   b. disposable sheath
2. Identify resident and explain what you plan to do.
3. Cover probe with protective sheath.
4. Insert covered probe under resident's tongue toward side of mouth.
5. Hold probe in position.
6. When buzzer signals that temperature has been determined, take reading and record on pad.
7. Discard sheath in wastepaper basket. Do not touch sheath.
8. Return probe to proper position and entire unit to charging stand. Wash hands.
9. Record the temperature on resident's chart and note the time it was taken.
10. Report any unusual variations in reading to the supervising nurse.

▪▪▪ PROCEDURE: Measuring Rectal Temperature Using Electronic Thermometer ▪▪▪▪▪▪▪▪▪▪▪▪▪▪▪▪▪

1. Wash hands and assemble the following equipment:
   a. electronic thermometer
   b. disposable sheath
   c. lubricant
2. Identify resident and explain what you plan to do.
3. Screen unit.
4. Lower back rest of bed. Ask resident to turn on his or her side. Assist if necessary.
5. Put the sheath over the tip of the thermometer and place a small amount of lubricant on the tip of the sheath.
6. Fold the top bedclothes back to expose anal area.
7. Separate buttocks with one hand. Insert sheath-covered probe about ½-inch into rectum. Hold in place. Replace bedclothes as soon as thermometer is inserted.
8. Read temperature when registered on digital display. Note on pad.
9. Remove probe and discard sheath.
10. Assist the resident to a comfortable position.
11. Wash hands and return equipment to proper location.
12. Record the temperature reading on the graph. Place an "R" after the reading.

▪▪▪ PROCEDURE: Measuring Axillary Temperature Using Electronic Thermometer ▪▪▪▪▪▪▪▪▪▪▪▪▪▪▪▪▪

1. Wash hands and assemble equipment as for procedure using oral thermometer, but substitute an oral electronic thermometer with an oral probe (blue) and disposable sheaths.
2. Identify resident and explain what you plan to do.
3. Wipe axillary area dry and place covered probe in place. Keep resident's arm close to the body. Hold probe in place until temperature records on digital display. Note on pad.
4. Remove thermometer probe and dispose of sheath. Return equipment.
5. Wash hands and record axillary temperature, placing AX after the reading on the graphic chart.

PULSE AND RESPIRATION ▪▪▪▪▪▪▪▪▪▪▪▪▪▪▪▪▪▪▪▪▪▪▪▪▪▪▪▪▪▪▪

The **pulse** and **respiration** of the resident are usually counted during the same procedure. Breathing is partially under voluntary control, that is, a person is able to stop breathing temporarily for a short period of time. This frequently happens when a resident realizes that breathing is being watched and being counted. The breathing pattern is altered unintentionally. To avoid this, the respirations are counted immediately following the pulse count. The resident's hand is kept in the same position and your fingers remain upon the pulse. Each complete respiration includes one **inspiration** followed by one **expiration**. Count respirations for one full minute. Count the pulse rate for one minute also.

Pulse is the pressure of the blood felt against the wall of an arterial blood vessel as the heart alternately beats (contracts) and rests (relaxes). It is more easily felt in those arteries that are fairly close to the skin surface and can be gently squeezed against a bone by the fingers. The pulse rate and its character provide a good indication of how the cardiovascular system is able to meet the body needs.

Radial Pulse_____

You will usually take the pulse over the **radial artery** (at the base of the wrist on the thumb side), figure 17–8. The age, sex, size, and condition of the resident may influence the **pulse rate** (regularity) and **volume** (fullness). Rate and character (**rhythm** and volume) should be noted when taking the pulse. Always place the tips of three fingers over the artery to determine the pulse. Never use your thumb. There is a pulse in your thumb that may be confused with the resident's pulse.

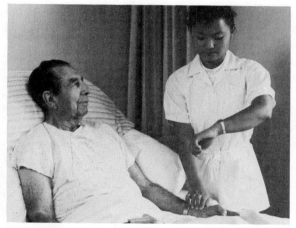

FIGURE 17–8. Count the pulse for one full minute.

PROCEDURE: Measuring the Radial Pulse

1. Wash hands and go to bedside. Identify resident and explain what you plan to do.
2. Place resident in a comfortable position, with arm resting across chest, palm of hand down.
3. Locate the pulse on the thumb side of the wrist with the tips of your first three fingers.
4. Exert slight pressure when a pulse is felt.
5. Using second hand of watch, count for 1 minute.
6. Record the rate and character of the pulse.

Apical Pulse_____

The heart rate is usually the same as the pulse rate. Sometimes, however, all the heartbeats are not strong enough to be transmitted and felt along the radial artery. This is called a **pulse deficit**. Pulse deficits are found in some forms of heart disease. If a pulse deficit (difference between the heart and pulse rate) is suspected, it may be necessary to determine the heart rate by checking the heart beats with a stethoscope placed on the chest over the **apex** or point of the heart. (The apex is the lowest point of the heart and can easily be located near the left nipple or under the left female breast.) This is called taking an **apical pulse**. The apical rate is then compared to the radial pulse rate. The average pulse rate is about 72 beats per minute (bpm). Pulse rates under 60 or over 90 should be reported. An unusually fast heartbeat is called **tachycardia**. An unusually low heartbeat is called **bradycardia**. Irregularities in rate, rhythm, or character should be reported at once.

▪▪▪ PROCEDURE: Measuring the Apical Pulse ▪▪▪▪▪▪▪▪▪▪▪▪▪▪▪▪▪▪▪▪▪▪▪

1. Wash hands and take stethoscope to bedside. Identify resident and explain what you plan to do.
2. Clean stethoscope earpieces with alcohol. Place the earpieces in ears.
3. Place the stethoscope diaphragm or bell over the apex of the heart.
4. Listen carefully for the heartbeat.
5. Count the beats for one minute.
6. Check radial pulse for one minute. Another health assistant may take the radial pulse at the same time that the apical pulse is being checked, figure 17–9.
7. Compare the results. Chart the apical pulse over the radial pulse. For example, $\frac{A108}{R82}$. Be sure to indicate character as well as rate differential. Pulse deficit may also be charted in this way: 26 (108 − 82 = 26).
8. Clean earpieces. Return stethoscope. Wash hands.
9. Report apical/radial differential to nurse.

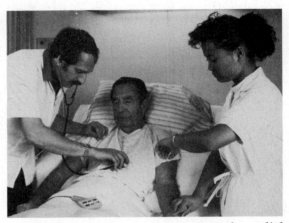

FIGURE 17–9. One person counts the radial pulse while another counts the apical pulse.

Respiration_____

Each respiration consists of one inspiration followed by one expiration.

The main function of **respiration** is to supply the cells in the body with oxygen and to rid the body of excess carbon dioxide. When respirations are inefficient, carbon dioxide gas accumulates in the bloodstream making the skin "dusky," bluish or **cyanotic**.

There are two parts to each respiration: one inspiration (inhalation) followed by one expiration (exhalation). The character of respirations must be noted as well as the rate. Respirations are described as *normal, shallow, deep, labored,* or *difficult.* The normal rate for adults is 13 to 18 per minute. If the rate is more than 25 per minute, it is said to be **accelerated** and should be reported.

The rate is determined by counting the rise and fall of the chest for one minute with a watch equipped with a second hand.

▪▪▪ PROCEDURE: Counting Respirations ▪▪▪▪▪▪▪▪▪▪▪▪▪▪▪▪▪▪▪▪▪▪▪▪▪

1. When the pulse rate has been counted, leave your fingers on the radial pulse.
2. Start counting the number of times the chest rises and falls during a period of one minute.
3. Note depth and regularity of respirations.
4. Record the time, rate, depth and regularity of respirations.

Special respiratory patterns include:

- dyspnea — difficult or labored breathing
- apnea — periods of no respirations
- Cheyne-Stokes — dyspnea followed by apnea followed by dyspnea
- **rales** — bubbling sounds as fluid collects in the air passageways. This is commonly seen in dying residents or those with respiratory or cardiac problems.

BLOOD PRESSURE

Blood pressure depends upon the amount of blood in the circulatory system, the force of the heartbeat, and the condition of the blood vessels. Arteries that have lost their elasticity or ability to stretch due to disease changes give more resistance, and so the pressure is greater. Blood pressure is also increased by:

- exercise
- eating
- stimulants
- emotional anxiety
- some drugs

Blood pressure is decreased by:

- **fasting** (not eating)
- rest
- **depressants** (drugs which slow down body functions)
- hemorrhage (loss of blood)

If the resident is resting, any reading between 60 and 90 **diastolic** (lower reading) is considered normal. Blood pressure rises slightly with age.

Hypertension is high blood pressure (greater than 140/90). Uncontrolled hypertension can lead to stroke. **Hypotension** is low blood pressure (below 100/70). Excessive hypotension can lead to shock. In either case, unusual or changed findings must be recorded and reported.

Blood Pressure Equipment

Blood pressure equipment includes the sphygmomanometer and the stethoscope, figure 17–10. The sphygmomanometer consists of a cuff with a rubber bladder connected to two tubes; one connected to the pressure control bulb and the other to the pressure gauge. The gauge may be a round dial or a column of mercury. Both are marked in numbers. Be sure to use a cuff of the proper size. Cuffs that are too wide or too narrow for the arm will give inaccurate readings. The width of the cuff should measure approximately two thirds the diameter of the resident's arm.

How to Read the Gauge

The gauges are marked with a series of large lines at 10-mm (millimeter) intervals. In between the large lines are shorter lines, each of which indicates 2 mm. For example, the small line above 80 mm is 82 mm, and the small line below 80 mm is 78 mm. For accuracy, the gauge should be at eye level when reading. The mercury column

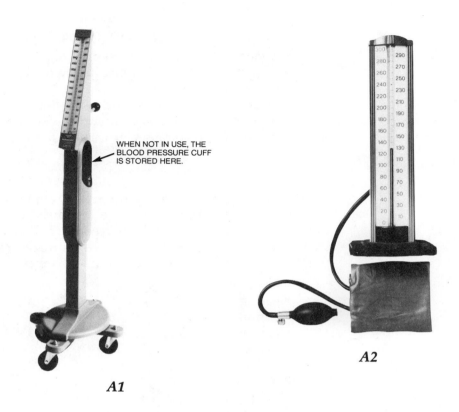

WHEN NOT IN USE, THE BLOOD PRESSURE CUFF IS STORED HERE.

A1

A2

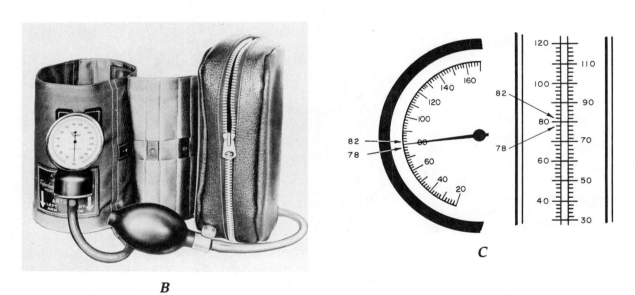

B

C

FIGURE 17–10. *Two types of blood pressure gauges are in use: A, the mercury gravity sphygmomanometer floor and table models, and B, the aneroid sphygmomanometer. C, the aneroid gauge (left) and the mercury gravity gauge (right).* (Floor model courtesy of W.A. Baum, Co., Inc.)

gauge must not be tilted. The level of the top of the column of mercury or the point of the dial is taken for the reading. Two readings are recorded:

- *systolic* — The loud sound heard as the tricuspid and bicuspid valves close. The larger number indicates when the first sound is heard, figure 17–11.
- *diastolic* — The soft sound heard when the semilunar heart valves close. The smaller number indicates when this change sound is heard.

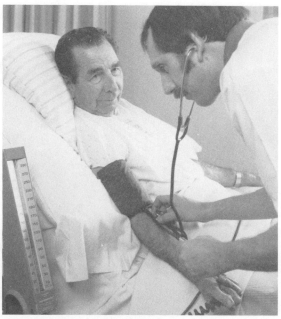

FIGURE 17–11. *Note the level of the mercury column when you hear the first regular beat.*

The blood pressure is recorded as an inverted fraction. For example, 112/68 means that 112 is the systolic pressure and 68 is the diastolic pressure. Remember, the **pulse pressure** is the difference between the systolic and diastolic pressures. In this example, it is 44.

PROCEDURE: Measuring Blood Pressure

1. Wash hands and collect the following equipment:
   a. sphygmomanometer
   b. stethoscope
2. Identify resident. Position comfortably and explain what you plan to do.
3. Place the resident's arm palm upward and support it on bed or table. The same arm should be used for all readings.
4. Roll resident's sleeve up about 5 inches above elbow. Be sure it is not tight on the arm.
5. Apply the cuff around the upper arm just above the elbow.
6. Wrap the rest of the arm band smoothly around the arm. Tuck the ends under a fold and hook or simply press if Velcro is used to secure.
7. Be sure that cuff is secure but not too tight.
8. Clean stethoscope earpieces with antiseptic solution and place in ears, figure 17–12.
9. Locate the brachial artery by placing fingers on the inner side of the arm just above the elbow.
10. Place stethoscope head directly over the artery.
11. Close valve attached to hand pump (air bulb) and inflate cuff until indicator registers 20 mm above where pulse ceases to be heard.

12. Open valve of pump and let air escape slowly until the first sound is heard.
13. Note reading at first regular sound on manometer as systolic pressure.
14. Continue to release the air pressure slowly until there is an abrupt change in the sound from very loud to very soft. In some situations, the last sound heard is taken as diastolic pressure. Note reading at second sound as diastolic.
15. Remove cuff and expel air.
16. Clean earpieces of stethoscope with antiseptic solution and return to proper place. Replace equipment.
17. Record time and blood pressure. The blood pressure is recorded as an inverted fraction with the systolic on top and the diastolic on bottom e.g., 100/70.

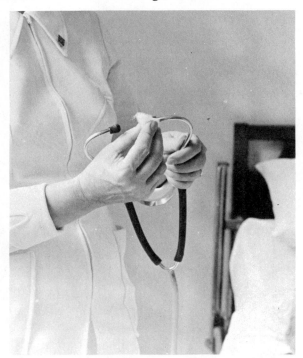

FIGURE 17–12. Clean the earpieces with alcohol before and after each use. (From Brooks, *The Nurse Assistant,* copyright 1978 by Delmar Publishers Inc.)

WEIGHING AND MEASURING THE RESIDENT ■■■■■■■■■■■■■■■■■

You must learn to read the scale correctly. There are two bars on the scale. The balance bar should hang free to start. The lower bar indicates weights in large 50-pound increments. The upper bar indicates smaller pound weights. The even numbered pounds are marked with numbers. The long line between even numbers indicates the odd number pounds. Each small line indicates one-quarter of a pound, or 4 ounces.

The two figures are added and recorded as the person's total weight. The sum is recorded according to facility policy in either pounds or **kilograms**. One kilogram equals 2.2 pounds. For example, the weight shown in figure 17–13 is determined as follows:

```
Large weight =  150 pounds
Small weight = + 8 pounds   or  158 ÷ 2.2 = 71.8 kilograms
       Total =  158 pounds
```

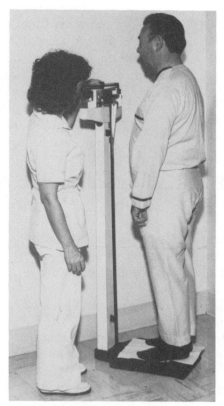

FIGURE 17–13. *Weighing the resident on an upright scale.*

Thus, the total weight is determined by adding the large and small weights, figure 17–14.

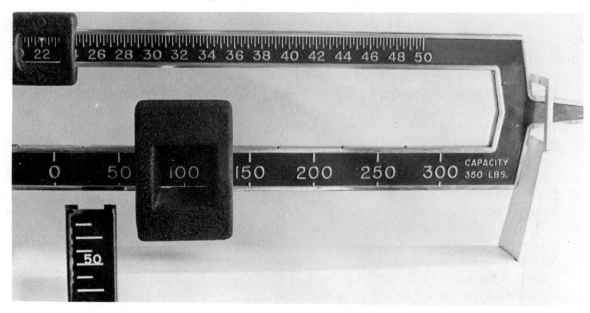

FIGURE 17–14. *The weight is determined by adding the large numbered pounds and the small numbered pounds.* (From Brooks, *The Nurse Assistant,* copyright 1978 by Delmar Publishers Inc.)

Measuring the resident may be done during the weighing procedure with an upright scale. The information is recorded in feet and inches or in **centimeters**, according to facility policy. There are 12 inches in 1 foot and 2.5 centimeters in 1 inch. For example, someone with a height of 62 inches might be recorded as 62 inches; 5 feet 2 inches (62 inches divided by 12); or 155 cm (62 × 2.5).

If the resident is ambulatory, an upright scale or floor scale can be used. If it is too difficult for the resident to stand safely, then a chair scale or overbed scale should be used, figure 17–15.

PROCEDURE: Weighing and Measuring a Resident Using an Upright Scale

1. Identify resident and explain what you plan to do. Escort the resident to the scale.
2. Place a paper towel on the platform of the scale.
3. Be sure the weights are at the extreme left and the balance bar hangs free.
4. Help the resident to remove shoes and to step onto the scale platform. Stand close by for support.
5. Move the large weight to the closest estimated weight.
6. Move the small weight to the right until the balance bar hangs free halfway between the upper and lower bar guide.
7. Add the two figures and record the total weight in pounds or kilograms, according to facility policy.
8. Raise the height bar until it rests level on the top of the resident's head, figure 17–16.
9. The reading is made at the movable point of the ruler. Record this information, according to facility policy, in inches, feet and inches, or centimeters.
10. Help the resident to step off the scale and to put on shoes.
11. Enter the height and weight in the appropriate place on the resident's record.

PROCEDURE: Weighing a Resident Using a Mechanical Lift

1. Wash hands and assemble equipment. If possible, obtain assistance from a coworker.
2. Check the slings and straps for frayed areas or poorly closing clasps.
3. Take scale to resident's bedside and screen the unit. Identify the resident and explain what you plan to do.
4. Lock the bed and roll resident toward you.
5. Position one-half sling beneath the body behind shoulders and buttocks.
6. Roll resident back onto the sling and position properly.
7. Attach suspension straps to sling. Check fasteners for security.
8. Position lift frame over bed with base legs in maximum open position and lock.
9. Elevate head of the bed and bring resident to a semi-sitting position.
10. Attach suspension straps to frame. Position resident's arms inside straps.
11. Secure restraint straps if needed.
12. Talking to resident, slowly lift the resident free of the bed.
13. Guide the lift away from the bed so that no part of the resident touches the bed.
14. Adjust weights to balance scale.
15. Note weight.
16. Lower resident to bed by releasing knob.
17. Detach hooks and roll resident toward you.
18. Fold sling under resident and roll resident away from you.
19. Reposition resident as you remove sling.
20. Position resident comfortably with call bell close at hand and side rails up.
21. Return equipment to proper location.
22. Wash hands.
23. Record and report findings.

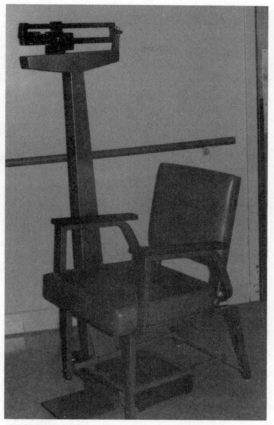

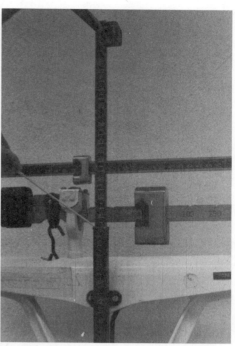

FIGURE 17–16. *Measuring the resident.*

FIGURE 17–15. *For those residents unable to stand, weight may be determined using a chair scale.*

▪▪▪ PROCEDURE: Measuring a Resident Who Must Remain in Bed ▪▪▪▪▪▪▪▪▪▪▪▪▪▪▪▪▪▪▪▪▪▪

1. Position him or her flat in bed with legs extended.
2. Mark the sheet at the top of the head and at the heels.
3. Use a tape measure to determine the distance between the two marks.
4. Record this figure as the resident's height.

TRANSFER AND DISCHARGE ▪▪▪▪▪▪▪▪▪▪▪▪▪▪▪▪▪▪▪▪▪▪▪▪▪▪▪▪▪▪

Be supportive during transfer and discharge.

Transfers and discharges require a physician's written order. Transfers to an acute hospital or other facility (figure 17–17) are handled as a discharge if the resident is to be absent for an extended period of time, and the record is closed. A return at a later date is treated as a new admission. If the transfer is only temporary, the room is left as it is until the resident returns, and his or her record is kept open.

Learn what the resident has been told about the reasons for the transfer. Residents will not always understand the reasons and may be confused and anxious. This can be a very stressful period for them.

If the discharge is to be permanent, gather the resident's personal belongings and check them against the inventory list. Assist the

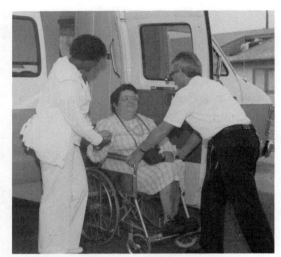

FIGURE 17–17. This resident is being transferred to another facility.

resident or family member to pack. Check the area carefully before and after the resident leaves, and then give the room a terminal cleaning. In the process of terminal cleaning, be sure to check for any articles that might have been left in the bathroom, drawers, or even under the bed. The nurse will supervise the discharge; however, be sure to ask if there are medications to go with the resident.

Let the resident know that you have enjoyed knowing and helping him or her. Accompany the resident to the door of the facility. Be sure to record the method of transportation as the resident leaves and the resident's reaction in leaving.

PROCEDURE: Transfer of the Resident

1. Identify resident and explain what is to be done. Be sure resident is clean and well groomed.
2. Gather all personal belongings.
3. Compare the articles against the original inventory.
4. Secure valuables in a sealed envelope, listing articles on the outside, and have the person receiving them sign with you. Give them to family member, if possible. Check with charge nurse for special instructions.
5. Escort the resident to the doorway of the facility.
6. Sign chart off, entering:
   a. time of transfer
   b. date of transfer
   c. method of transport
   d. destination of transfer
   e. resident's reaction(s)
   f. your signature

VOCABULARY

accelerated	diastolic	mercury
apex	expiration	pulse
apical pulse	fasting	pulse deficit
bradycardia	hypertension	pulse pressure
centimeter	hypotension	pulse rate
cyanotic	inspiration	radial artery
depressants	kilogram	rales

respiration   systolic   trapeze
rhythm   tachycardia   vital signs
sphygmomanometer   thermometer   volume
stethoscope

SUGGESTED ACTIVITIES

1. Practice admitting residents under supervision in your facility.

2. Practice weighing and measuring your classmates.

3. Practice taking vital signs until you develop skill and accuracy.

4. Practice transferring and discharging of residents.

5. Discuss the psychological stresses that accompany admission, transfer, or discharge of residents.

REVIEW

A. Brief Answer/Fill in the Blanks

1. The first impression made at the time of admission is _____.

2. Vital signs include

    a. _____

    b. _____

    c. _____

    d. _____

3. Your initial observations are important as a basis for later _____.

4. A blood pressure of 106/70 is charted. The number 106 represents the _____ pressure and the number 70 represents the _____ pressure.

5. A rectal temperature registers _____ degree(s) higher than an oral temperature of the same resident.

6. In addition to the rate, the pulse should be checked for _____ and _____.

7. The character of respirations are described as normal, _____, _____, _____, or _____.

8. If a resident must remain in bed but needs to be weighed, you would use an _____ scale.

9. Some facilities record height in centimeters. A height of 5 feet 1 inch would be recorded as _____.

10. A resident who weighs 142 pounds might have this information recorded as _____ kilograms.

B. Matching. Match the words on the left with the correct term on the right.

1. _____ low blood pressure

2. _____ fullness (amount)

3. _____ moist respirations

Continued

a. sphygmomanometer
b. tachycardia
c. thermometer
d. volume

Continued

4. _____ not eating

5. _____ rapid heart rate

6. _____ slow heart rate

7. _____ used to determine blood pressure

8. _____ used to determine temperature

9. _____ high blood pressure

10. _____ difference between radial and apical pulse rates

e. fasting
f. hypotension
g. bradycardia
h. hypertension
i. pulse deficit
j. rales

C. **Identification.** Read the temperature indicated on the thermometers (a, b, and c) shown.

a. _____

b. _____

c. _____

A

B

C

CLINICAL SITUATION

Mrs. Fiona Smythe, age 86, is being admitted to your facility, and you are assigned to her care. List three actions that you will take to help this lady make an easier transition to the status of resident.

Answer: _____

_____

_____

_____

LESSON 18 Applying Heat and Cold

OBJECTIVES

After studying this lesson, you should be able to:

- State the effects of heat and cold applications.
- Give reasons why applications of heat and cold may be ordered.
- List equipment used for heat and cold treatments.
- Describe precautions in carrying out heat and cold application procedures.
- Define and spell all the vocabulary words and terms.

Applications of hot and cold require a physician's order and must be carefully carried out in order to prevent injury to the resident. Some facilities permit only licensed people to perform hot and cold applications, so be sure to check your policy manual for direction.

Elderly persons are more sensitive to heat and cold.

Older people have less sensitivity to changes in temperature and can be easily burned if temperatures are too high. They may experience tissue damage if the temperature is too low or if the application is left on too long.

SAFETY

The diminished sensitivity to pain makes the older person at greater risk for injury. Heat is especially dangerous, so it is very important to:

1. Frequently check the area being treated with either hot or cold applications.
2. Report unusual changes. You should check for excessive redness or discoloration and report any complaints of discomfort or pain. Do not rely on the resident's ability to inform you of any problems; check carefully yourself. The resident may not be aware that a problem exists.
3. Discontinue the treatment promptly as ordered.

Applications of heat and cold may be either moist or dry, figure 18-1. Moisture makes both heat and cold more penetrating, therefore, moist heat or moist cold is more likely to cause injury. Extra care must be taken to protect the resident when moist treatments are employed. Be sure you know the:

1. exact method to be used
2. correct temperature
3. proper length of time the heat or cold application is to be performed

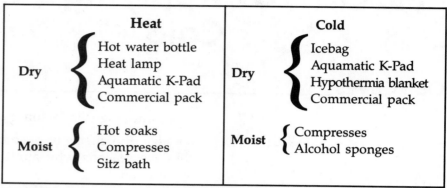

FIGURE 18–1. *Summary of heat and cold applications.*

COMMERCIAL PREPARATIONS

Commercially prepared packs for dry application of heat and cold are available and simple to use. They may be available in your facility for short term local applications. A single blow activates the heat or cold and the units are discarded after one use.

APPLICATION OF HEAT

Heat applications may be ordered to:

- relieve muscle spasms
- reduce pain
- promote healing
- combat local infection
- improve mobility prior to exercise periods

The value of heat treatments (**diathermy**) lies in the fact that heat dilates blood vessels, bringing more blood to the area, which promotes inflammation and healing. Heat is very soothing when there is pain. There must be a specific order for a heat treatment.

Cautions_____

- Constant heat must be carefully monitored.
- Moisture intensifies the effect of heat. Use extra caution.
- Never allow a resident to lie on a constant heat unit since heat may be trapped and build up to dangerous levels.
- Temperature of a constant heat unit should be between 95° and 100°F.
- Always use a bath thermometer to check solution temperatures.
- Always remove a part being soaked before adding hot solution.
- Always stay with the resident during the treatment.
- Protect areas not being treated from excessive exposure.

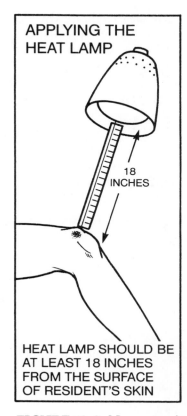

FIGURE 18-2. Never permit the heat lamp to be closer than 18 inches from the resident's skin.

The figure shows:
APPLYING THE HEAT LAMP
18 INCHES
HEAT LAMP SHOULD BE AT LEAST 18 INCHES FROM THE SURFACE OF RESIDENT'S SKIN

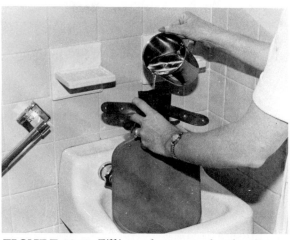

FIGURE 18-3. Filling a hot water bottle. (From Brooks, The Nurse Assistant, copyright 1978 by Delmar Publishers Inc.)

Method: Dry Heat___

- **Aquamatic K-Pads** — plastic pads of heated fluid-filled coils that maintain a constant temperature.
- **Heat Lamps** — intense dry heat. The lamp should never be closer than 18 inches from the resident's skin, figure 18-2. Use a tape measure or ruler to be sure of the distance. Never use more than a 40 to 60 watt bulb.
- **Hot Water Bottles** — dry heat. These are infrequently used in care facilities but are often used in home care, figure 18-3. Hot water bottles should be checked carefully for leaks, since the plastic or rubber tends to become brittle and crack over time.
- **Electric Heating Pads** — dry, constant heat. Check carefully for frayed cords or broken wires. This form of heat application will probably not be used in your facility but, again, may be seen in the home situation.

▧▧▧ PROCEDURE: Applying an Aquamatic K-Pad ▪▪▪▪▪▪▪▪▪▪▪▪▪▪▪▪▪▪▪▪▪▪

1. Wash hands and assemble the following equipment:
   a. K-Pad and control unit (figure 18–4)
   b. covering for pad
   c. distilled water
2. Identify resident and explain what you plan to do.
3. Place the control unit on the bedside stand.
4. Remove the cover and fill the unit with distilled water to fill line.
5. Screw the cover in place and loosen it one-quarter turn.
6. Cover the pad and place it on the resident.
7. Be sure that the tubing is coiled on the bed to facilitate the flow.
8. Do not allow tubing to hang below the level of the bed.
9. Turn on the unit. Set temperature at 95° to 100°F and remove key.
10. Leave pad in place for prescribed time, checking resident frequently.
11. Remove pad, replacing it according to facility policy. Assist resident to comfortable position.
12. Wash hands.
13. Record the procedure on the resident's chart.

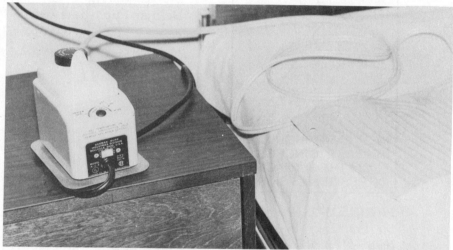

FIGURE 18–4. A covered K-Pad may be used to provide continuous warmth to an area.

▧▧▧ PROCEDURE: Applying a Heat Lamp ▪▪▪▪▪▪▪▪▪▪▪▪▪▪▪▪▪▪▪▪▪▪▪▪

1. Wash hands and assemble the following equipment:
   a. bath blanket
   b. heat lamp
   c. tape measure
2. Identify resident and explain what you plan to do.
3. Screen unit.
4. Position resident and drape with bath blanket so that only the area to be treated is exposed.
5. Position the lamp at least 18 inches from the resident.
6. Check distance with the tape measure.
7. Turn lamp on, noting time.
8. Check resident every 5 minutes, observing the skin carefully for signs of redness or burning.
9. Turn off lamp and discontinue procedure after prescribed time.
10. Assist resident to a comfortable position.
11. Adjust bedding and remove drape.
12. If procedure is to be repeated, fold and leave bath blanket in bedside table.
13. Leave unit tidy.
14. Clean and return equipment according to facility policy.

15. Wash hands.
16. Report and record procedure, including:
    a. time started
    b. length of treatment
    c. your observations

PROCEDURE: Applying Hot Water Bag

1. Wash hands and assemble the following equipment in the utility room:
   a. hot water bag
   b. cover
   c. container for hot water
   d. thermometer
   e. paper towels
2. Fill container with water and test for correct temperature, which should be approximately 115°F unless otherwise ordered.
3. Fill hot water bag one third to one half full to avoid unnecessary weight.
4. Expel air by placing hot water bag horizontally on flat surface, holding neck of bag upright until water reaches neck.
5. Close the top when all air has been expelled.
6. Wipe bag dry with paper towels and turn upside down to check for leakage.
7. Place cover on hot water bag so that the resident's skin does not come in contact with rubber or plastic.
8. Take equipment to bedside on tray.
9. Identify resident and explain what you plan to do.
10. Apply hot water bag to the affected area as ordered. Caution resident not to lie on the hot water bag.
11. Check the resident's condition at 15 to 20 minute intervals.
12. When heat has been applied for the proper amount of time, remove bag. Observe area.
13. Empty bag. Clean and replace according to facility policy. Place cover in laundry hamper.
14. Report any unusual observations immediately to supervising nurse.
15. Wash hands.
16. Record procedure on the resident's chart.

Method: Moist Heat

- **Hot Soaks** — For a hot soak, the resident, or a body part, is immersed in a tub filled with water at a specific temperature.
- **Wet Compresses** — Wet compresses are moistened with a solution and placed on the affected area. An **Asepto syringe** may be used to add water to the compresses to keep them moist. The compresses can be kept warm by covering them with an Aquamatic K-Pad. Each time the pad is removed and replaced, be careful to reposition the protective covering.
- **Sitz Bath** — This type of soak applies moist heat to the rectal and perineal (the area between the rectum and the external genitalia in both men and women) areas. The Sitz bath is often ordered to promote healing of hemorrhoids or after surgery.
  Three styles of sitz units are:
  — stationary tub
  — sitz chair
  — portable unit

PROCEDURE: Assisting with the Hot Arm Soak

1. Wash hands and assemble the following equipment on a tray:
   a. bath thermometer
   b. pitcher
   c. arm soak basin

   Collect and bring to the bedside (along with equipment):
   a. large plastic sheet
   b. bath blanket
   c. bath towel

2. Identify the resident and explain what you plan to do.
3. Screen unit and place equipment on overbed table.
4. Cover resident with bath blanket.
5. Fanfold bedding to foot of bed.
6. Expose arm to be soaked.
7. Elevate the head of the bed to a sitting position, if permitted.
8. Help resident to move to far side of bed, opposite the arm to be soaked.
9. Be sure side rail is up and secure.
10. Cover bed with plastic sheeting and towel.
11. Fill arm soak basin half full with water at prescribed temperature (usually 100°F). Check temperature with bath thermometer if available.
12. Take arm soak basin from overbed table and position on bed protector.
13. Assist resident to place arm gradually in basin.
14. Check temperature every 5 minutes.

15. Use pitcher to get additional water and add to arm soak basin to maintain prescribed temperature. *Note:* Be sure to remove arm before adding hot solution.
16. Discontinue procedure at end of prescribed time by lifting resident's arm out of basin. Place basin on overbed table and gently pat resident's arm dry with towel.
17. Remove plastic sheeting and towel.
18. Adjust bedding and remove bath blanket. If treatment is to be repeated, fold bath blanket and place in bedside table.
19. Lower head of bed and make resident comfortable.
20. Leave unit tidy and call bell within reach.
21. Take equipment to utility room. Clean and store according to hospital policy.
22. Wash hands.
23. Record and report procedure, including:
   a. area treated
   b. length of treatment
   c. your observations

PROCEDURE: Assisting with the Hot Foot Soak

1. Wash hands and assemble the following equipment on a tray:
   a. bath thermometer
   b. solution as ordered in container
   c. extra pitcher of hot water
2. Place the tray on the overbed table.
3. Also bring the following equipment to the bed:
   a. large rubber or plastic sheet
   b. 2 bath blankets
   c. 2 bath towels
   d. tub or basin of appropriate size
   e. filled hot water bottle
4. Screen unit. Identify resident and explain what you plan to do.
5. Have resident flex knees. Loosen the top bedclothes at the *foot* of the bed and fold them back toward the top of the bed, just below resident's knees.
6. Make a bed protector by placing the rubber sheet across the foot of the bed. Place bath blanket folded in half, top half fanfolded toward foot of bed, over rubber sheet. Place towel on blanket and a hot water bottle at lower edge of towel.

7. Raising resident's feet, draw rubber sheet, blanket and bath towel up under the legs and feet of resident. Bring upper half of bath blanket over feet.
8. Fill tub half full of water and place it lengthwise at the foot of bed. Temperature should be 105°F unless otherwise ordered. Check temperature with bath thermometer.
9. Raising the resident's feet with one hand, draw tub under them and gradually immerse feet. Place a towel between the edge of the tub and the legs.
10. Draw the bath blanket up over the knees and fold it over from each side. Bring back top covers over foot of bed to retain heat.
11. Replenish water as necessary to maintain desired temperature.
12. Discontinue treatment within 15 or 20 minutes.
13. Remove the resident's feet from tub and move them to the towel with hot water bottle under towel. Cover feet.
14. Remove tub to table or chair.
15. Dry and powder feet.
16. Remove bath blanket, rubber sheet, and towel.

17. Draw down top bedclothes and tuck in at foot.
18. Clean and replace equipment according to facility policy.
19. Wash hands.
20. Report and record procedure, including:
    a. area treated
    b. length of treatment
    c. your observations

PROCEDURE: Applying a Moist Compress

1. Wash hands and assemble the following equipment on a tray:
   a. Asepto syringe
   b. bath thermometer
   c. bed protector
   d. basin containing prescribed solution at temperature ordered
   e. binder or towel
   f. compresses
   g. pins or bandage
   h. hot water bag filled with water at ordered temperature
2. Identify resident and explain what you plan to do.
3. Bring tray to the bedside and screen the unit.
4. Expose only the area to be treated.
5. Protect bed and resident's clothing with bed protector (Chux).
6. Moisten the compresses; remove excess liquid. Apply to treatment area.
7. Secure the dressings with bandage or binder, making sure compresses are in contact with skin.
8. Help resident to maintain a comfortable position throughout the treatment.
9. Keep compresses moist or hot water bag hot or cold, as prescribed.
10. Check skin several times each day.
11. Remove compresses when ordered and discard.
12. Clean and replace equipment according to facility policy.
13. Wash hands.
14. Record the treatment on the resident's chart.

PROCEDURE: Assisting with the Sitz Bath (Portable Unit)

1. Wash hands and assemble the following equipment and take to the bathroom:
   a. bath thermometer
   b. bath towel, face cloth
   c. bath blanket
   d. clean gown
   e. safety pin
   f. portable sitz unit, figure 18–5
2. Adjust temperature of bathroom to between 78° to 80°F. Clean tub. Go to resident's room.
3. Identify resident. Explain what you plan to do and take resident to bathroom.
4. Fill unit to level given by unit's directions.
5. Adjust water temperature to 105°F.
6. Check temperature with bath thermometer.
7. Remove resident's robe and slippers and assist to sit. Leave slippers on.
8. Cover resident's shoulders with a bath blanket. Hold in place with a safety pin.
9. Place cool compresses on resident's forehead to prevent headache.
10. Stay with resident during procedure.
11. Allow some water to run out of unit; replace it to maintain constant temperature.
12. Assist resident to stand after 10 to 20 minutes.
13. Help resident to dry by patting, not rubbing, and put on clean gown.
14. Assist resident to return to bed.
15. Clean unit. Replace it according to facility policy.
16. Wash hands and record procedure on resident's chart.

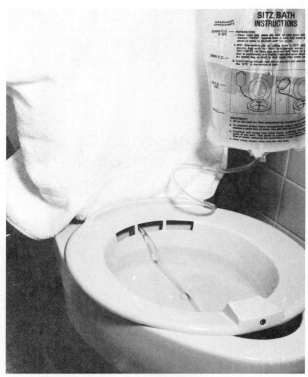

FIGURE 18–5. *The temperature of water for the Sitz bath is about 105°F.*

APPLICATION OF COLD

Applications of cold (**hypothermia**) are given only with a physician's order. Local cold applications:

- constrict blood vessels and reduce swelling
- decrease sensitivity to pain
- reduce temperature

Cautions_____

1. Excessive cold can damage body tissues. Remember, moisture intensifies the effect of cold just as it does heat. Therefore, extreme caution must be used in the application of moist cold.
2. Report color changes such as blanching or cyanosis.
3. Report feelings of numbness or discomfort experienced by resident.
4. Stop the cold treatment if shivering should develop. Cover resident with blanket and report immediately to the nurse.

Method: Dry Cold____

- **Thermal blankets** — These are large, fluid-filled blankets. The temperature of the fluid may be raised or lowered as the blanket is wrapped around the resident. The blanket can be used to lower or raise the resident's body temperature; however, they are most often used in care facilities to lower the body temperature. This process is called hypothermia.
- **Ice bags** — Ice bags should never be filled more than two thirds full. Never place them directly on the affected area, since the weight will cause discomfort. Make sure that there is a cloth covering, figure 18–6.

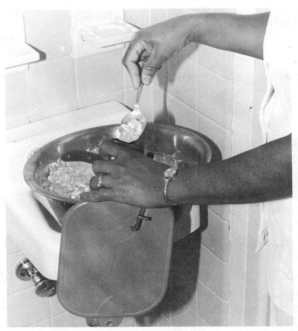

FIGURE 18–6. After filling the ice bag, be sure to check for leaks and cover the bag before applying it to the affected area. (From Brooks, The Nurse Assistant, copyright 1978 by Delmar Publishers Inc.)

▮▮▮ PROCEDURE: Applying a Disposable Cold Pack ▮▮▮▮▮▮▮▮▮▮▮▮▮▮▮▮▮▮▮▮▮▮▮▮▮▮

1. Wash hands and assemble the following equipment:
   a. commercially prepared disposable cold pack (read instructions)
   b. cloth covering (towel, hot water bag cover)
   c. tape or rolls of gauze
2. Identify the resident and explain what you plan to do.
3. Screen unit.
4. Place cold pack in cloth covering.
5. Expose area to be treated. Note condition of area.
6. Strike or squeeze cold pack to activate chemicals.
7. Place covered cold pack on proper area, and secure with tape or gauze.
8. Note time of application.
9. Leave resident in comfortable condition with signal cord within easy reach.
10. Return to bedside every 10 minutes and check area being treated for discoloration or numbness. If either occurs, discontinue treatment and report to supervisor.
11. If no adverse symptoms occur, leave pack in place for 30 minutes.
12. Remove pack and note condition of area.
13. Apply new pack if treatment is to be continued.
14. Remove cover and discard used pack according to facility policy.
15. Put cover in laundry bag.
16. Leave resident comfortable and unit tidy.
17. Wash hands.
18. Record and report procedure, including:
    a. type of treatment
    b. length of treatment
    c. your observations

▥▥▥ PROCEDURE: Applying an Ice Bag ▦▦▦▦▦▦▦▦▦▦▦▦▦▦▦▦▦▦▦▦▦▦▦▦

1. Wash hands and assemble the following equipment in the utility room:
   a. ice bag or collar
   b. paper towels
   c. ice cubes or crushed ice
   d. spoon or similar utensil
   e. cover (usually muslin)
2. If ice cubes are used, rinse them in water to remove sharp edges.
3. Fill ice bag half full, using ice scoop or large spoon, figure 18–7. Avoid making bag too heavy.
4. Expel air by resting ice bag on table in horizontal position with top in place but not screwed on. Squeeze the bag until air has been expelled.
5. Fasten top securely.
6. Wipe dry with paper towels.
7. Test for leakage.
8. Place muslin cover on ice bag. Never permit rubber or plastic to touch resident's skin.
9. Take equipment to bedside on tray.
10. Identify resident and explain what you plan to do.
11. Apply ice bag to the affected part for pre-scribed period with metal away from resident.
12. Refill bag before all ice is melted.
13. Check skin area at least every ten minutes.
14. Report to supervising nurse immediately if skin is discolored or white or if resident reports that skin is numb.
15. After discontinuing procedure, wash ice bag with soap and water; drain and screw top on loosely after use.
16. Wash hands and record procedure on the resident's chart.

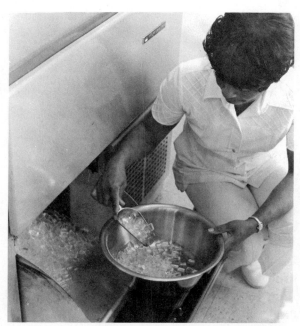

FIGURE 18–7. *When preparing a cooling bath or soak, use an ice scoop to put the cubes into a basin.* (From Brooks, *The Nurse Assistant,* copyright 1978 by Delmar Publishers Inc.)

Method: Moist Cold_

• **Wet compresses** — The same cautions apply to cold as to hot compresses. They may be kept wet with an Asepto syringe and cold by placing a covered ice cap against the area.

• **Cooling sponge bath** — A sponge bath with cool water or alcohol solution is used primarily to lower resident's temperature when there is fever.

▪▪▪ PROCEDURE: Giving a Tepid Bed Bath ▪▪▪▪▪▪▪▪▪▪▪▪▪▪▪▪▪▪▪▪▪▪▪

1. Wash hands and assemble the following equipment:
   a. 2 bath towels
   b. 2 bath blankets
   c. 1 washcloth
   d. basin of tap water (ice cubes, if ordered)
   e. 1 covered, filled ice bag
   f. 5 covered, filled hot water bottles
2. Identify resident and explain what you plan to do.
3. Screen unit for privacy and to prevent drafts.
4. Take the resident's temperature and record.
5. Fanfold top bedclothes to foot of bed.
6. Position bath blanket under resident.
7. Cover the resident with the other bath blanket.
8. Remove resident's gown.
9. Water should be about 70°F.
10. Apply ice bag to head.
11. Apply hot water bags to feet, groin, and axilla.
12. Sponge with wash cloth, exposing only one area at a time.
13. Cover sponged area; allow to air dry.
14. Sponge strokes in direction of heart for approximately 20 minutes.
15. Bathe entire body, avoiding the eyes and genitals. Remove ice bag and hot water bottles.
16. Replace gown and top bedding.
17. Remove bath blankets and discard.
18. Clean equipment according to facility policy.
19. Take vital signs 10 minutes after sponge bath.
20. Record and report procedure.

VOCABULARY

Aquamatic K-Pad	hypothermia
Asepto syringe	perineal
diathermy	Sitz bath
hot soak	wet compress

SUGGESTED ACTIVITIES

1. Practice applying hot and cold applications.
2. Investigate the availability of disposable single unit packs for heat and cold application in your facility.
3. Practice operating the electric Aquamatic K-Pad.
4. Practice filling an ice bag and hot water bag properly.

REVIEW

Brief Answer/Fill in the Blanks

1. Hot and cold treatments require a physician's _____.
2. Two ways of reducing body temperature are _____ and _____.
3. Dry heat may be provided by use of _____, electric heating pads, and _____.
4. Moist heat is usually _____ penetrating than dry heat.

5. The Sitz bath applies heat to the _____ and the _____ area.

6. An ice bag or hot water bag should be filled _____ full.

7. Plastic and rubber may be irritating to a resident's skin; therefore, equipment made of these materials should always be_____.

8. Extreme caution should be used in heat treatments so as not to cause _____.

9. When using a heat lamp, the source of heat must be at least _____ inches from the resident. The bulb should not be higher than _____ watts.

10. The resident receiving a heat lamp treatment must have the area checked every _____ minutes.

CLINICAL SITUATION

Ms. Kudakas is assigned to your care. She is ill with a fever and, despite antibiotics and drugs to reduce her temperature, her fever remains high. Your orders are to give her a tepid bed bath. List the equipment you would prepare to carry out the procedure.

Answer: _____

_____

_____

LESSON 19 Musculoskeletal System

OBJECTIVES

After studying this lesson, you should be able to:

- Name the parts and function of the musculoskeletal system.
- Recognize normal musculoskeletal changes as they relate to the aging process.
- State the dangers of immobility.
- Carry out passive range of motion (ROM) exercises.
- Demonstrate proper body mechanics as you position, ambulate, and transfer residents.
- Define and spell all the vocabulary words and terms.

The musculoskeletal system is composed of the bones, skeletal muscles, **joints, tendons,** and **ligaments**. It provides form, strength, and protection to the body and permits the body to move.

BONES

There are 206 bones in the human body, figure 19–1. All of the bones are not alike. Some are:

Learn the names of major bones. Many body structures take their names from them.

- long bones, like the bones of the arms and legs
- short bones, like the bones of the fingers and toes
- irregular bones, like the bones that form the spinal column
- flat bones, like the pelvic bones and shoulder blades

Each type of bone has a name, and many other body structures take their name from that of the nearby bone. For example, the thigh bone, in the upper leg, is the **femur**. Close by are the:

- femoral nerve
- femoral artery
- femoral vein

Learning the names of the bones isn't nearly as difficult as it first seems. A line drawn down the center of the body, dividing it into half, demonstrates that the bones found on one side are matched by bones on the other side. (Already the number of bones to learn has been cut in half.) There are twelve pairs of **ribs**, all with the same name (rib), for a total of 24 bones. The finger and toe bones number 56 and are called **phalanges**. Study figure 19–1 and you will easily learn the names of the major bones.

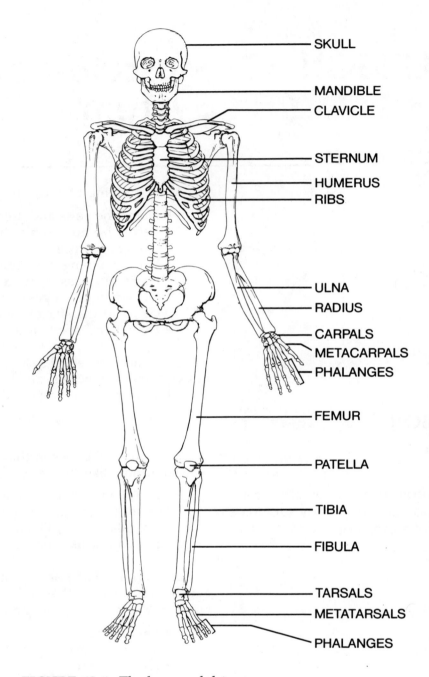

FIGURE 19–1. *The human skeleton.*

Bones give strength to the body, protect the delicate body organs, are a source of red blood cells and some white cells, and produce cells which are important in blood clotting.

SKELETAL MUSCLES

There are over 500 muscles in the body, figure 19–2. They work in groups to bring about body movement. There are three types of muscles:

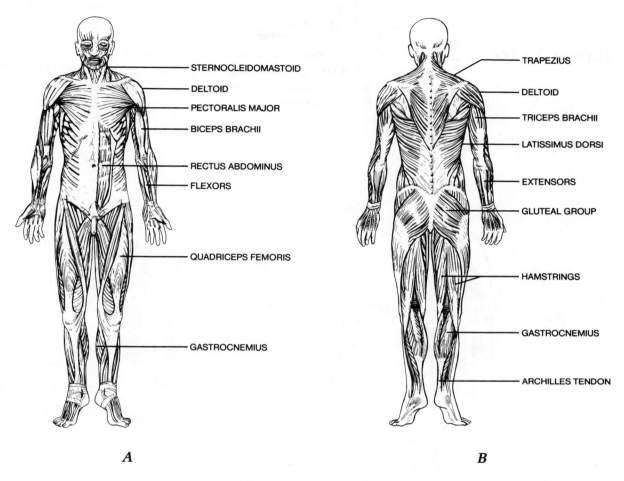

STERNOCLEIDOMASTOID

DELTOID

PECTORALIS MAJOR

BICEPS BRACHII

RECTUS ABDOMINUS

FLEXORS

QUADRICEPS FEMORIS

GASTROCNEMIUS

TRAPEZIUS

DELTOID

TRICEPS BRACHII

LATISSIMUS DORSI

EXTENSORS

GLUTEAL GROUP

HAMSTRINGS

GASTROCNEMIUS

ARCHILLES TENDON

A

B

FIGURE 19–2. *Major muscles.*

1. Cardiac muscle, found only in the heart wall.
2. Skeletal muscles, also called **voluntary muscles** because you can cause them to constrict or relax with your conscious thought.
3. Visceral muscles, which are also called **involuntary muscles** because we do not usually consciously control them.

The involuntary muscles make up the walls of organs like the stomach and guard body openings like those of the digestive and urinary tract. Involuntary muscles are usually controlled automatically for us in a special part of the brain.

Muscles are named by location, shape, or action. Could you guess where the quadriceps femoris is located? If you placed it near the thigh bone (femur), you would be correct.

Muscles have three parts:

- **origin**, or beginning
- **belly**, or middle part
- **insertion**, or ending

The origin and belly of a muscle are found on one side of a joint and the insertion is attached on the other side. Skeletal muscles are attached to the bones by tough, fibrous bands called **tendons**.

Action of Muscles_____

When the muscle shortens, it pulls the point of insertion toward the point of origin, changing the position of the bones, figure 19-3. It is in this way that movements such as walking, sitting or holding a pencil are possible.

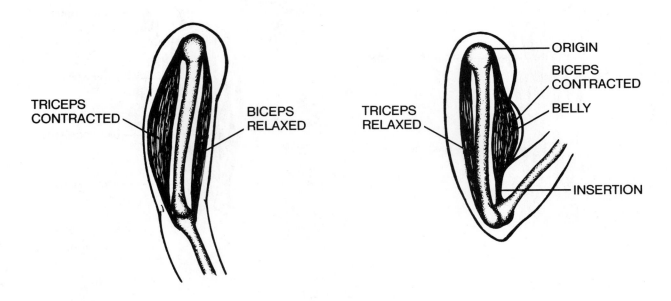

FIGURE 19-3. *Notice that as one muscle group contracts, another relaxes.*

JOINTS ▪▪▪▪▪▪▪▪▪▪▪▪▪▪▪▪▪▪▪▪▪▪▪▪▪▪▪▪▪▪▪▪▪▪▪▪▪

Joints are found at the points where two bones come together (touch, or **articulate**). For example, the elbows, knees and hips are joints. **Ligaments** are fibrous bands that help support the points of articulation. Movements in joints depend upon the way in which the joint is formed.

There are three types of joints:

Joint formation determines the type of movement.

1. **Synarthrotic joints**. These are immovable joints. The bones of the skull do not move after maturity, figure 19-4.
2. **Amphiarthrotic joints**. These are slightly movable joints such as the joints of the backbone (spinal column).
3. **Diarthrotic joints**. These are freely movable joints such as those formed by the bones of the arms and legs, fingers and toes, figure 19-5. Diarthrotic joints are more easily injured and are protected by a joint capsule. Two examples are the ball joint and hinge joint, figure 19-6.

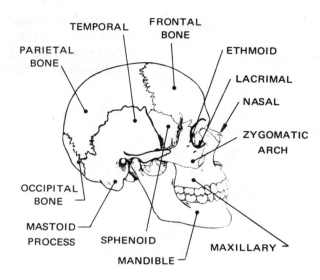

FIGURE 19-4. *The bones of the skull form immovable joints after growth is completed.*

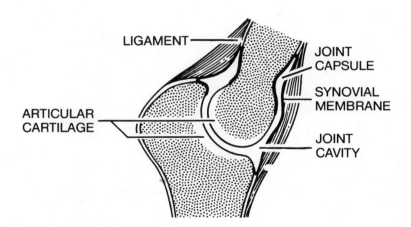

FIGURE 19-5. *Diarthrotic joint.*

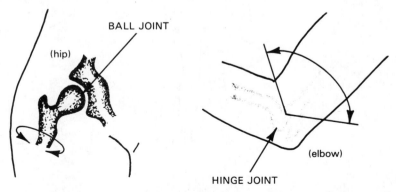

FIGURE 19-6. *Two types of diarthrotic joints are the ball joint and the hinge joint.*

Types of joint movements (figure 19–7):

- **Extension** — increasing the angle between two bones
- **Rotation** — twisting motion
- **Abduction** — moving away from the midline
- **Adduction** — moving toward the midline

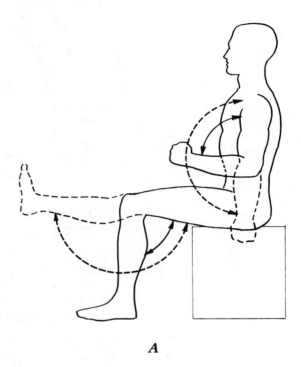

A

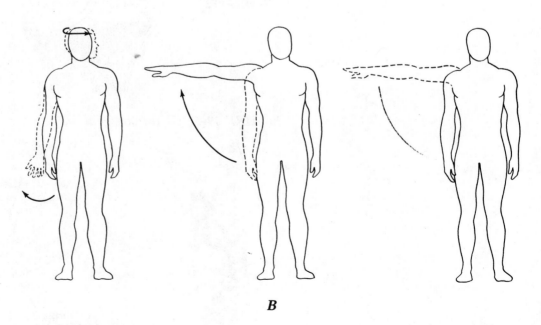

B

FIGURE 19–7. *Types of joint movements. A, Flexion and extension; B, rotation (left), abduction (center), and adduction (right).*

IMMOBILITY ▪▪▪

Lack of movement (**mobility**) leads to many serious problems, so residents should be encouraged to be as active as possible. When residents are unable to move themselves, the staff must assist by carrying out the program of exercises.

There are four problems which can develop from inactivity. They are:

Inactivity leads to serious problems.

1. *Contractures.* Unused muscles tend to shorten, causing permanent **flexion** of joints called **contractures**. Contractures can often be avoided by conscientious positioning, by carrying out regular routine exercises, and by encouraging as much activity as possible.
2. *Decreased respiration and circulation.* Proper exercise improves ventilation and stimulates blood flow through the body.
3. *Loss of bone calcium.* Loss of minerals, including calcium, from the bones makes the bones more fragile and easily broken.
4. *Renal calculi.* Kidney stones (**renal calculi**) are formed as blood calcium levels increase and the kidneys try to eliminate these salts from the body.

RANGE OF MOTION (ROM) EXERCISES ▪▪▪▪▪▪▪▪▪▪▪▪▪▪▪▪▪▪▪▪▪▪▪▪▪▪

Range of motion exercises should permit each of the resident's joints to be exercised. There are three types:

- **Active exercise** is performed by the resident, figure 19–8.
- **Passive exercises** are performed by someone else when a resident cannot carry out such movement.
- **Resistive exercises** are performed in response to resistance that is offered by a therapist, figure 19–9.

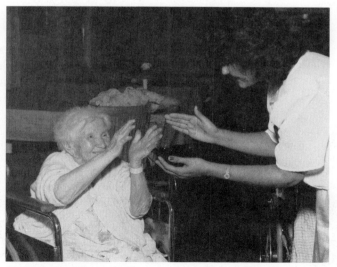

FIGURE 19–8. Active exercise is performed by the resident.

Complete ROM exercises may be carried out with the resident in bed. Some exercises can be carried out with the resident seated.

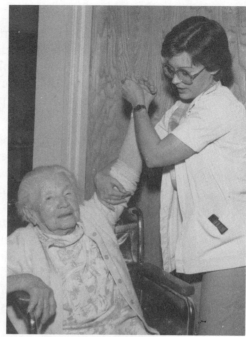

FIGURE 19–9. Passive resistive exercises are performed in response to resistance offered by the therapist.

These exercises are usually performed in the morning after A.M. care or in the evening, but they may be carried out at other times. Points you should keep in mind include:

Report if ROM exercise is resisted or causes discomfort.

- Be sure you have specific instructions as to the type of motions to be carried out.
- Always be gentle as you do each exercise, supporting the area above and below the moving joint.
- Carry out each exercise three times.
- Do not complete an exercise if the resident complains of pain or discomfort or if there is resistance in the joint movement.
- Position yourself close to the resident, using good body mechanics.
- Do not expose the resident unnecessarily during the procedure.

Some terms you will want to keep in mind as you learn range of motion exercises are:

- *Suppination* — Turning the forearms so that the palms face up
- *Pronation* — Turning the forearms so that the palms face down
- *Flexion* — Decreasing the angle between two bones
- *Extension* — Increasing the angle between two bones
- *Eversion* — Turning the foot so that the sole of the foot faces outward
- *Inversion* — Turning the foot so that the sole of the foot faces inward

▪▪▪ PROCEDURE: Range of Motion (ROM) Exercises ▪▪▪▪▪▪▪▪▪▪▪▪▪▪▪▪▪▪▪▪

ROM for the Neck

1. *Rotation.* Support the head and turn gently from side to side, figure 19–10A.
2. *Lateral flexion.* Support the head. Bend head toward right shoulder and then left, figure 19–10B.
3. *Flexion.* Support the head. Bring chin toward chest, figure 19–10C.
4. *Extension.* Return head to straight position. Adjust pillow under head and shoulders.
5. *Hyperextension.* Place pillow under shoulders and gently support head in a backward tilt.

ROM for Upper Extremities: Shoulder and Elbow

Note: Perform these motions on one side and repeat on the other side

1. *Shoulder: Abduction.* Supporting the elbow and wrist, bring entire arm out at a right angle to body, figure 19–11A.
2. *Shoulder: Adduction.* Supporting the elbow and wrist; bring entire arm back against body.
3. *Shoulder: Flexion.* With shoulder in abduction, flex elbow and raise entire arm over head, figure 19–11B.

4. *Elbow: Flexion.* Supporting upper arm and wrist, bend elbow toward shoulder, figure 19–11C.
5. *Elbow: Extension.* Supporting upper arm and wrist, straighten elbow out, figure 19–11D.
6. *Elbow: Suppenation.* Position arm flat on bed with palm of hand up, figure 19–11E.
7. *Elbow: Pronation.* With arm flat on bed, rotate forearm until palm of hand is down, figure 19–11F.

ROM for Upper Extremities: Wrist and Fingers

1. *Wrist: Flexion.* Supporting arm and hand, flex wrist, figure 19–12A.
2. *Wrist: Extension.* Supporting wrist, arm and hand, straighten wrist, figure 19–12B.
3. *Wrist: Ulnar Deviation.* Point hand in suppination toward thumb side.
4. *Wrist: Radial Deviation.* Point hand in suppination toward little finger side, figure 19–12C.
5. *Fingers: Flexion.* Cover resident's fingers and make a fist, figure 19–13A.
6. *Fingers: Extension.* Slip your fingers over resident's fingers and gently straighten them out, figure 19–13B.

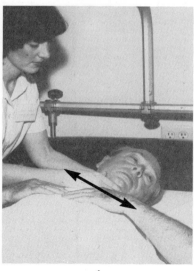
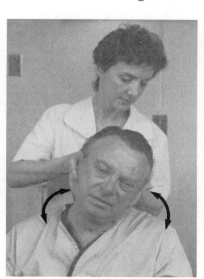
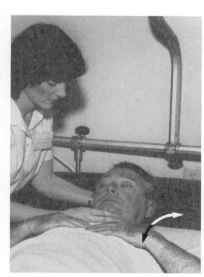

A   *B*   *C*

FIGURE 19–10. *ROM exercises for the neck.*
A. Neck rotation. Support head and turn gently from side to side.
B. Lateral neck flexion. Support head. Bend head toward right shoulder and then left.
C. Anterior flexion. Support head and bring chin toward chest.

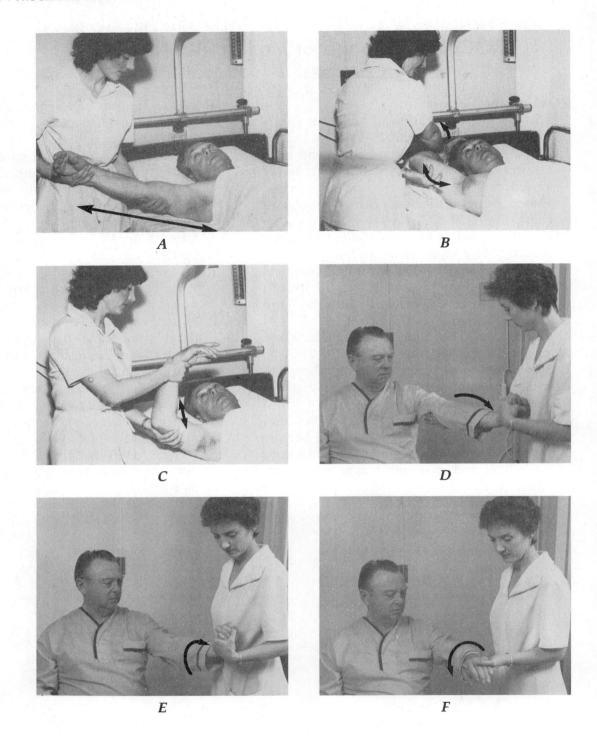

FIGURE 19–11. *ROM exercises for the shoulder and elbow.*

A. *Abduction. Supporting the elbow and wrist, bring the entire arm out at right angles from the body.*

B. *Shoulder flexion. With shoulder in abduction, flex elbow and raise entire arm over head.*

C. *Flexion of elbow. Supporting upper arm and wrist, bend elbow toward shoulder.*

D. *Elbow extension. Supporting upper arm and wrist, straighten elbow.*

E. *Supination. Supporting wrist and elbow, turn palm up.*

F. *Pronation. Supporting wrist and elbow, turn palm down.*

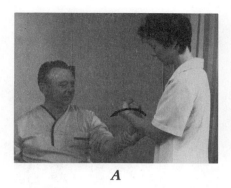
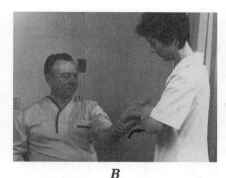
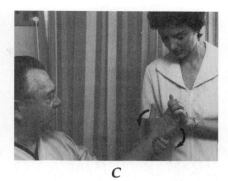

A

B

C

FIGURE 19–12. ROM exercises for the wrist.
A. Flexion. Supporting arm and hand, flex wrist.
B. Extension. Supporting arm and hand, extend wrist.
C. Ulnar/radial deviation. Move wrist toward ulna, then toward radius.

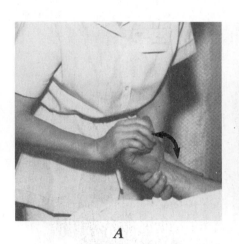
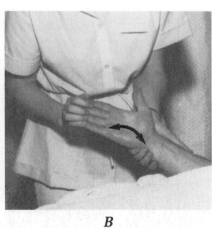
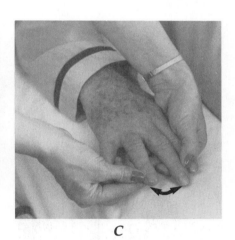

A

B

C

FIGURE 19–13. ROM exercises for the fingers.
A. Flexion. Cover resident's fingers and curl them — making a fist.
B. Extension. Slip fingers over flexed fingers and straighten fingers out.
C. Abduction and adduction.

7. *Fingers: Opposition.* Touch the thumb to each fingertip.
8. *Fingers: Abduction.* Move each finger in turn, including thumb, away from the middle finger.
9. *Fingers: Adduction.* Move each finger in turn, including thumb, toward the middle finger, figure 19–13C.

ROM for Lower Extremities: Hip and Knee

1. *Hip: Abduction.* Supporting knee and ankle, move entire leg away from body center, figure 19–14A.
2. *Hip: Adduction.* Supporting knee and ankle, move entire leg back, figure 19–14B.
3. *Hip: Flexion.* Supporting knee and ankle, flex knee and hip, figure 19–14C.
4. *Hip: Extension.* Supporting knee and ankle, straighten hip and knee, figure 19–14D.
5. *Hip: Rotation (Medial).* Supporting ankle and thigh, flex knee and rotate leg medially (toward midline of body), figure 19–14E.
6. *Hip: Rotation (Lateral).* Supporting ankle and thigh, flex knee and rotate leg laterally (away from midline of body), figure 19–14F.
7. *Knee: Flexion.* Supporting ankle and thigh, bend knee as you raise the leg from the bed.
8. *Knee: Extension.* Supporting ankle and thigh, straighten knee out as you lower leg to the bed.

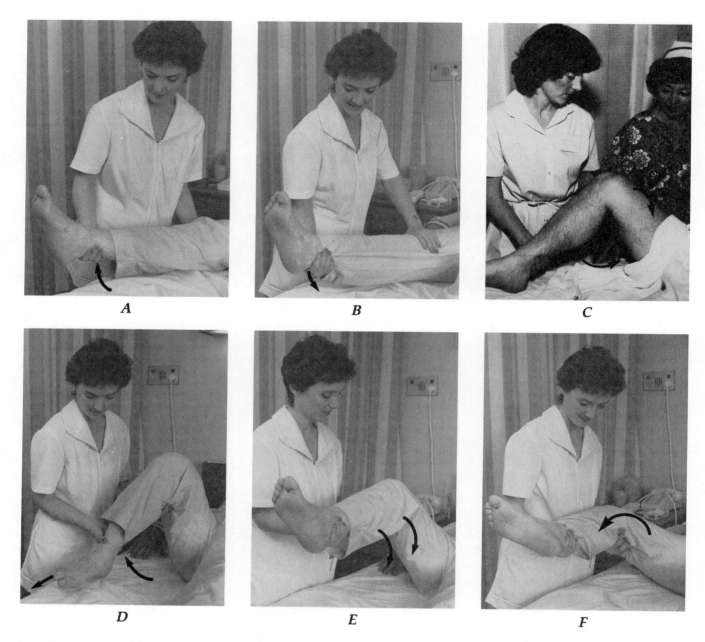

A

B

C

D

E

F

FIGURE 19–14. *ROM exercises for the hip.*
A. *Abduction. Supporting knee and ankle, move entire leg away from body center.*
B. *Adduction. Supporting knee and ankle, move entire leg back toward body center.*
C. *Flexion. Supporting knee and ankle, flex knee and hip.*
D. *Extension. Supporting ankle and thigh, straighten out knee as you lower leg to the bed.*
E. *Medial rotation. Supporting ankle and thigh, flex knee and bring leg toward midline.*
F. *Lateral rotation. Supporting ankle and thigh, rotate hip laterally, turning leg away from midline.*

ROM for Lower Extremities: Ankle, Foot and Toes

1. *Ankle: Dorsal Flexion.* Supporting ankle and toes, bring toes toward knee, figure 19–15A.
2. *Ankle: Plantar Flexion.* Supporting ankle and toes, bring toes toward foot of bed, figure 19–15B.
3. *Foot: Eversion.* Grasp foot and gently turn outward, figure 19–15C.

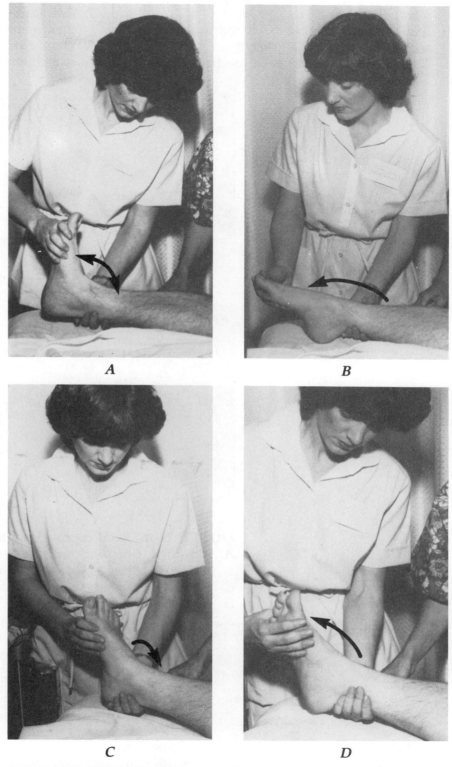

FIGURE 19–15. ROM exercises for the ankle.
A. Dorsiflexion. Supporting ankle, draw toes toward knee.
B. Plantar flexion. Supporting ankle, point foot away from knee.
C. Foot eversion. Grasp foot and gently turn outward.
D. Foot inversion. Grasp foot and gently turn inward.

4. *Foot: Inversion.* Grasp foot and gently turn inward, figure 19–15D.
5. *Toes: Abduction.* Move each toe away from second toe, figure 19–16A.
6. *Toes: Adduction.* Move each toe back toward second toe, figure 19–16B.
7. *Toes: Flexion.* Place fingers over toes, bending them gently, figure 19–16C.
8. *Toes: Extension.* Place fingers over toes, straightening them out gently, figure 19–16D.

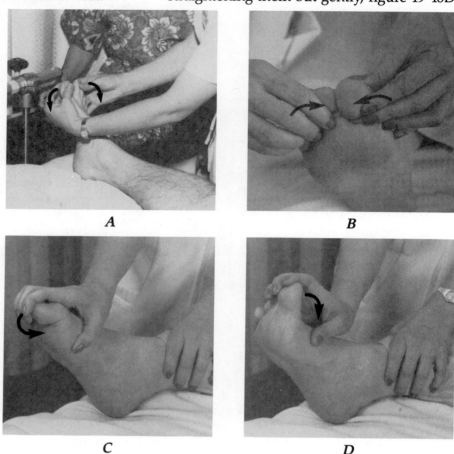

A   *B*

C   *D*

FIGURE 19–16. ROM exercises for the toes.
A. Abduction. Bring each toe away from the second toe.
B. Adduction. Bring each toe toward the second toe.
C. Flexion. Place fingers over toes, bending toes gently.
D. Extension. Place fingers over toes, and straighten out gently.

SENESCENT CHANGES

Changes in the aging musculoskeletal systems result in:

- poorer response to stimuli
- diminished ability to maintain posture and balance
- awkward walking patterns
- slowed recovery from sudden movements or changes in position
- difficulty and pain when moving, as a result of diseases of the bones such as osteoporosis and arthritis

Osteoporosis is a condition, most often seen in older women, that results in weakened, more easily broken bones, figure 19–17A. **Arthritis** is inflammation of the joints, figure 19–17B.

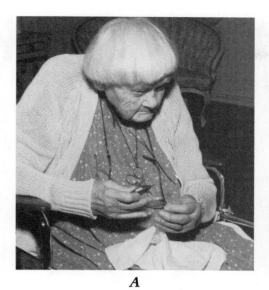
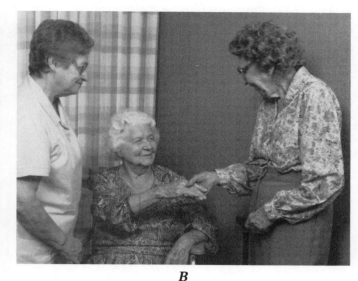

A B

FIGURE 19–17. Senescent changes.
A. Note the spinal curvature of this woman with osteoporosis.
B. There is a loss of height due to osteoarthritic changes in this woman's standing posture.

Conditions affecting other body systems also can make moving about difficult. For example, the shortness of breath experienced by a resident with respiratory disease, the rapid fatigue seen in the resident with multiple sclerosis or heart disease can make the effort of moving seem not worthwhile.

Foot problems that are common in the elderly, such as bunions, flat feet, corns, calluses, and thickened toenails, can make walking very painful. Attention must be paid to these problems so that corrective care can be given. Properly fitting shoes are a must. More attention is given to these later in the lesson.

REHABILITATION

Rehabilitation is the process of becoming as independent in self-care as possible. All residents will not be able to achieve the same levels of rehabilitation, but it is the job of all staff members to help each person reach the highest level of which he or she is capable. A positive attitude is necessary for successful rehabilitation.

Rehabilitation is assisting residents to assist themselves.

Part of the rehabilitation process includes efforts to help residents move about more freely with or without assistance. Remember, older persons frequently become residents just because their mobility is so limited that they cannot completely care for themselves.

Many residents will need assistance either from the staff or from mechanical aids to move about and carry out the activities of daily living, figures 19–18 and 19–19. Remember that safe, successful ambulation requires a good sense of balance and strength, both of which may be lacking in the elderly resident, figure 19–20. Be ready to assist if needed. Use proper body mechanics yourself and encourage them in the resident. For example, when you assist the resident from her

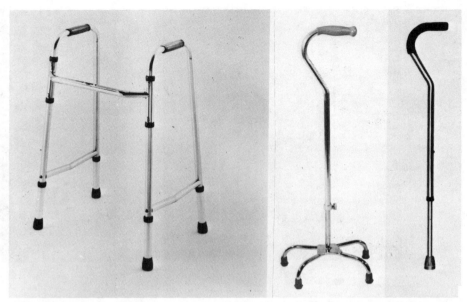

FIGURE 19–18. Walkers and canes add a measure of safety to ambulation.

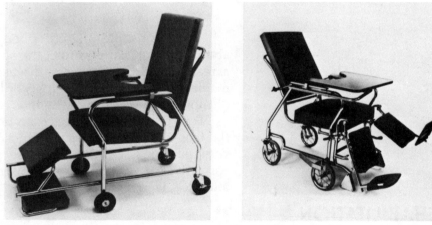

FIGURE 19–19. These geri chairs are designed to provide position changes while offering maximum support. Courtesy of Invacare Corporation.

- Loss of muscle tone and strength
- Increase in intramuscular fat
- Glycogen (energy) storage diminished
- Response to stimuli lessened
- Smooth muscle walls of organs lose strength
- Disks (pads) between vertebra thin
- Rib cage more rigid
- Bone more porous and brittle

FIGURE 19–20. Musculoskeletal system changes associated with aging.

bed to a wheelchair do the following things to improve her body mechanics and assist you in the process:

1. Ask the resident to put her arms around your neck with one hand on top of the other. Place your hands under her armpits, figure 19–21A, keeping your back straight but not rigid, and bending at the knees.
2. As you straighten your legs and stand up, you will be pulling the resident up with you. You will notice immediately that the resident's hand-clasp position distributes her weight over a larger area of your body. She is, in fact, helping to lift herself, figure 19–21B.
3. Pivot to the left or right (depending on where the chair is) bringing the resident to the edge of the wheelchair. When the back of her legs touch the chair, reverse step #1 and lower her slowly to a sitting position in the chair, figure 19–21C.

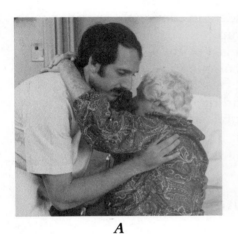 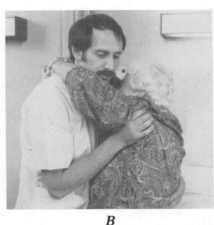 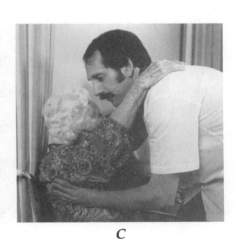

A   B   C

FIGURE 19–21. Assisting the resident to get out of bed.
A. Lower bed and face resident. Keep your back straight.
B. Supporting resident under the arms, straighten up, assisting resident to standing position.
C. Pivot resident and seat in wheel chair with locked wheels.

Ambulatory Aids____

Ambulatory aids that are frequently used include:

- canes
- wheelchairs
- walkers
- crutches

These aids must be kept in good repair and used properly. Check frequently for defects such as broken cane or walker tips, frayed straps, and worn parts. Report any defects before allowing the resident to use the aid. Each aid is fitted for a specific resident and is usually labeled for identification.

Safety belts (**gait belts**) are bands of fabric fastened around the resident's waist during ambulation. They provide a sense of security. Be sure the belt is not too tight for comfort but snug enough to offer support. Hold on to the belt at the back.

At all times, check body position (**alignment**). The principle of good alignment applies to the resident who is walking or being turned and repositioned in bed or as well as to one who is seated in a geri-chair or wheelchair.

▪▪▪ PROCEDURE: Assisting Resident Who Ambulates with a Cane or Walker ▪▪▪▪▪▪▪▪▪▪▪▪▪▪▪▪

1. Wash hands; secure correct aid (cane or walker).
2. Check aid for worn areas or loose parts.
3. Identify patient and explain what you plan to do.
4. Lower bed to lowest horizontal position; lower side rail.
5. Raise head of bed and assist resident to a sitting position.
6. Assist resident with robe and slippers or other clothing.
7. Have resident swing legs over edge of bed to allow feet to rest on floor.
8. If necessary, apply a transfer belt around resident's waist.
9. Place walker or cane within easy reach.
10. Assist resident to a standing position.
11. Have resident grasp walker or cane to maintain balance.
12. Walk beside resident, grasping transfer belt for additional support.
13. After ambulation, return resident to bed by reversing the procedure.
14. Leave resident in comfortable position with side rails up.
15. Wash hands.
16. Record completion of task on chart, including:
    a. Date and time
    b. Procedure: ambulation with cane (or walker)
    c. Resident reaction

▪▪▪ PROCEDURE: Assisting Resident to Get Out of Bed and Ambulate ▪▪▪▪▪▪▪▪▪▪▪▪▪▪▪▪

1. Wash hands.
2. Check orders for ambulatory aid.
3. Secure correct aid, such as cane or walker, and check for defects. (Report any defects and replace if necessary.)
4. Identify resident and explain what you plan to do.
5. Have slippers and robe or other clothing ready.
6. Place a chair at right angles beside the bed, facing the head of the bed; screen unit.
7. Explain how the resident can help.
8. Lower side rails.
9. Drape the resident with a bath blanket and fanfold top bedcovers to foot of bed.
10. Gradually elevate the head of the bed.
11. Allow resident to sit up in bed for a few minutes; note color, pulse, and response.
12. Help resident to dress or put on robe.
13. Lower bed to lowest position.
14. Put on resident's shoes or slippers.
15. Give instructions to swing the legs over the side of bed. (*Note:* If resident becomes dizzy, return resident to bed, secure side rails and report to nurse.)
16. Help resident to stand for a few minutes. (*Note:* If resident becomes weak or tired, pivot to the left or right, and seat resident in chair or return resident to bed.) Note that the direction that you pivot depends on what side of the bed you are on.
17. Transfer your arm behind the resident's waist and turn so you face in the same direction.
18. Assist resident to transfer weight to aid (cane or walker).
19. Follow, walking behind and to one side, until you are sure resident is stable, figure 19–22.
20. Observe frequently.
21. Report and record completion of task.

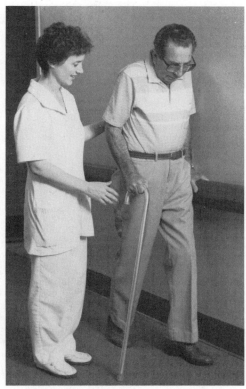

FIGURE 19–22. Be prepared to assist, but allow the resident to develop confidence.

PROCEDURE: Assisting Resident Who Is Out of Bed to Ambulate

1. Check that orders permit ambulation.
2. Wash hands.
3. Secure aids, such as canes or walkers, if needed.
4. Check aids for defects.
5. Identify resident and explain what you plan to do and how the resident can help.
6. Assist resident slowly to standing position.
7. Keep one hand under the resident's bent arm for support.
8. Adjust aids.
9. If gait belt is used, check for security.
10. Walk behind and to one side of resident during ambulation.
11. Encourage resident to use hand rails.
12. Watch for signs of fatigue. If resident becomes fatigued, assist to sit.
13. Talk to resident during procedure and be on guard for anything in the way that might contribute to a fall.
14. Washes hands.
15. Report and reocrd completion of task.

Assisting During a Fall_____

If a resident that you are assisting starts to fall, you must protect both the resident and yourself, figure 19–23.

PROCEDURE: Care of Falling Resident

1. Keep your back straight and base broad as you assist falling resident.
2. Ease resident to the floor, protecting head.
3. Stay with resident.

4. Call for help.
5. Do not move resident until he or she has been examined.

6. Assist in returning resident to bed.
7. Wash hands.
8. Report and record incident on resident's chart.

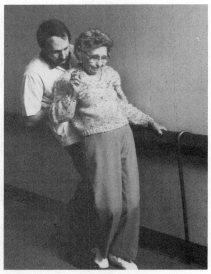

FIGURE 19–23. Protect the falling resident and yourself by going down with the resident.

TRANSFER ACTIVITIES

Size up the job.
Get assistance.
Use mechanical aids.
Use good body mechanics.

Good alignment must be maintained for the resident in bed just as it must during ambulation or when the resident is seated in a geri-chair or wheelchair. During position changes and transfer activities, both your own body mechanics and those of the resident need attention. Postural supports can help residents who have difficulty maintaining proper alignment. Check them frequently to be sure alignment is correct and that the support has not become too restrictive.

Remember to always size up the task first and employ mechanical aids or ask for help whenever it is needed. Aids such as the Hoyer lift must be in safe mechanical condition and you must be thoroughly familiar with their operation before using them. Lift sheets, which are half sheets (draw sheets) placed under the resident from shoulders to hips, can make moving a heavy or helpless resident easier.

POSITIONING

Residents in bed or seated can be positioned and supported in ways that promote mobility and improve body functioning. Positions should be changed at least every two hours, and more often if possible. Properly applied postural supports include:

- pillows
- rolled towels
- bath blankets

Remember, when making position changes to:

- use good body mechanics
- support the resident in proper alignment
- use postural supports as needed (check frequently)
- inspect the resident's skin for any signs of redness or breakdown and report findings
- check bed linen for moisture and change as needed
- talk with the resident
- offer fluids, unless **counterindicated** (not permitted)

There are five basic positions:

1. **horizontal recumbent**
2. **prone**
3. **semi-Fowler**
4. **Sims'**
5. **Knee-chest**

Each position with proper supports is illustrated in Lesson 20.

PROCEDURE: Assisting Resident into Chair or Wheelchair

1. Wash hands.
2. Identify the resident and explain what you plan to do and how the resident can help. Has robe and slippers nearby.
3. Screen the unit to provide privacy.
4. Cover the chair or wheelchair with a bath blanket.
5. Place chair or wheelchair near the head of bed facing the foot of the bed; lock the wheelchair and raise foot rests. (*Note:* Whenever possible, position chair or wheelchair so that it is secure against a wall or solid furniture to ensure that it will not slide backward.
6. Elevate head of bed and lock wheels. Lower the bed to lowest horizontal position.
7. Drape resident with a bath blanket and fanfold top bedclothes to foot of bed.
8. Assist the resident to a sitting position by placing your arm (the one closest to the head of the bed) around the resident's shoulders. Place your other arm under the resident's knees and pivot (rotate) the resident toward the side of the bed slowly and smoothly, figure 19–24A. Remain facing the resident to prevent a fall.
9. Assist the resident in putting on robe and slippers.
10. Still facing the resident, check to be sure he or she is ready to stand.
11. Have resident place feet on floor with both hands on your shoulders, figure 19–24B. Place your hands on either side of the resident's underarms. Raise resident slightly and help resident to slide off edge of bed gradually to a standing position, figure 19–24C.
12. Keeping hands in same position, help resident to turn slowly until the resident's back is toward the chair.
13. Have another person hold chair, or move to side of resident, placing one foot behind front leg of chair. Lower resident gradually to a sitting position in chair, bending at your hips and knees, figure 19–24D. Keep your back straight. Arrange robe or blanket smoothly. If the resident is in a wheelchair, place both feet on the foot rests and lock the wheelchair securely.
14. Cover resident with bath blanket. Stay with the resident until you are sure there are no adverse side effects. Report anything unusual to supervising nurse.
15. Leave signal cord and drinking water in reach. Make sure bed and unit are tidy.
16. Wash hands, record and report completion of task to your supervisor.

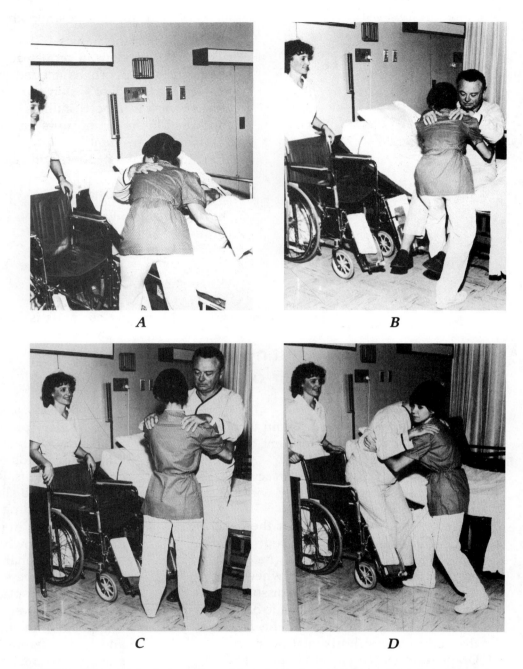

A

B

C

D

FIGURE 19–24. Assisting the resident from the bed to the wheelchair. Note that the assistant maintains a broad base of support.

PROCEDURE: Assisting Resident into Bed from Chair or Wheelchair

1. Wash hands. Identify resident and explain what you plan to do.
2. Screen the unit for privacy.
3. Check to see that the bed is in the lowest horizontal position and that the wheels are locked. Raise head of bed, fanfold top bedclothes to the foot, and raise opposite side rail.
4. Position chair or wheelchair at foot of the bed. Lock wheels of wheelchair and lift foot rests.

5. Have resident place feet flat on floor.
6. Remove bath blanket, fold, and return to bed-side stand.
7. Stand in front of the resident. Keep your back straight and your base of support broad.
8. Place your hands on either side of the resident's chest. Have resident place his or her hands on your shoulders. Assist resident to stand.
9. Pivot the resident toward the bed slowly and smoothly. Assist resident to sit on edge of bed.
10. Remove robe and slippers.
11. Place one arm around the resident's shoulders and one arm under the resident's legs and swing the resident's legs onto the bed.
12. Lower head of bed and assist resident to move into center of bed.
13. Draw top bedding over resident. Remake bed if necessary.
14. Make resident comfortable with signal cord within reach.
15. Wash hands.
16. Report completion of your assignment.

PROCEDURE: Lifting Resident Without Lift Sheet

1. Wash hands.
2. Ask someone to help.
3. Identify resident and explain what you plan to do and how resident can help.
4. Stand on one side of bed, with assisting person on opposite side of bed.
5. Elevate bed to working height and lock wheels.
6. Drop side rails.
7. Stand close to bed.
8. Face head of bed, knees flexed, feet separated, and back straight.
9. Slip one hand and arm under resident's head and shoulders.
10. Place other hand and arm under resident's buttocks.
11. Instruct assisting person to assume a similar position.
12. On the count of three, together with assisting person, lift resident, moving toward head of bed, figure 19–25.
13. Position resident comfortably.
14. Leave call bell at hand.
15. Lower bed and secure side rails.
16. Wash hands and report completion of task.

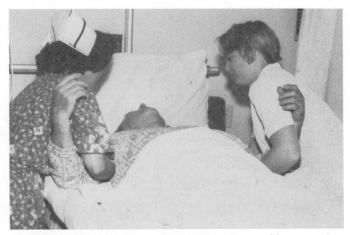

FIGURE 19–25. When the resident is unable to assist, two persons can support and move him to the head of the bed.

PROCEDURE: Lifting Resident Using Lift or Draw Sheet

1. Wash hands.
2. Ask someone to assist.
3. Identify resident and explain what you plan to do and how the resident can help.
4. Stand on one side of the bed, with assisting person on opposite side of bed.
5. Elevate bed to working height and lock bed wheels.
6. Drop side rails.
7. Roll lift sheet close to resident's body.
8. Grasp rolled sheet with hand closest to resident.
9. Face head of bed, flex knees, feet separated and back straight.
10. Place the other hand under the resident's head and neck.
11. Instruct assisting person to assume similar position.
12. On the count of three, together with assisting person, lift sheet and resident, moving toward head of bed, figure 19–26.
13. Position resident comfortably, leaving lift sheet in place.
14. Leave call bell at hand.
15. Lower bed and secure side rails.
16. Wash hands and report completion of task.

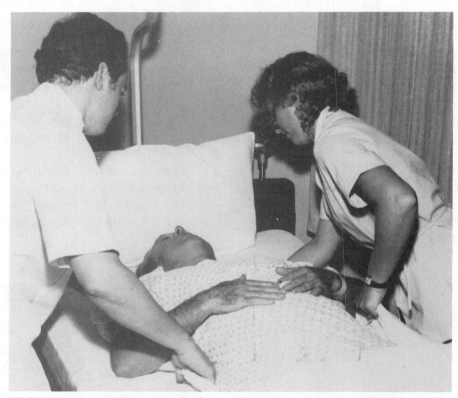

FIGURE 19–26. Keep your back straight. With draw sheet rolled close to the resident's body, lift and move smoothly to the head of the bed.

PROCEDURE: Turning Resident Toward You

1. Wash hands.
2. Identify resident and explain what is to be done.
3. Elevate bed to working height and lock wheels.
4. Cross resident's far leg over other leg.

5. Place hand nearest head of bed on resident's far shoulder. Place other hand on the resident's hip on the far side. Brace yourself against the side of the bed.
6. Roll resident toward you slowly, gently, and smoothly, figure 19–27. Help resident bring upper leg toward you and bend comfortably.
7. Raise side rail. Be sure that it is secure.
8. Go to the opposite side of the bed.
9. Place hands under resident's shoulders and hips. Pull toward the center of the bed. This helps the resident maintain the side-lying position.

10. Make sure resident's body is properly aligned and safely positioned.
11. If the resident is unable to move independently, position legs and support with pillows. If resident has an indwelling catheter, make sure the tubing is not between the legs in order to prevent undue stress on it.
12. A pillow may be placed behind the resident's back. Secure it by pushing the near side under the resident to form a roll.
13. Wash hands and report completion of task.

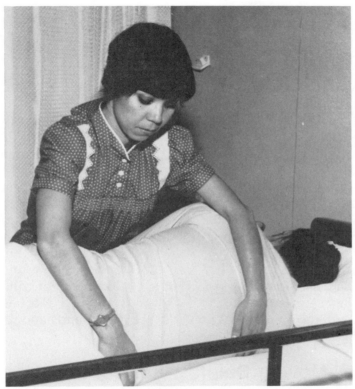

FIGURE 19–27. As the resident is turned toward you, slip your hands to the back for support.

◼◼◼ PROCEDURE: Turning Resident Away from You ◼◼◼◼◼◼◼◼◼◼◼◼◼◼◼◼◼◼◼◼◼◼◼◼◼◼◼

1. Wash hands.
2. Identify resident and explain what you plan to do.
3. Lock bed and raise side rail on the opposite side of the bed. Raise bed to working horizontal height.
4. Have resident bend knees, if able. Cross resident's arms on chest.

5. Place your arm nearest to head of bed under resident's head and shoulders, and your other hand and forearm under small of the back of resident. Bend your body at hips and knees, keeping back straight. Gently pull resident toward you.
6. Place your forearms under resident's hips and pull them toward you.

7. Move resident's ankles and knees toward you by placing one hand under the resident's shoulder and one under the knees.
8. Cross resident's near leg over other leg at ankles.
9. Roll resident away from yourself, slowly and carefully, by placing one hand under the resident's shoulder and one hand under the hips.
10. Place hands under resident's head and shoulders and move him or her back toward center of bed.
11. Move resident's hips toward center of bed.

12. Place pillow for support behind resident's back.
13. Make sure that resident's body is in good alignment. Support upper legs with pillow.
14. Raise side rail on near side of bed and return bed to lowest position. (*Note:* A turning sheet (folded large sheet or half sheet) may be placed under heavy or helpless resident to make moving easier. To be effective, the turning sheet must extend from above the shoulders to below the hips.)
15. Wash hands and report completion of task.

PROCEDURE: Assisting Resident to Move to Head of Bed

1. Wash hands.
2. Identify resident and explain what you are planning to do and how the resident may assist.
3. Lock wheels of bed. Raise bed to high horizontal position and lower side rail nearest to you.
4. Remove the pillow and place on chair.
5. Facing the head of the bed, position resident's foot that is farthest away from the edge of the bed approximately twelve inches in front of other foot.
6. Place your arm that is closest to head of bed under resident's head and shoulders and lock other arm with resident's arm.
7. Instruct resident to bend knees and press in with heels as you lift resident's shoulders.

Move resident smoothly toward head of bed on a count of three. An alternate method is as follows:
   a. Place pillow at the head of the bed on its edge.
   b. Have resident grasp head of bed with both hands.
   c. Slip your hands under resident's back and buttocks.
   d. Have resident press in with heels, and assist resident to raise hips and move to head of bed.
8. Replace pillow under resident's head and make resident comfortable.
9. Lower bed and raise side rail.
10. Wash hands and report completion of task.

PROCEDURE: Moving Helpless Resident to Head of Bed

1. Wash hands.
2. Ask a coworker to assist from opposite side of the bed.
3. Identify resident and explain what you plan to do. (*Note:* Do this even if the resident seems unresponsive.)
4. Lock wheels of bed. Raise bed to high horizontal position and lower side rails.
5. Remove pillow and place on chair, or place on its edge at the head of the bed, for safety.
6. Lift top bedclothes and expose draw sheet. Loosen both sides of draw sheet.
7. Roll edges close to sides of resident's body.

8. Facing head of bed, grasp the roll with the hand closest to the resident.
9. Position your feet twelve inches apart with the foot forward that is farthest from the bed edge.
10. Place free hand and arm under resident's neck and shoulders, cradling head from both sides.
11. Bend your hips slightly.
12. Together, with assisting person, on a count of three, raise resident's hips and back with the draw sheet while supporting head and

shoulders. Move resident smoothly toward the head of the bed.
13. Replace pillow under resident's bed.
14. Tighten and tuck in draw sheet.
15. Check resident for proper body alignment.
16. Adjust bedclothes.
17. Raise side rails and lower bed.

18. Wash hands and report and record completion of task. (All repositioning and turning of residents should be recorded on the resident's chart). *Note:* Do not leave the resident lying on his back for prolonged periods of time unless turning is contraindicated.

PROCEDURE: Log-Rolling Resident

1. Wash hands.
2. Ask another assistant to help you.
3. Identify resident and explain what you plan to do.
4. Screen unit.
5. Elevate bed to waist-high horizontal position and lock wheels. Side rails should be securely raised.
6. Lower side rail on side opposite that to which resident will be turned. Both assistants should be on the same side of the bed.
7. Move the resident as a unit toward you.
8. Place a pillow lengthwise between resident's legs. Fold resident's arms over his or her chest.
9. Raise side rail and check for security.

10. Go to the opposite side of bed and lower side rail.
11. At a specified signal, draw resident toward yourself and assisting person in a single movement, keeping resident's spine, head, and legs in straight position.
12. Place additional pillows behind resident to maintain alignment. A small pillow or folded blanket may be placed under resident's neck and head. Leave pillow between legs and position small pillows or folded towels to support resident's arms.
13. Check resident for comfort, alignment, and support. Leave call bell within reach.
14. Raise side rail and lower bed. Remove screen.
15. Wash hands and report completion of task.

To log-roll resident to opposite side, use the turning sheet previously placed under the resident and:

1. Remove positioning pillows.
2. Reaching over resident, grasp and roll turn sheet toward resident.
3. Position yourself beside resident so that you can keep resident's shoulders and hips straight.
4. Position assisting person so that he or she can keep resident's thighs and lower legs aligned.

If turning sheet is not in position, you should place your hands on far shoulder and hip of resident, while assisting person positions hands on resident's far thigh and lower leg.

PROCEDURE: Transferring Dependent Resident from Stretcher to Bed

1. Wash hands.
2. Identify resident and explain what you are going to do.
3. Lock wheels of bed and raise to horizontal position equal to height of stretcher. Fanfold top bedclothes to foot of bed.

4. Enlist help from two other assistants.
5. Position one assistant next to opposite side of bed and one at the foot of the stretcher. The third person will be positioned on opposite side of stretcher.

6. Position stretcher against bed. Lock wheels and lower side rails of stretcher.
7. Loosen stretcher restraints and bath blanket that covers resident.
8. Roll turning sheet close to resident's body.
9. Assistant on opposite side of bed uses both hands to grasp turning sheet. Lift and draw resident onto bed.
10. Assistant opposite stretcher places one arm for support under head and shoulders of resident and, with the other hand, grasps turning sheet to guide resident. (*Note:* All assistants must coordinate their activities and move together as signal is given.)
11. Move stretcher out of the way.
12. Using the turning sheet, position resident in bed.
13. Pull top bedclothes up over resident and slip bath blanket from underneath.
14. Raise side rails and check to be sure that they are secure.
15. Return bed to lowest horizontal position.
16. Wash hands.
17. Report and record transfer of resident.

PROCEDURE: Lifting Resident Using Mechanical Lift

1. Wash hands and assemble equipment. If possible, obtain assistance from coworker.
2. Check slings and straps for frayed areas or poorly closing clasps.
3. Take lift to resident's bedside and screen unit.
4. Identify resident and explain what you plan to do.
5. Place wheelchair or chair at right angles to foot of bed, facing head of bed.
6. Lock bed and roll resident toward you, figure 19–28A.
7. Position slings beneath body behind shoulders and buttocks. Be sure that sling is smooth, figure 19–28B.
8. Roll resident back onto sling and position properly, figure 19–28C.

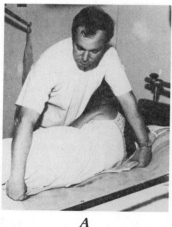
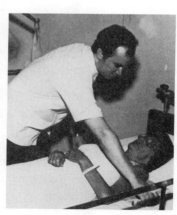
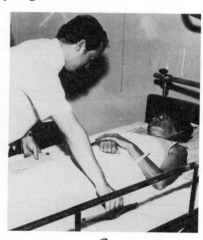

A   B   C

FIGURE 19–28. Lifting a person using a mechanical lift.
A. Roll the resident toward you and place the sling under her body.
B. Make sure top of sling is positioned under the shoulders.
C. Position sling smoothly under the hips.
D. Grasp the shifter handle in one hand and place the opposite hand on the steering handle on the mast for balance. Stay close to the bed.
E. Move the handle to your right to release the lock pin, then bring the handle toward you in a complete half circle. Lock legs in full open position.
F. Hook straps from inside to out.
G. Lift resident free of bed.
H. Swing resident into wheelchair.

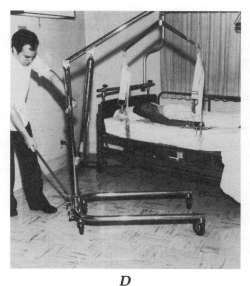

D

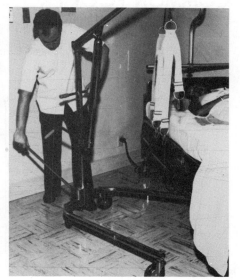

E

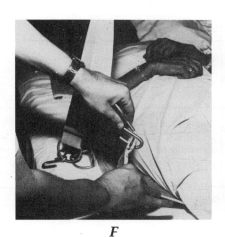

F

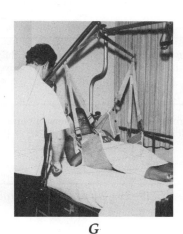

G

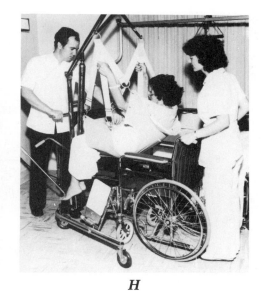

H

FIGURE 19–28 (continued)

9. Attach suspension straps to sling. Check fasteners for security.
10. Position lift frame over bed with base legs in maximum open position and lock, figure 19–28D and E.
11. Elevate head of the bed and bring resident to semi-sitting position.
12. Attach suspension straps to frame. Position resident's arms inside straps, figure 19–28F.
13. Secure restraint straps, if needed.
14. Talking to resident, slowly lift him or her free of the bed, figure 19–28G.
15. Guide lift away from the bed.
16. Position resident close to chair or wheelchair (with wheels locked).
17. Slowly lower resident into chair or wheelchair, figure 19–28H. Pay particular attention to the position of resident's feet.
18. Unhook suspension straps and remove lift.
19. If resident is to remain in chair or wheelchair for a period of time, make comfortable and secure before leaving.
20. Wash hands.
21. Record procedure on resident's chart.

COMMON FOOT PROBLEMS ▨▨▨▨▨▨▨▨▨▨▨▨▨▨▨▨▨▨▨▨▨▨▨▨▨▨

There are some relatively common foot problems you will encounter while working with the elderly resident. These problems are detailed in figure 19–29.

Condition	Disease Process	Treatment	Special Care
Thickened toenails	Nails become thickened and may become ingrown or curved.	Trimmed straight across; severe cases treated by podiatrist.	Soak prior to cutting; cut straight across; wisps of cotton placed under nail encourage proper growth.
Flatfoot (pes planus)	Foot arches flatten as muscles decrease in size (atrophy).	Surgery may be used on occasion; corrective shoes.	Make sure that shoes are on when ambulating; check that shoes are in good repair; report any pain.
Bunions (hallux valgus)	Joints become misaligned, inflamed, and tender as bony overgrowth develops.	Specially fitted shoes or protective pads over affected joints; surgery to remove excess bone.	Same as above.
Hammertoes (digiti flexis)	Toes become tightly flexed; corns form on top surface of toes.	Surgery and/or specially fitted shoes.	Same as above.
Corns (heloma) Calluses (tyloma)	Hardened tissues form in areas of pressure and friction.	Removal by a podiatrist; pads or soft rings to reduce pressure.	Apply pads or rings to areas before putting on shoes; report condition to nurse.

FIGURE 19–29. Common foot problems.

SPECIAL ORTHOPEDIC CARE ▨▨▨▨▨▨▨▨▨▨▨▨▨▨▨▨▨▨▨▨▨▨▨▨

Orthopedic care is the care given to residents who are suffering from disorders and deformities of the locomotor apparatus including:

- muscle disease
- bone disease
- joint disease (see figure 19–30)

SPECIAL PROBLEMS ▨▨▨▨▨▨▨▨▨▨▨▨▨▨▨▨▨▨▨▨▨▨▨▨▨▨▨▨▨

Fractures_____

A fracture is a break or loss of continuity of a bone, figure 19–31. Sometimes the bone is broken completely through (*complete*) and sometimes the bone is only partially broken (*incomplete*). Greenstick fractures are seen mostly in young children. In a greenstick fracture the bone doesn't break completely through.

Condition	Disease Process	Treatment	Special Care
Osteoarthritis	Breakdown (degeneration) of joints. Weight-bearing joints such as ankles, knees, and hips are most commmonly involved. Movement is painful and condition is progressive.	Medication to relieve pain; physiotherapy to maintain mobility; light massage and heat; ambulatory aids to reduce pressure in joints; weight reduction; surgery in selected cases.	Give positive, emotional support; carry out heat treatments, massage, and ROM exercises, as ordered.
Osteoporosis	Defective bone formation and maintenance. Bones become brittle and are easily broken. Complications: fractures, kidney stones, and loss of height and posture. More common in females than males.	Keep resident as active as is possible; diet adequate in protein and vitamins C and D, and calcium; maintain adequate fluid intake; hormone therapy.	Encourage food and fluid intake. Assist in exercise. Report pain; apply support as needed. Emotional support must not be overlooked.
Rheumatoid Arthritis	Inflammation of joint lining (synovium). Joint changes cause painful muscle spasm, flexion and deformities. Signs and symptoms may temporarily disappear (remission). Flareups may be related to emotional stress.	Drugs to reduce pain and inflammation; heat treatments for comfort; exercise when inflammation subsides; surgery in selected cases.	Provide emotional support. Make self-help devices such as long shoe horns and grab bars available. Carry out heat treatments and ROM exercises, as ordered.

FIGURE 19–30. Common geriatric orthopedic problems.

Types of fractures commonly seen in the elderly are:

- simple fracture
- compound fracture
- comminuted fracture
- compression fracture
- spiral fracture

Simple Fracture. Bones do not protrude through the skin, and although broken they remain in good position.

Compound Fracture. Fragments of broken bone protrude through skin.

Comminuted Fracture. Bones are broken into many pieces.

Compression Fracture. The internal spongy bone is crushed without necessarily making a break in the hard bone outer covering. This type of fracture occurs most often in the vertebral bodies.

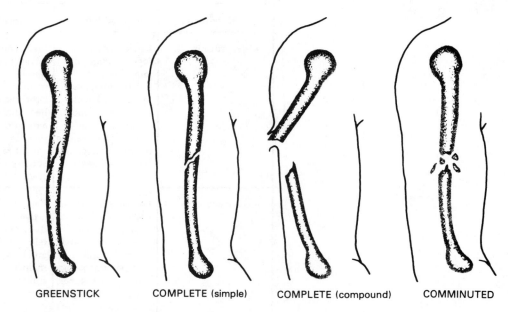

GREENSTICK   COMPLETE (simple)   COMPLETE (compound)   COMMINUTED

FIGURE 19–31. Types of fractures.

Spiral Fracture. The bone is broken in a twisted manner.

Fractures can be treated by **traction**, which pulls the broken ends of the bones slightly apart and maintains the position until healing occurs, or by repositioning the broken ends and then using a cast or splint to hold the position until healed, figure 19–32.

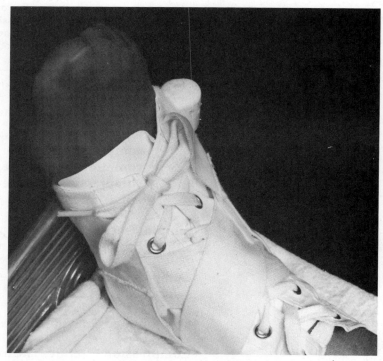

FIGURE 19–32. Fracture areas may be supported with traction, casts, or braces.

POST-FRACTURE CARE

If surgery is needed to repair the fracture, the resident will be transferred to an acute hospital for the procedure called open reduction. Upon return to the facility, rehabilitative support will be needed. During the rehabilitation process, the resident will need a great deal of emotional support and encouragement. Special exercises will be prescribed for the injured area and ROM exercises should be performed on the non-affected joints.

Care of Resident with Cast

A simple fracture may need only a cast or splint to support the area until healing is complete. If the cast is applied in the facility, you will have to give special care to the resident. Special precautions are:

- Allow wet cast to air-dry (figure 19–33).
- Do not put pressure on wet cast. Any pressure applied to the cast can leave permanent indentations that can press against resident's skin.
- Keep the part in the cast elevated and uncovered until dry.
- Frequently check area for signs of circulatory impairment: blueness (cyanosis) in color, coldness to touch, or swelling (edema), odor, drainage, and complaints of pain or tingling in the area. Report at once.
- Closely observe skin areas around cast edges for signs of irritation.

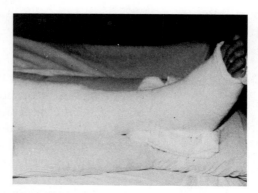

FIGURE 19–33. Keep cast uncovered and support in good alignment until completely dry.

Continue to check around cast area for circulation and areas of irritation. An arm cast will need to be supported with a sling. Residents with a leg cast may need a wheelchair or crutches for support.

PROCEDURE: Care of Resident in Cast

1. Provide over-bed trapeze, if available.
2. Handle the cast material by supporting the area with the palms of the hands.
3. Maintain good alignment with pillows under the cast.
4. Keep the cast uncovered.
5. Check the area for circulation by noting warmth, color and pulse.
6. Report coldness, color change or numbness immediately.

7. Observe for drainage and odors.
8. Turn resident frequently to permit air to circulate.

9. Pad rough edges to prevent irritation.
10. Report and record observations.

Traction_____

When caring for a resident in traction, you should:

- review the traction lines with your supervisor until you are sure you know the purpose of each, figure 19–34.
- be careful not to disturb the weights or permit them to swing, drop, or rest on any surface.
- keep the resident in good alignment and see that his or her body is properly acting as countertraction (for example, resident's feet pressed against the foot of the bed will decrease the amount of countertraction).
- check under belts for areas of pressure or irritation.
- make sure that straps of halters and belts are smooth, straight, and properly secured.
- carry out ROM exercises of unaffected parts.

 ## PROCEDURE: Care of Resident in Traction ▪▪▪▪▪▪▪▪▪▪▪▪▪▪▪▪▪▪▪▪▪▪▪▪▪▪▪▪▪▪▪▪▪▪▪

1. Examine traction lines to find the primary traction lines.
2. Locate support lines.
3. Do not disturb weights or permit them to swing.

4. Check under belts for areas of pressure or irritation.
5. Make sure that straps, belts, or halters are smooth, straight, and properly secured.

Amputation_____

Amputation is the removal of a limb or other body part, such as a breast. Amputations are common in residents with long-standing diabetes mellitus and disease of the blood vessels that serve the outer body areas (peripheral vascular disease). The portion of the extremity remaining after the amputation is called the **stump**. The stump should be carefully inspected for bleeding, infection, or signs of irritation. The artificial limb or part is called a **prosthesis**. It will be designed and fitted for each amputee. Make sure that you know how to apply the prosthesis and that it fits properly.

Amputees need a great deal of emotional support as they learn to deal with their new prosthesis. A positive, realistic attitude on the part of the staff can make the adjustment easier. Some residents may complain of pain in the part that has been amputated. This is called **phantom pain**. Be sure to report complaints of phantom pain to the nurse.

OTHER ORTHOPEDIC CONDITIONS ▪▪▪▪▪▪▪▪▪▪▪▪▪▪▪▪▪▪▪▪▪▪▪▪▪▪

Osteoporosis_____

Osteoporosis is an orthopedic disease that causes the bones to become brittle and porous as minerals are lost. Brittle bones fracture easily and deformities occur as softened bone collapses. Typically, compression fractures of the vertebral bodies are found, leading to **kyphosis** (flexing of vertebral column), shortened stature, and fractures.

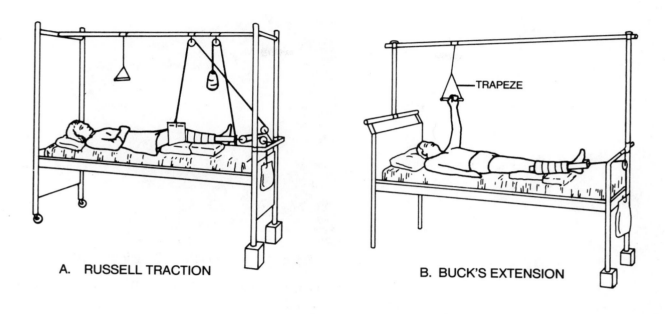

A. RUSSELL TRACTION   B. BUCK'S EXTENSION

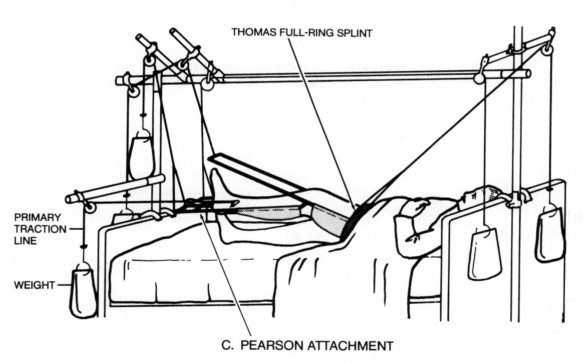

C. PEARSON ATTACHMENT

FIGURE 19–34. Types of traction: A, Russell; B, Buck's extension; C, Pearson's attachment.

Calcium leaves the bone via the bloodstream and is excreted from the body in the urine and feces. The accumulation of calcium in the urine makes kidney stones more probable. Residents with advanced osteoporosis experience extreme pain when they attempt weight bearing and are in constant danger of new fractures, figure 19–35.

Osteoporosis occurs in postmenopausal women, due to hormone deficiencies. It is found in between 30 and 80 percent of women over age 65. However, in both men and women, it may also be due to

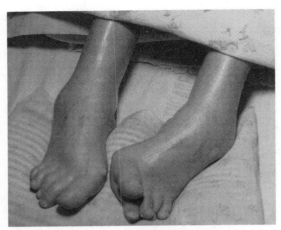

FIGURE 19–35. Note the deformed feet and overlapping toes that make walking impossible.

inactivity and is then referred to as **senile osteoporosis**. Senile osteoporosis is usually diagnosed when in the advanced stage and is associated with pain or stress fractures.

Signs and Symptoms. Some residents suffering from osteoporosis complain of aching pains, particularly in the back. Frontal or cervical headaches are common. These residents exhibit fear and insecurity in walking. Psychologically, they may appear depressed, irritable, and pessimistic. They are easily fatigued.

Treatment. The condition is treated by keeping the resident active. Adequate support must be provided in the form of corsets or braces. Exercises are prescribed to improve the musculature. Periods of weight bearing are increased by walking or standing between parallel bars. Progressive resistive exercises are also used.

Arthritis

The term *arthritis* means joint inflammation. The two most common types are:

- rheumatoid arthritis
- osteoarthritis

Rheumatoid Arthritis

Rheumatoid arthritis usually first develops in persons between age 35 and 45. Its effects are carried into the senior years, resulting in deformity and permanent damage. Onset may also be late, not starting until the eighth or ninth decade. It affects women two to three times as often as men. The cause of rheumatoid arthritis is unknown.

Signs and Symptoms. The symptoms of rheumatoid arthritis include pain, heat and swelling in the joints and early morning stiffness. These symptoms come and go.

Treatment. Early treatment gives the best results. Drugs are used during the active disease periods to relieve inflammation and pain. Dry or moist heat gives comfort to many residents. Warm baths (104°F) or paraffin baths (126° to 130°F) are sometimes ordered. Periods of active disease are alternated with periods when the disease is in remission.

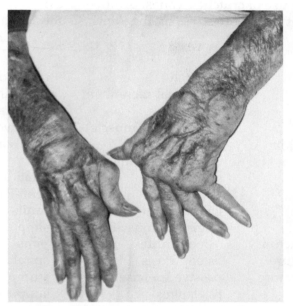

FIGURE 19–36. *Rheumatoid arthritis has severely damaged the finger joints.*

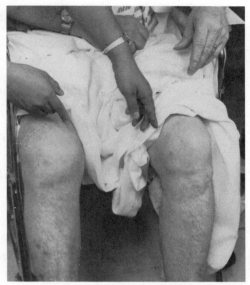

FIGURE 19–37. *Note the swelling of the right knee. The inflammation is due to osteoarthritis.*

After the symptoms of pain, fatigue, and weakness subside, exercises may be started. During the active phase it is important to continue ROM exercises of all unaffected joints. Deformities of the hips can be prevented by making sure that the resident spends part of each day lying on the abdomen.

A great deal of emotional support is required by the resident with rheumatoid arthritis. Self-help devices such as long shoehorns, grab bars, elastic shoelaces, and long pick-up forceps can be of assistance as the resident carries out the activities of daily living.

Osteoarthritis

The other common form of arthritis is **osteoarthritis**, figure 19–37. All joints undergo some degree of degeneration with age, and most residents over 60 years of age have some symptoms. These residents are often overweight, and the joints affected are those that receive the greatest trauma and strain, such as the knees and lower back.

Each time the affected joint is moved, the friction against the joint surface results in further destruction, until the bone is damaged.

Symptoms. Symptoms may be minimal. Pain in the joints is aggravated by changes in temperature and humidity. Affected joints are tender and swollen. Pain may be **referred**. For example, pain in the hips may be felt in the groin. Motion in affected joints is limited.

Treatment. The treatment of osteoarthritis includes medication to relieve pain and reduce inflammation if it is present, physiotherapy, light massage, and heat. At all times the staff must have a confident, positive, supporting attitude.

Physiotherapy must be carried on indefinitely, with ROM exercises performed several times daily. Special exercises to build up muscular strength may be prescribed. Good posture in and out of bed should be encouraged. Mechanical stress on joint surfaces can be minimized by the use of crutches, canes, orthopedic collars, and arch supports. Weight puts more stress on the joints, so obesity should be reduced.

VOCABULARY

abduction	gait belt	referred pain
active exercise	horizontal recumbent	rehabilitation
adduction	position	renal calculi
alignment	insertion (of muscle)	resistive exercise
amphiarthrotic joint	inversion	rheumatoid arthritis
amputation	involuntary muscle	ribs
arthritis	joint	rotation
articulation	kyphosis	semi-Fowler's position
belly (of muscle)	ligament	senile osteoporosis
cast	origin (of muscle)	simple fracture
comminuted fracture	osteoarthritis	Sims' position
compound fracture	osteoporosis	spiral fracture
compression fracture	passive exercise	stump
contracture	phalanges	suppination
diarthrotic joint	phantom pain	synarthrotic joint
eversion	pronation	tendons
extension	prone position	traction
femur	prosthesis	voluntary muscle
flexion	range of motion	
fracture	(ROM) exercises	

SUGGESTED ACTIVITIES

1. Examine a skeleton or diagram to become familiar with the major bones.

2. Practice with a partner the movements possible at different joints.

3. Working in pairs, practice the basic techniques of proper body mechanics.

4. Under supervision, position residents and give care to residents who need ambulatory assistance.

REVIEW

A. Brief Answer/Fill in the Blanks

1. The musculoskeletal system is composed of the bones, muscles, _____, _____, and _____.

2. Skeletal muscles have three parts. They are the origin, _____, and _____.

3. Decreasing the angle between two bones is called_____.

4. Three dangers of immobility include _____, _____ and _____.

5. ROM exercises take joints through all their possible _____.

6. The older person has more _____ recovering once a fall is started.

7. Common foot problems experienced by the elderly include _____, _____, _____, hammertoes and thickened, curved toenails.

8. Rehabilitation is the process of helping residents become as _____ as possible in caring for themselves.

9. Another word used to describe proper body position is proper _____.

10. An artificial limb or part is called a _____.

B. Identification. Write the names of bones indicated by number on the diagram below.

1.	5.	9.
2.	6.	10.
3.	7.	11.
4.	8.	12.

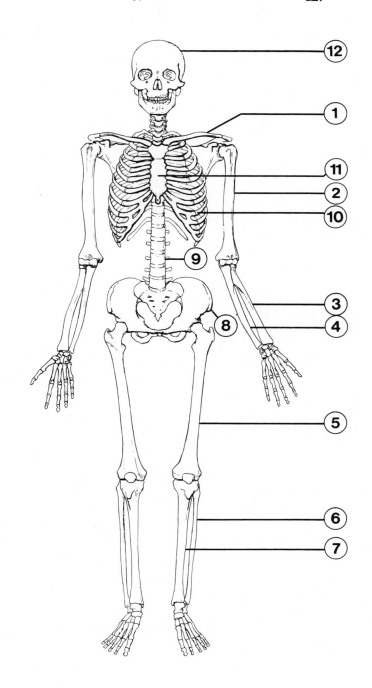

C. **Latin to English.** Give the common name for each of the following bones:

1. femur _____   3. tibia _____   5. clavical _____

2. scapula _____   4. sternum _____   6. carpal _____

CLINICAL SITUATION

Mr. Murphy has just been admitted to the facility. He is 6 feet 4 inches tall, with a heavy frame. He is 78 years old and two months post-stroke, and he is unable to use his left arm or leg. You are assigned to his care and must move him up in bed. Describe your actions, using the principles of good body mechanics.

Answer: _____

_____

_____

LESSON 20 The Integumentary System

OBJECTIVES

After studying this lesson, you should be able to:

- Name the parts and function of the integumentary system.
- Recognize changes in the integument as they relate to the aging process.
- Describe procedures related to skin care.
- Give hand, foot, and hair care.
- Define and spell all the vocabulary words and terms.

The **integumentary system** consists of the skin, the oil and sweat glands of the skin and hair, the nails, and the environmental sense organs.

The outermost layers of the skin makeup the **epidermis**, figure 20–1. Underneath the epidermis is the **dermis**, and underneath the dermis is the **subcutaneous tissue** that attaches the skin to the muscles.

EPIDERMIS

The skin is continuously being worn off and renewed.

The epidermis consists of dead outer cells that are constantly being shed as new cells move upward from the dermis. There are no blood vessels in the epidermis, so injury to this level does not produce bleeding. Nerve endings do reach into this outer covering. The nerves form sense organs that keep us in contact with changes in the environment. Nerve endings called **receptors** receive information about temperature; other receptors receive information about pressure or pain.

DERMIS

The dermis contains many blood vessels and nerve fibers and two kinds of glands:

- **sweat glands**
- **oil glands**

Sweat Glands

The sweat glands produce perspiration. This perspiration reaches the skin surface through tubes or ducts that end in openings called **pores**. Heat from deep within the body is brought to the skin by blood vessels. This heat is transferred to the perspiration. The perspiration reaches the skin surface through the pores and is lost, along with

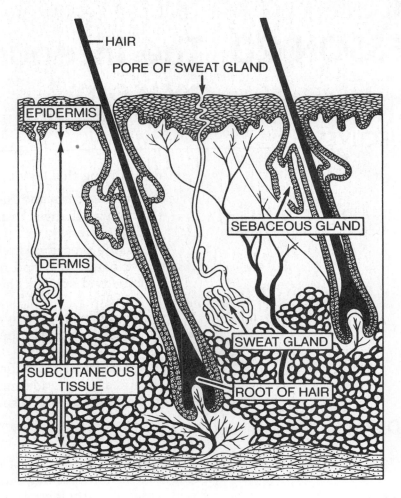

FIGURE 20–1. The skin.

the heat, to the atmosphere. The heat of the body can be controlled by enlarging (**dilating**) or narrowing (**constricting**) blood vessels in the skin.

Oil Glands

Oil glands lubricate the hairs that are found in the skin. Hair is located over almost all the body surfaces except for the palms of the hands and the soles of the feet. Oil glands help keep the hairs flexible.

Skin Functions. The functions of the skin include:

- protection — forms a continuous membraneous covering and regulates body temperature
- storage — stores fat and vitamins
- eliminations — water and salts are lost in perspiration
- sensory perceptions — nerve endings keep us aware of environmental changes

THE AGING SKIN

As the individual ages, there are changes in the integumentary system (figure 20–2) just as there are changes in all the other parts of the body. These changes include:

1. Sweat glands decrease in activity.
2. Loss of elasticity and fatty tissue causes wrinkling. The eyelids tend to drop and the skin is drier as oil glands slow down their secretions.
3. Areas of pigmentation seem more pronounced, and the skin takes on a more sallow or yellowish, less pink coloration. Skin tabs and moles are more common.
4. The hair loses its color, becoming first gray and then white. Less oil causes the hair to become duller and lifeless. The amount of hair, especially in men, diminishes.
5. Nails on both fingers and toes thicken, becoming more brittle and often splitting.

- Skin glands produce less oil.
- Skin tabs, moles, and warts are present.
- There is loss of elasticity and fat.
- Skin is drier, scaly and thin.
- Fingernails and toenails thicken.
- Skin circulation is poorer.
- Dimished hair loses color.
- Sweat glands diminish activity.

A

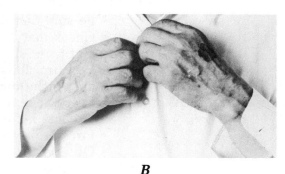

B

FIGURE 20–2. Aging changes in the skin.

GENERAL CARE OF THE INTEGUMENT

Injuries of the elderly skin are slower to heal. Too frequent bathing, especially with soaps, can rob the skin of what little lubrication is still present. The skin of the older person receives less blood flow and, hence, less nutrition than that of younger persons.

Care must always be taken to handle the elderly skin very gently. This is true when bathing, dressing, or turning a resident. The elderly skin is very sensitive and must be protected.

A complete bath two or three times a week is usually sufficient to maintain cleanliness. Too frequent bathing can lead to dryness and itching, referred to as "bath itch." Many facilities require a daily partial bath, with particular attention to incontinent residents.

Mild lotions can be applied to dry, roughened areas. This is especially important for elbows, hands, and feet. Skin areas that touch, such as the area between the legs, under the arms and breasts, under the scrotum, and between the buttocks, should be sponged, patted dry and lightly dusted with talcum. Care should be taken not to use too much powder, since it may cake and cause irritation.

Do not allow perspiration, urine, or feces to remain on sensitive skin surfaces. They are highly irritating if left in contact and the skin surfaces quickly break down.

BATHING RESIDENTS

Partial baths, bed baths, and tub or shower baths are all ways to meet resident cleanliness needs, but the most stimulating form of bathing for residents is a whirlpool bath that is given in a **Century tub**. There are three reasons why the whirlpool bath is so beneficial for the resident:

1. The temperature of the water can be regulated to an optimum 97°F.
2. The movement of the water stimulates circulation.
3. Being surrounded by warm circulating water is both relaxing and invigorating.

Safety Factors

The following general safety factors must be considered when giving a tub or shower bath:

Bathing can be dangerous and fatiguing. Obey safety rules.

- Be sure that there is adequate help.
- Check that all safety aids such as hand rails, shower seats, and hydraulic lifts are in proper working order.
- Wipe up all water spilled on the floor immediately so that no one, including yourself, will slip and fall.
- Keep the temperature of the room comfortable and see that the area is free of drafts.
- Provide privacy during the bathing process.
- Observe the skin for any changes or irregularities. Be careful not to disturb or injure any warts or moles that are present. Be sure to report anything unusual that you notice.
- Protect resident from fatigue by making adequate provisions for transporting residents to and from the tub room and carrying out the bathing procedure as efficiently as possible.

PROCEDURE: Giving a Bed Bath

1. Wash hands and assemble the following equipment:
   a. Bed linen
   b. Bath blanket
   c. Laundry bag or hamper
   d. Bath basin
   e. Bath thermometer
   f. Soap and soap dish

g. Washcloth

h. Face towel

i. Bath towel

j. Hospital gown or the resident's night clothes

k. Alcohol or lotion, powder

l. Equipment for oral hygiene

m. Nail brush and emery board

n. Brush and comb

o. Bedpan or urinal and cover

2. Identify resident and explain what you plan to do and how the resident can help you.

3. Make sure that any windows and door are closed to prevent chilling the resident.

4. Screen unit.

5. Put towel and linen on chair in order of use. Place laundry hamper so that it is convenient.

6. Offer bedpan or urinal. Empty and clean before proceeding with bath. Wash hands.

7. Lower the back of bed and siderails if permitted.

8. Loosen top bedclothes. Remove and fold blanket and spread. Place bath blanket over top sheet and remove sheet by sliding it out from under the bath blanket.

9. Leave one pillow under resident's head. Place other pillow on chair.

10. Remove resident's nightwear and place in laundry hamper. If resident is receiving an intravenous (IV) infusion remove nightwear as follows:

a. Loosen gown from neck.

b. Slip free arm from gown.

c. Make sure that resident is covered by bath blanket.

d. Slip gown away from body toward arm with IV line in place.

e. Gather gown at arm and slip downward over arm and line, being careful not to disturb line.

f. Gather material of gown in one hand so that there is no pull or pressure on line and slowly draw gown over tip of fingers.

g. With free hand, lift IV line free of standard and slip gown over IV bottle.

11. Fill bath basin two thirds full with water at 105°F.

12. Assist resident to move to the side of the bed nearest you.

13. Fold face towel over upper edge of bath blanket to keep blanket dry.

14. Form a mitten by holding washcloth around hand, figure 20–3. Wet washcloth; wash eyes, using separate corners of cloth for each eye, figure 20–4. Do not use soap near eyes.

15. Rinse washcloth and apply soap if resident desires. Squeeze out excess water.

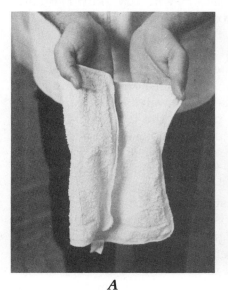 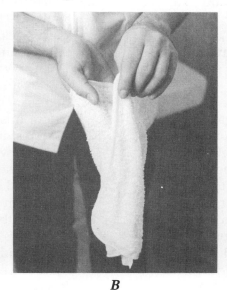 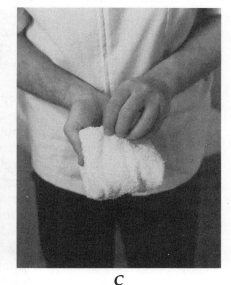

A   *B*   *C*

FIGURE 20–3. *Making a bath mitt.*

A. Wrap wash cloth around one hand.

B. Bring free and over palm.

C. Grasp folded end and tuck into palm.

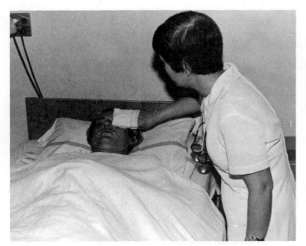

FIGURE 20–4. Using a clean washcloth, wash each eye from nose outward. Rinse cloth after washing each eye. (From Brooks, *The Nurse Assistant*, copyright 1978 by Delmar Publishers Inc.)

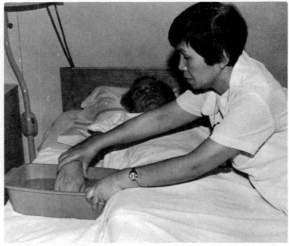

FIGURE 20–5. Allow resident to soak each hand in warm water for a few minutes. (From Brooks, *The Nurse Assistant*, copyright 1978 by Delmar Publishers Inc.)

16. Wash and rinse resident's face, ears, and neck. Use towel to dry.
17. Expose resident's far arm. Protect bed with bath towel placed underneath arm. Wash, rinse, and dry arm and hand. Be sure **axilla** (armpit) is clean and dry. Apply deodorant and powder if resident requests them or needs them. Repeat for other arm.
18. If necessary, care for hand and nails as follows:
    a. Wash each hand carefully, figure 20–5. Rinse and dry. Push back cuticle (base of fingernails) gently with towel while wiping the fingers.
    b. Clean under nails and shape with emery board. Be careful not to file nails too close. If resident is diabetic, do not cut nails, but inform the nurse if attention is needed.
19. Put bath towel over resident's chest, and then fold blanket to waist. Under towel, wash, rinse, and dry chest. Rinse and dry folds under breasts of female resident carefully to avoid irritating skin. Powder lightly if necessary. Do not allow powder to cake.
20. Fold bath blanket down to pubic area. Wash, rinse, and dry abdomen. Unfold bath blanket and cover abdomen and chest. Slide towel out from under bath blanket.
21. Ask resident to flex knee if possible. Fold bath blanket up to expose thigh, leg, and foot. Protect bed with bath towel, and put bath

basin on towel. Place resident's foot in basin, figure 20–6. Wash and rinse leg and foot. When moving leg, support leg properly.
22. Lift leg and move basin to other side of bed. Dry leg and foot. Dry well between toes.
23. Repeat for other leg and foot. Take basin from bed before drying leg and foot.
24. Care for toenails as necessary. Apply lotion to feet of resident with dry skin. File nails straight across. Do not round edges. Do not push back the cuticle, because it is easily injured and infected.
25. Change water and check for correct temperature with bath thermometer. It may be necessary to change water, if it becomes cold, before this point in the resident's bath.
26. Help resident to turn on side away from you and to move toward center of bed. Place towel lengthwise next to resident's back. Wash, rinse, and dry neck, back, and buttocks. Use long, firm strokes when washing back.
27. A back rub is usually given at this time. (See procedure given later in this lesson.)
28. Help resident to turn on back.
29. Place towel under buttocks and upper legs. Place washcloth, soap, basin, and bath towel within convenient reach of resident. Instruct resident to wash genitalia, assisting if necessary. (You must assume responsibility for this procedure if resident has difficulty. Many times residents are reluctant to

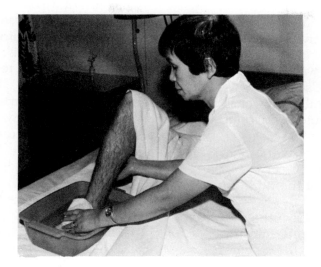

FIGURE 20-6. *If possible, soak each foot as you wash resident's leg.* (From Brooks, *The Nurse Assistant*, copyright 1978 by Delmar Publishers Inc.)

acknowledge the need for help.) When assisting female resident, always wash from front to back, drying carefully. When assisting male resident, carefully wash and dry penis, scrotum, and groin area. (See procedures given later in this lesson.)

30. Carry out ROM exercises as ordered. (See Lesson 19 for proper procedure.)

31. Cover pillow with towel and comb or brush hair. Oral hygiene is usually given at this time. (See procedures given later in this lesson.)

32. Place used towels and washcloth in hamper.

33. Provide clean gown. If resident has an IV, then put on gown as follows:
    a. Gather sleeve on IV side in one hand.
    b. Lift IV bottle free of standard, maintaining height.
    c. Slip bottle through sleeve from inside and rehang.
    d. Guide the gown along the IV tubing to bed.
    e. Slip gown over hand. Do this very carefully so as not to disturb infusion site.
    f. Position gown on infusion arm, and then insert opposite arm.

34. Clean and replace equipment, according to facility policy.

35. Put clean washcloth and towels in bedside stand or hang, according to facility policy.

36. Change bed linen, following occupied bed procedure. Put soiled linen in laundry hamper.

37. Leave resident in comfortable position. Raise side rails. Place signal cord or call bell and water within reach of resident. Replace furniture, and leave unit orderly. Wash hands. Turn out ceiling light, if used.

38. Report completion of tasks and any important observations to the nurse.

▪▪▪ PROCEDURE: Assisting With Tub Bath or Shower ▪▪▪▪▪▪▪▪▪▪▪▪▪▪▪▪▪▪▪▪▪▪▪▪

1. Wash hands and assemble the following equipment:
   a. soap
   b. wash cloth
   c. 2 to 3 bath towels
   d. bath blanket
   e. resident's gown, robe and slippers
   f. bath thermometer
   g. bath powder
   h. chair or stool
   i. bath mat

2. Identify resident and explain what you plan to do.
3. Take the supplies to the bathroom and prepare it for the resident. Make sure tub is clean.
4. Full tub half full with water at 95° to 105°F or adjust shower flow. Use your elbow to test the water temperature if a shower is being given. The water should feel comfortably warm.
5. Assist resident to bathroom and help them with robe and slippers.
6. Place towel in bottom of the tub to prevent resident from slipping.
7. Help resident undress. Give the male resident a towel to wrap around midriff. Cover resident with bath blanket when going to and from shower, figure 20-7.
8. Assist resident into tub or shower.
9. Wash resident's back. Observe skin for signs of redness or breaks. Resident may be left alone to wash genitalia. If resident shows any signs of weakness, remove plug and let water drain out, or turn off shower. Allow resident to rest until feeling better before making any attempt to assist him or her out of tub or shower. Keep resident covered with bath towel to avoid chilling.
10. Hold bath blanket around resident when he or she is stepping out of tub. A male resident may choose to remove wet towel under bath blanket.
11. Assist resident to dry, powder, dress, and return to unit.
12. Return supplies to proper areas.
13. Clean bathtub. Wash hands.
14. Report completion of task to nurse.
15. Record on chart:
    a. date
    b. time
    c. tub bath/shower
    d. resident's reaction

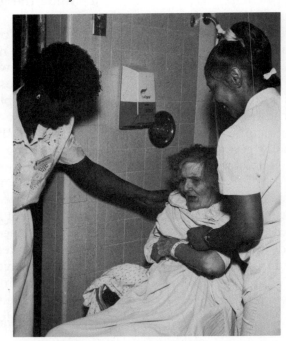

FIGURE 20—7. To prevent chilling, keep resident covered with a bath blanket until he or she is in the shower.

PROCEDURE: Bathing Resident in a Century Tub

1. To prepare bath before transporting resident, figure 20–8:
   a. Check to be sure that tub is clean.

   b. Fill tub with water at 97°F to approximately 8 inches from the top.

c. Check that room temperature is approximately 70°F.

d. Add one capful of liquid soap.

2. Wash hands and assemble the following equipment:

    a. talcum powder

    b. deodorant

    c. 2 bath towels

    d. 1 bath blanket

    e. resident's clothing

3. Take Saf-Kary chair to bedside.

4. Identify resident and explain what you plan to do.

5. Screen unit.

6. Assist resident to undress.

7. Position resident in Saf-Kary chair; secure safety straps and cover resident with a bath blanket, figure 20–9.

8. Transport resident to tub room.

9. Replace bath blanket with two towels. Fold blanket for later use.

10. Position chair with back against lift arms.

11. Step on "up" pedal of lift to engage seat on Saf-Kary chair.

12. Check to see that both pins are engaged in lift arm slots.

13. Latch safety latches.

14. Raise seat to maximum height.

15. Rotate seat on lift arm 90 degrees so resident faces you.

16. Facing resident, slowly guide chair to tub edge so resident is parallel and over tub edge.

17. Lift resident's feet and guide over tub edge toward lower well of tub.

18. Lower resident into tub by stepping gently on down pedal. Water should be chest high. *Note:* If resident has an indwelling catheter, drape tubing over tub edge so that drainage is below bladder level.

19. Press turbine button, activating whirlpool for 5 minutes.

20. Wash face and upper body.

21. Step on up pedal, raising resident until feet are level with whirlpool outlet.

22. Dry upper body.

23. Raise lift to maximum height.

24. Pull chair and resident toward you, rotating seat as you lift feet from tub. Dry feet.

25. Cover resident with bath blanket.

26. Raise safety latch on Saf-Kary chair.

27. Apply deodorant and talcum powder. Help resident to dress.

28. Slowly lower Saf-Kary until chair is flat on floor.

29. Return resident to unit. Replace supplies.

30. Return to tub room and clean tub according to facility policy.

31. Report and record completion of task.

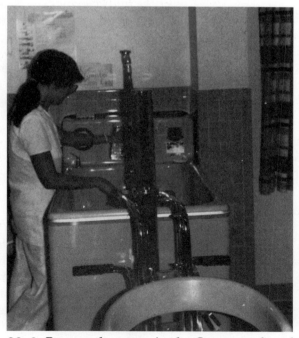

20–8. Prepare the water in the Century tub and adjust the whirlpool activity before lowering the resident.

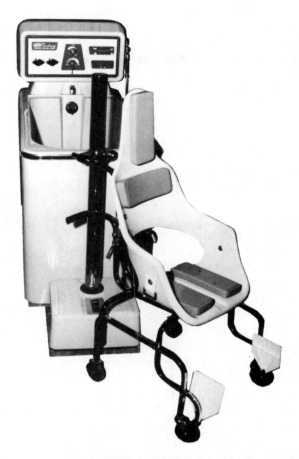

FIGURE 20–9. Chair can be elevated and moved over the tub, lowering the resident into the water. (Courtesy of Century Manufacturing Company)

Partial Bath _____

A partial bath assures cleaning of the hands, face, axilla, buttocks, and genitals. It is very refreshing. Many residents will be able to help with the bath process and, whenever possible, should be encouraged to do so.

▪▪▪ PROCEDURE: Giving a Partial Bath ▪▪▪▪▪▪▪▪▪▪▪▪▪▪▪▪▪▪▪▪▪▪▪▪▪▪▪▪▪▪▪▪

1. Wash hands and assemble the following equipment:
   a. bed linen
   b. bath blanket
   c. bath thermometer
   d. soap and soap dish
   e. washcloth
   f. face towel
   g. bath towel
   h. gown or robe
   i. laundry bag or hamper
   j. bath basin
   k. alcohol or lotion; powder
   l. equipment for oral hygiene
   m. nail brush and emery board
   n. brush, comb, and deodorant
   o. bedpan or urinal and cover
   p. paper towels or bed protector
2. Identify resident and explain what you plan to do.
3. Make sure that any windows and door are closed to prevent chilling resident.

4. Screen unit.
5. Put towels and linen on chair in order of use. Place laundry hamper so that it is convenient.
6. Offer bedpan or urinal (see Lesson 23). Empty and clean before proceeding with bath. Wash hands.
7. Elevate head rest, if permitted, to comfortable position.
8. Loosen top bedclothes. Remove and fold blanket and spread. Place bath blanket over top sheet and remove sheet by sliding it out from under bath blanket.
9. Leave one pillow under resident's head. Place other pillow on chair.
10. Assist resident to remove gown and place gown in laundry hamper. Wrap bath blanket around resident.
11. Place paper towels or bed protector on overbed table.
12. Fill bath basin two thirds full with water at 105°F and place on overbed table.
13. Push overbed table comfortably close to resident.
14. Place towels, washcloth and soap on overbed table within easy reach.
15. Instruct resident to wash as much as he or she is able and that you will return to complete the bath.
16. Place call bell within easy reach. Ask resident to signal when ready.

17. Wash hands and leave unit.
18. Wash hands and return to unit when resident signals.
19. Change bath water. Complete bathing those areas the resident couldn't reach. Make sure the face, hands, axilla, buttocks, back, and genitalia are washed and dried.
20. Give a back rub with lotion or alcohol and powder.
21. Assist the resident in applying deodorant and/or powder and fresh gown.
22. Cover pillow with towel and comb or brush hair. Assist with oral hygiene if needed.
23. Clean and replace equipment according to facility policy.
24. Put clean washcloth and towels in stand or hang according to facility policy.
25. Change bed linen, following occupied bed procedure. Discard soiled linen in laundry hamper.
26. Leave resident comfortably positioned with side rails up and bed in lowest horizontal position. Place call bell and water within easy reach of the resident.
27. Replace furniture. Leave unit in order. Turn out ceiling light if used.
28. Wash hands.
29. Report completion of tasks and any important observations to the nurse.

■■■ PROCEDURE: Giving Female Perineal Care ■■■■■■■■■■■■■■■■■■■■■■■■■

1. Wash hands and assemble the following equipment:
   a. bath blanket
   b. bedpan and cover
   c. graduate pitcher
   d. cotton balls
   e. disposable gloves
   f. bed protector or bath towel
   g. ordered solution (if other than water)
   h. plastic bag to dispose of used cotton balls
   i. perineal pad and belt, if needed
2. Identify resident and explain what you plan to do.
3. Fill pitcher with warm water (or ordered solution) at approximately 100°F and take to bedside.
4. Screen unit.

5. Lower side rail and position bed protector (or towel) under resident's buttocks.
6. Fanfold spread to foot of bed.
7. Cover resident with bath blanket and fanfold sheet to foot of bed.
8. Position resident on bedpan.
9. Put on disposable gloves.
10. Have resident flex and separate knees.
11. Draw bath blanket upward to expose perineal area only.
12. Unfasten perineal pad if in use. Touch only the outside. Note amount and color of discharge. Fold with the insides together and place in plastic bag.
13. Holding pitcher of water approximately 5 inches above pubis, allow all the water to flow downward over vulva and into bedpan.

14. Dry vulva using cotton balls in the following manner:
    a. Use each cotton ball once only and dispose of it into plastic bag.
    b. Bring one or more cotton balls down one side of vulva from pubis to perineum until dry.
    c. Repeat on opposite side of vulva. Remember, use each cotton ball only once and discard.
    d. Dry area over center of vulva.
15. Remove and discard disposable gloves.
16. Ask resident to raise hips. Carefully remove bedpan; cover, and place on chair.
17. Apply perineal pad if needed and secure to belt. Never touch fingers to inside of pad. Apply from front to back, then fasten belt.
18. Remove bath towel or disposable pad and dispose according to facility policy.
19 .Unfold sheet and spread and draw up over resident. Remove bath blanket.
20. Fold bath blanket and store in bedside stand.
21. Make resident comfortable and leave unit tidy.
22. Clean equipment and discard all disposables according to facility policy.
23. Wash hands.
24. Report completion of task and observations to nurse.

▓▓▓ PROCEDURE: Giving Male Perineal Care ■■■■■■■■■■■■■■■■■■■■■■■■■■

1. Wash hands and assemble the following equipment:
   a. bath blanket
   b. urinal and cover
   c. soap, washcloth and towel
   d. disposable gloves and plastic bag
   e. bed protector or bath towel
   f. ordered solution (if other than water)
2. Identify resident and explain what you plan to do.
3. Fill basin with warm water at approximately 100°F.
4. Screen unit.
5. Lower side rail and position bed protector (or towel) under resident's buttocks.
6. Fanfold spread to foot of bed.
7. Cover resident with bath blanket and fanfold sheet to foot of bed.
8. Offer urinal. Empty after use and wash hands.
9. Put on disposable gloves.
10. Have resident flex and separate knees.
11. Draw bath blanket upward to expose perineal area only.
12. Make a mitt with washcloth.
13. Using soap and water, wash pubis, penis, and scrotum. Gently draw foreskin back and clean glans. Dry and reposition prepuce.
14. Turn resident on side away from you. Wash, rinse, and dry area under scrotum and around anus.
15. Reposition resident.
16. Remove and discard disposable gloves.
17. Remove bath towel or disposable pad and dispose of according to facility policy.
18. Unfold sheet and spread and draw up over resident. Remove bath blanket.
19. Fold bath blanket and store in bedside stand.
20. Make resident comfortable and leave unit tidy.
21. Clean equipment and discard disposables according to facility policy.
22. Wash hands.
23. Report completion of task and observations to nurse.

SKIN CONDITIONS ■■■■■■■■■■■■■■■■■■■■■■■■■■■■■■■■■■■■■■■

Because the skin is exposed to the environment, it is subject to easy injury. Changes in the structure of the skin are referred to as skin **lesions**. Skin lesions must be described accurately. Review figure 20–10 for the names and descriptions of some of the most common skin lesions seen in the elderly.

- **Macule** — flat, discolored spot
- **Papule** — small, raised solid spot
- **Pustule** — raised spot filled with pus
- **Vesicle** — blister-like raised spot filled with serous fluid
- **Wheal** — large, raised, solid, irregular area frequently associated with itching
- **Excariation** — scratched area
- **Crust (scab)** — area of dried secretions
- **Ulceration** — shallow, crater-like area
- **Decubiti** — skin ulcerations known as "bedsores"
- **Bath itch** — pinpoint red spots
- **Senile lentigines** (singular: *lentigo*) — yellowish or brown skin discolorations
- **Senile keratoses** (singular: *keratosis*) — roughened, scaly, slightly raised wart-like lesions
- **Petechiae** — small, pinpoint hemorrhages

FIGURE 20–10. Common skin lesions.

Cancers

Cancers of the skin are fairly common in the older individual. Be sure to report any changes you note in the size or shape of a wart or mole or indications of inflammation (redness) around the area of a wart or mole.

Senile Lentigines

Areas of skin pigmentation seem to become more pronounced with advancing years. *Senile lentigines* are sometimes called liver spots, although they are not related to liver function and are thought to be due to response to environment exposure, figure 20–11. They appear as yellowish or brownish spots on exposed skin surfaces.

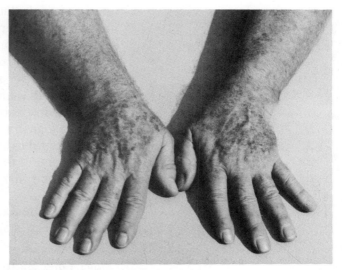

FIGURE 20–11. Senile lentigines.

Senile Keratoses

Senile keratoses are roughened, wart-like lesions thought to be formed in response to sun damage.

Decubitus Ulcers_____

You can prevent skin breakdown.

Decubiti, or pressure sores, are a serious problem at any time and especially so in the advancing years. Decubitus ulcers are shallow crater-like lesions that develop when prolonged pressure is exerted against tissues, which causes collapse of the tiny tissue blood vessels. Skin surfaces receiving less nourishment quickly break down.

Situations Leading to Breakdown

Decubiti can frequently be prevented by conscientious care and attention. In order to prevent decubiti, you must be alert to avoid situations that contribute to their formation, figure 20–12.

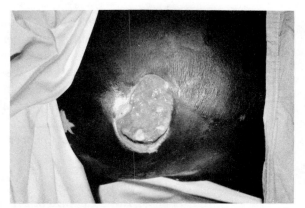

FIGURE 20–12. Untreated pressure areas quickly involve deeper tissue.

Tissues can become trapped between the mattress, wheelchair or geri-chair and the bony parts of the body. To prevent breakdown:

- Change resident position at least every two hours to reduce pressure in any one area (figure 20–13.).
- Immediately remove feces, urine or moisture of any kind which is very irritating to the skin. Keep the skin clean and dry.
- Encourage residents sitting in geri-chairs or wheelchairs to raise themselves or change position every 10 minutes to relieve pressure or do this yourself.
- Encourge proper nutrition and adequate fluids.
- Keep linen dry and wrinkle-free.
- Check for improperly fitted or worn braces and restraints.
- Check nasogastric tubes and urinary catheters to be sure they are positioned in such a way as not to be a source of irritation. Keep nasal and urinary openings clean and free of drainage. These areas must be checked frequently and carefully.

Signs of Tissue Breakdown. The tissue breakdown occurs in three stages. Action at each stage can prevent additional damage. These stages are:

1. *Stage One.* Signs of impending skin breakdown include redness or blue-gray discoloration of the skin surface over a pressure point.
   Action: Remove the pressure and gently massage around the outside of the affected area to help prevent the development

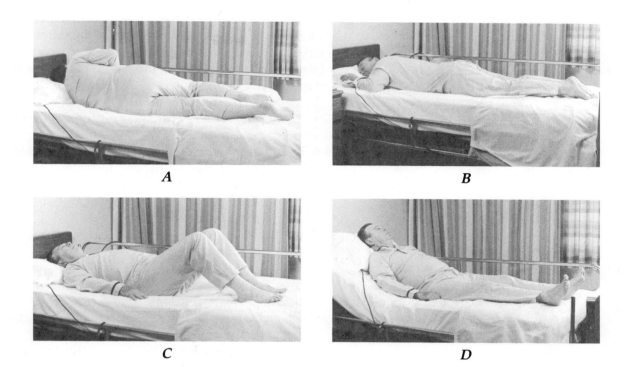

FIGURE 20–13. *Residents are turned to and supported on one of these four basic positions every 1 to 2 hours:*

A. *Sims' position.*
B. *Prone position.*
C. *Dorsal recumbent position.*
D. *Semi-Fowler position.*

of a bedsore. Make sure you notify the nurse. If, however, this first stage of involvement is neglected, further and deeper damage occurs.

2. *Stage Two.* This stage of the breakdown process is signaled by reddened skin with blister-like lesions. Sometimes the epidermis will be broken. The area around the site is reddened.

Action:
• Gently massage outside the reddened area.
• Keep the area around the breakdown clean and dry.
• Relieve all pressure over the affected area by using mechanical aids.
• Encourage the resident to eat and drink.
• Keep the broken area covered as ordered.
• Carry out heat lamp treatments as ordered.
• Report indications of infection such as odor or drainage, bleeding and changes in size.

Note: In each situation that the skin is broken, the area will be covered with a **dry sterile dressing** (DSD) or some other protective covering, such as Op-site or duoderm. These are two clear plastic-like coverings which permit air to reach the tissues but keeps the tissues dry, thus promoting healing.

Holding a DSD in place without causing additional injury is not easy. The elderly skin may be sensitive to regular tape, so elastoplast, paper tape or cellophane may be better to use. Be careful to loosen the tape with saline before lifting the tape when the dressing is changed. Other measures that may be ordered include:

- Antiseptic sprays, antibiotic ointments and dressings to control infection.
- Techniques which dry the area and promote healing are commonly employed. These include:
  — exposure to ultraviolet radiation
  — sunlight
  — low oxygen concentrations

3. *Stage Three.* This stage of the process is where the deeper tissues breakdown, figure 20–14.
Action
- Care is carried out as in stage two but continued faithfully if the third stage develops.
- When there is dead tissue, ointments which remove the dead tissue (*debride*) from the area may be ordered.
- Daily whirlpool baths help keep the area clean.
Note: In severe cases surgery may be needed to close the ulcerated area.

The nursing assistant must be constantly on the alert for signs of impending skin breakdown. Remember those residents who must

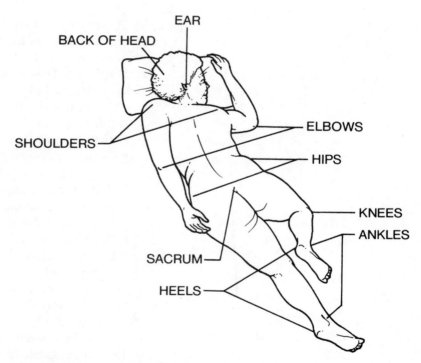

FIGURE 20–14. Areas at greatest risk for decubiti.

remain in bed and those who must sit in geri-chairs or wheelchairs are at the highest risk. Their position must be changed at least every two hours.

Encourage residents to participate to whatever extent is possible in their own care. Follow the established routines for turning and repositioning residents faithfully. It is far easier to prevent decubiti than to heal them.

BACK RUB

Regular back care is given after the bath. It may also be given following the use of the bed pan or after changing a resident's position. A good back rub takes 3 to 5 minutes. When performed properly, with long, smooth strokes, it stimulates the resident's circulation and aids in preventing skin breakdown. It is also soothing and refreshing.

PROCEDURE: Giving a Back Rub

1. Wash hands and assemble the following equipment:
   a. basin of water (105°F)
   b. bath towel
   c. soap and alcohol or lotion
   d. body powder
2. Identify resident and explain what you plan to do.
3. Screen unit. Raise bed to comfortable working height.
4. Place lotion in basin of water to warm.
5. Turn the patient on his or her side with back toward you.
6. Expose and wash back.
7. Pour a small amount of lotion into one hand. Apply to skin and rub with gentle but firm strokes. Give special attention to all bony prominences.
8. Begin at base of spine:
   a. With long, soothing strokes rub up the center of back, around the shoulders, and down sides of back and buttocks, figure 20–15.
   b. Repeat previous step 4 times, using long, soothing upward stroke and circular motion on downstroke.
   c. Repeat, but on downward stroke rub in small circular motion with palm of hand. Include areas over coccyx (over base of spine).
   d. Repeat long, soothing strokes on muscles for 3-5 minutes.
   e. Dry area well.
   f. If pressure areas are noted, report to nurse.
9. Straighten draw sheet.
10. Change resident's gown if needed. Position resident comfortably.
11. Replace equipment. Wash hands.
12. Reports completion of task.

MECHANICAL AIDS

Mechanical aids are used to reduce pressure, figure 20–16. Examples are:

- sheepskin pads (or artifical sheepskin)
- foam and egg-crate pads and pillows
- bed cradles (foot cradles)
- alternating pressure mattresses
- flotation mattresses
- egg-crate foam mattresses

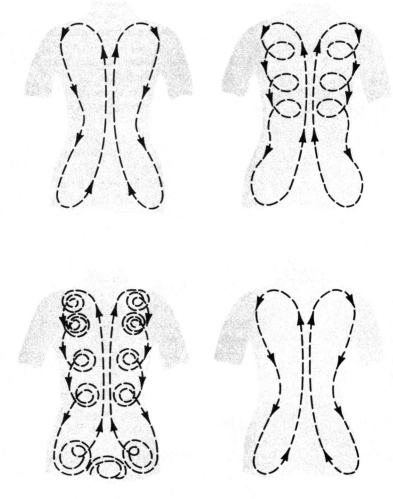

FIGURE 20–15. *Types of movements used in a complete back rub.*

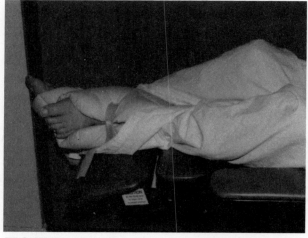

FIGURE 20–16. *Foot protectors pad areas that are prone to breakdown.*

Sheepskin pads (or artificial sheepskin). These absorb moisture and reduce friction when placed under the resident, figure 20–17.

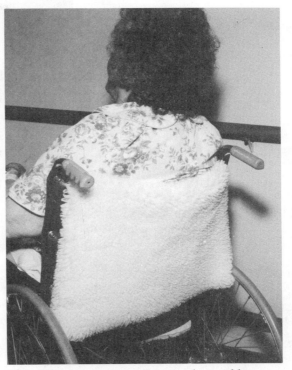

FIGURE 20–17. Sheepskin can be used between resident and bed or wheelchair as padding.

Foam and egg-crate pads and pillows. These are used to bridge areas to reduce pressure. Rubber or hard doughnut-shaped pads may not be effective since, although they shield the affected areas, they create pressure by their own shape.

Use mechanical aids to reduce pressure.

Bed cradles (foot cradles). These can lift the weight of bedding but must be carefully positioned and padded, because injury can occur if the resident strikes them.

Alternating pressure mattresses. These mattresses are used in some facilities. Air pressure is reduced in certain areas of the mattress every 5 minutes on an alternating basis. The pressure alteration reduces pressure against the body so that no skin area is subject to pressure for more then 5 minutes at a time.

Flotation mattresses. These are water beds with controlled temperature. The weight of the resident's body displaces water to the extent that pressure is consistently equalized against the skin. Sheets should not be tucked tightly over flotation mattresses, as this will restrict the function of the mattress.

Egg-crate foam mattress. This type of mattress is in common use in long term care facilities, figure 20–18. The weight of the body is equally distributed when the mattress is placed under the resident.

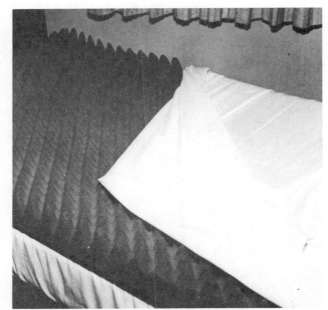

FIGURE 20–18. *The weight of the body is more evenly distributed over the egg-crate type of surface.*

Each of these aids reduces pressure but nothing can take the place of vigilent nursing observation and care.

HAIR CARE

The hair should be brushed and neatly arranged each day (figure 20–19) and whenever necessary. A neat appearance improves everyone's morale. In many facilities, barber and hair dressing services are available right in the facility. When you care for a resident's hair:

- handle the hair gently as you brush and comb
- note any unusual appearance of scalp or hair
- brush or comb one section at a time, gently untangling snags
- clean brush and comb before returning to resident's drawer

Clean neat hair improves appearance and morale.

If barber and hair services are available, your responsibility may include daily care and making sure that the resident is safely transported to and from the hair dressing room for special services such as a shampoo or set. Shampoos may be given once a week or once or twice a month. If beauty services are not available, the staff will give shampoos. More advanced cosmetology services such as hair cutting are not performed by the nursing staff. A cosmetologist or a family member should perform this service.

The shampoo is most safely given during the shower with the resident seated or when the resident is in bed, figure 20-20. Make sure that there are no drafts and, when possible, use a hair dryer to be sure that the hair is thoroughly dry.

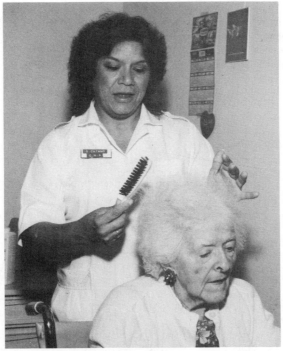

FIGURE 20–19. The hair should be neatly arranged each day.

PROCEDURE: Giving a Bed Shampoo

1. Wash hands and assemble the following equipment and supplies:
   a. Shampoo tray — plastic sheeting which has the top and 2 sides forming a drain may be used if regular tray is not available.
   b. washcloth
   c. 3 bath towels
   d. bath blanket
   e. basin of water (105°F)
   f. safety pin
   g. 2 bed protectors
   h. waterproof covering for pillow
   i. large basin to collect used water
   j. portable hair dryer if available
   k. hairbrush and comb
   l. small, empty pitcher or cup
   m. large pitcher of water (115°F) — used if additional water is needed
2. Screen unit.
3. Identify patient and explain what you plan to do.
4. Place chair beside head of bed. Cover seat with bed protector. Place large, empty basin on chair.
5. Arrange on bedside stand within easy reach:
   a. basin of water (105°F)
   b. pitcher of water (115°F)
   c. washcloth
   d. 2 bath towels
   e. shampoo
   f. empty pitcher
6. Replace top bedding with bath blanket.
7. Ask resident to move to side of bed nearest you.
8. Replace pillow case with waterproof covering.
9. Cover head of bed with bed protector, well under resident's shoulders.
10. Loosen neck ties of gown.
11. Place towel under resident's head and shoulders. Brush hair free of tangles, working snarls out carefully.
12. Bring towel down around resident's neck and shoulders and pin. Position pillow under shoulders so that head is tilted slightly backward.

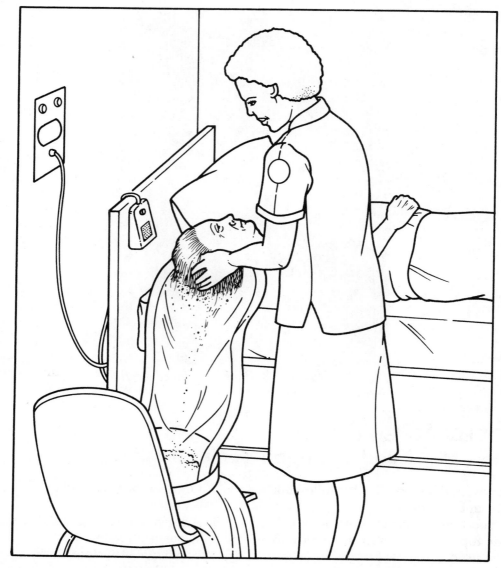

FIGURE 20–20. When residents must remain in bed, a shampoo may still be given.

13. Raise bed to high horizontal position.
14. Raise resident's head and position shampoo tray so that drain is over the edge of bed directly above basin in chair.
15. Give resident washcloth to cover eyes.
16. Re-check temperature of water in basin. Using small pitcher, pour a small amount of water over hair until thoroughly wet. Use one hand to help direct the flow away from the face and ears.
17. Apply a small amount of shampoo, working up lather. Work from scalp to hair ends.
18. Massage scalp with tips of fingers. Do not use fingernails.
19. Rinse thoroughly, pouring from hairline to hair tips and directing flow into drain. Use water from pitcher if needed but be sure to check temperature of water before use.
20. Repeat procedure a second time.
21. Lift resident's head. Remove tray and bed protector. Adjust pillow and slip a dry bath towel underneath head.
22. Place tray on basin and wrap hair in towel. Be sure to dry face, neck, and ears as needed.
23. Dry hair with towel. If available and not counterindicated, a portable hair dryer may be used to complete the drying process. Brushing the hair as you blow dry facilitates drying. Be sure to keep the dryer moving and not too close to the hair.
24. Comb hair appropriately and remove protective pillow cover. Replace with cloth cover.

25. Lower height of bed to comfortable working position.
26. Replace bedding and remove bath blanket. Help resident assume comfortable position and lower bed to lowest horizontal position. Length of procedure may tire resident, so allow resident to rest undisturbed.
27. Empty water from collection basin.
28. Clean equipment according to facility policy and return to proper area.
29. Be sure that unit is left in proper order. Wash hands.
30. Report and record procedure, including:
    a. date and time
    b. bed shampoo
    b. resident's reaction

▓▓▓ PROCEDURE: Giving Daily Care of Hair ▓▓▓▓▓▓▓▓▓▓▓▓▓▓▓▓▓▓▓▓▓▓▓▓▓

1. Wash hands and assemble the following equipment:
   a. towel
   b. comb and brush
   c. alcohol or petroleum jelly
2. Identify resident and ask him or her to move to the side of bed nearest you or resident may sit in chair if permitted.
3. Screen unit.
4. Cover pillow with towel.
5. Part or section hair and comb with one hand between scalp and end of hair.
6. Brush carefully and thoroughly.
7. Have resident turn so hair on back of head may be combed and brushed. If hair is snarled, working section by section, apply alcohol to oily hair or petroleum jelly to dry hair as needed. Unsnarl hair, beginning near ends and working toward scalp.
8. Complete brushing and arrange attractively. Braid long hair to prevent repeated snarling.
9. Clean and replace equipment according to facility policy. Wash hands.
10. Report completion of task.

FACIAL HAIR ▓▓

Men feel better groomed when they are shaved regularly. This is a procedure that you will carry out during the morning care. For safety, use an electric razor or rotary razor.

▓▓▓ PROCEDURE: Shaving Male Resident ▓▓▓▓▓▓▓▓▓▓▓▓▓▓▓▓▓▓▓▓▓▓▓▓▓▓▓▓▓

1. Wash hands and assemble the following equipment:
   a. Electric shaver or safety razor
   b. Shaving lather or pre-shave lotion for electric razor
   c. Basin of water (115°F)
   d. Face towel
   e. Mirror
   f. After-shave lotion or powder
2. Identify resident and explain what you plan to do (figure 20–21.) Let resident help as much as possible.
3. Screen unit.
4. Raise the head of the bed. Place equipment on overbed table.
5. Place face towel across resident's chest.
6. Moisten face and apply lather. Otherwise, applies pre-shave lotion.
7. Starting in front of ear, hold skin taut and bring razor down over cheek toward chin. Repeat until lather on cheek is removed and area has been shaved. Repeat on other cheek. Use firm short strokes, rinsing razor frequently.
8. Lather neck area and stroke up toward the chin in a similar manner.
9. Wash face and neck and dry thoroughly.
10. Apply after-shave lotion or powder if desired.
11. If the skin is nicked, apply pressure directly over the area and then an antiseptic. Report incident to nurse.
12. Clean and replace equipment. Wash hands.
13. Reports completion of task.

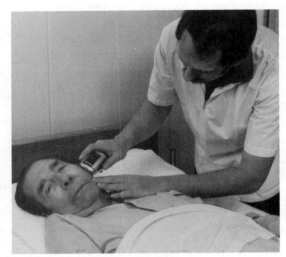

FIGURE 20–21. It is safest to shave residents with a rotary razor.

Older women have an increase in the growth and coarseness of hairs on their chin and upper lip. Many women find this very distressing. Tweezers can be used to remove some of the hairs, but a more permanent method is to have the hairs removed professionally with an electric needle. Some women may require a shave. In some facilities nursing assistants are not permitted to shave women residents. Be sure to check the policy of your facility.

HAND CARE

Fingernails are routinely cleaned during the morning care. Use a soft brush and orangewood stick to gently clean under the nails. Fingernail care can also be carried out as a separate procedure. Soak the hands in warm soapy water. Creams can be used to soften the cuticles which can then be gently pushed back with a towel. When cutting the fingernails, follow the curve of the finger and then file any rough edges. Polish can then be applied. Be careful not to injure the corners of the fingers when cutting the nails.

PROCEDURE: Giving Hand and Fingernail Care

The procedure described below can be carried out independently or can be modified and incorporated with the bath procedure.
1. Wash hands and assemble the following equipment:
   a. basin
   b. soap
   c. bath towel and washcloth
   d. lotion
   e. plastic protector
   f. nail clippers
   g. nail file
   h. orangewood stick
2. Identify resident and explain what you plan to do.
3. Screen unit.
4. Elevate head of bed, if permitted, and adjust overbed table in front of resident. If resident is allowed out of bed, assist to transfer to a chair and position overbed table waist-high across lap.
5. Place plastic protector over bedside table.

6. Fill basin with warm water at approximately 105°F and place on overbed table.
7. Instruct resident to put hands in basin and soak for approximately 20 minutes. Place towel over basin to help retain heat. Add warm water if necessary. Remember to remove the resident's hands before adding water.
8. Wash hands. Push cuticles back gently with washcloth.
9. Lift hands out of basin and dry with towel.
10. Use nail clippers to cut fingernails straight across. Do not cut below tips of fingers. Keep nail cuts on protector to be dicarded.
11. Shape and smooth fingernails with nail file.
12. Pour small amount of lotion in your palms and gently smooth on resident's hands.
13. Empty basin of water. Gather equipment. Clean and store according to facility policy.
14. Return overbed table to foot of bed. If resident has been sitting up for the procedure, assist into bed.
15. Lower head of bed and make resident comfortable. Leave call bell within easy reach. Make sure bed is in lowest position and side rails are up and secure.
16. Leave unit tidy. Wash hands.
17. Report completion of your task and any observations to nurse.

FOOT CARE

Report thickened and deformed toenails to the nurse.

Residents should be given routine foot care, which includes bathing, massage of the feet, and attention to the toenails. Proceed carefully:

- Dry feet carefully after soaking in warm water.
- Give special attention to drying between the toes.
- Carefully inspect the feet and apply lotion to dry areas.
- Check the resident's toenails. If the nails are very thick or curved, refer situation to nurse.

A podiatrist may need to give the care. The podiatrist will care for the toenails of residents who have poor circulation or diabetes or those whose nails are deformed.

Part of good foot care includes being sure that slippers or shoes fit well and are securely laced so that they offer optimum support.

PROCEDURE: Giving Foot and Toenail Care

1. Wash hands and assemble the following equipment:
   a. wash basin
   b. soap
   c. bath mat
   d. lotion
   e. disposable bed protector
   f. bath towel and washcloth
   g. orangewood stick
2. Identify resident and explain what you plan to do.
3. If permitted, assist resident out of bed and into chair.
4. Place bath mat on floor in front of resident.
5. Fill basin with warm water (105°F). Put basin on bath mat.
6. Remove slippers and allow resident to place feet in water. Cover with bath towel to help retain heat.
7. Soak feet approximately 20 minutes. Add warm water as necessary. Lift feet from water while warm water is being added.
8. At end of soak period, wash feet with soap. Use washcloth to scrub roughened areas. Rinse and dry. Note any abnormalities such as corns or callouses.
9. Remove basin, covering feet with towel.
10. Use orangewood stick to gently clean toenails. If nails are long and need to be cut,

report this fact to the nurse. Do not undertake this task yourself.
11. Dry feet.
12. Pour lotion into palms of hands. Hold hands together to warm lotion and apply to feet.
13. Assist resident with slippers and to return to bed unless ambulatory.

14. Make resident comfortable.
15. Gather equipment, clean, and store according to facility policy. Leave unit tidy.
16. Wash hands.
17. Report completion of task and your observations to nurse.

ORAL HYGIENE

The elderly need good oral hygiene just as much as younger people. Regular cleansing by brushing and flossing should be carried out routinely when the resident has any teeth of his/her own. Visits by a dentist can help maintain existing dental function.

PROCEDURE: Assisting Resident to Brush Teeth

1. Wash hands and assemble the following equipment:
   a. emesis basin
   b. toothbrush
   c. toothpaste
   d. glass of cool water
   e. mouth wash, (if permitted)
   f. hand towel
   g. bed protector
   h. dental floss
2. Identify resident and explain what you plan to do and what the resident can do to help.
3. Screen unit.
4. Elevate head of bed. Help resident into comfortable position.
5. Lower side rails and position overbed table across resident's lap.

6. Cover table with plastic protector and place emesis basin and glass of water on table.
7. Place towel across resident's chest.
8. Be prepared to help as resident brushes and flosses teeth.
9. After resident has brushed teeth, push overbed table to foot of bed. Remove towel and fold and place on table.
10. Lower head of bed. Help resident to assume comfortable position and adjust bedding. Raise side rails.
11. Gather equipment, clean, and store according to facility policy. Discard soiled linen in proper receptacle.
12. Wash hands. Leave unit tidy.
13. Report completion of task and your observations to nurse.

PROCEDURE: Cleaning and Flossing Resident's Teeth

1. Wash hands and assemble the following equipment:
   a. emesis basin
   b. toothbrush
   c. toothpaste
   d. glass of cool water
   e. mouth wash, if permitted
   f. hand towel
   g. bed protector
   h. dental floss
2. Identify resident and explain what you plan to do.

3. Screen unit.
4. Elevate head of bed. Help resident into a comfortable position.
5. Lower side rails and position overbed table across resident's lap.
6. Place towel or bed protector across resident's chest.
7. Place toothpaste on moistened toothbrush.
8. Clean all surfaces of each tooth. Use a sweeping motion working from gum line to tip of tooth.
9. Have resident rinse mouth into emesis basin.

10. Select a piece of dental floss about 12 inches long. Wrap ends of dental floss around middle fingers, leaving center area free.
11. Ask resident to open his or her mouth.
12. Gently insert floss between each tooth down to, but *not into*, gum line.
13. Ask resident to rinse mouth using emesis basin.
14. Wipe resident's face dry with towel.
15. Push overbed table to the foot of bed.
16. Position resident comfortably. Be sure that water and call bell are close at hand.
17. Raise and secure side rails.
18. Gather equipment, clean, and store according to facility policy. Discard soiled linen in proper receptacle.
19. Wash hands. Leave unit tidy.
20. Report completion of task and your observations to nurse.

Dentures

Many residents have artificial dentures. Care for the dentured resident includes:

- cleaning dentures daily under cool running water
- storing dentures in a safe place when out of the resident's mouth
- checking the resident's mouth daily for signs of irritation
- checking resident's lips for cracking and dryness
- applying creams, petroleum jelly, or glycerin to lips for excessive dryness

Partial plates, which are removable but attached by small metal clips, should be given the same care as artificial dentures.

PROCEDURE: Caring for Dentures

1. Wash hands and assemble the following equipment:
   a. tissues
   b. emesis basin
   c. denture brush
   d. toothpaste or tooth powder
   e. mouthwash, if permitted
   f. gauze squares
   g. denture cup
2. Identify resident and explain what you plan to do.
3. Screen unit.
4. Allow resident to clean own dentures if able to do so. If resident cannot, give tissue to resident and ask him or her to remove dentures, figure 20–22. Assist if necessary.
5. Place dentures in denture cup padded with gauze squares. Take to bathroom or utility room.
6. Put toothpaste or tooth powder on denture brush. Place dentures in palm of hand and hold them under gentle stream of warm water. Brush until all surfaces are clean. *Note:* Dentures may be soaked in a solution with a cleansing tablet before brushing, if necessary.
7. Rinse dentures thoroughly under cold running water. Never use hot water. Rinse denture cup.
8. Place fresh gauze squares in denture cup. Place dentures in cup and take them to bedside.
9. Assist resident to rinse mouth with mouthwash, if permitted. Otherwise use water.
10. Use tissue or gauze to hand wet dentures to resident. Insert if necessary.
11. Clean and replace equipment according to facility policy. Wash hands.

Store dentures in denture cup inside the bedside stand when not in use. Some residents prefer storing dentures dry while others prefer to store dentures in a special solution.

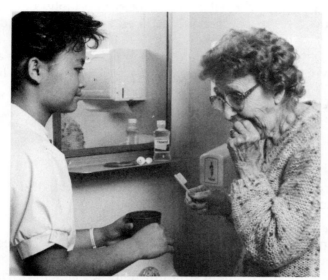

FIGURE 20–22. *You may need to assist the resident with denture care.*

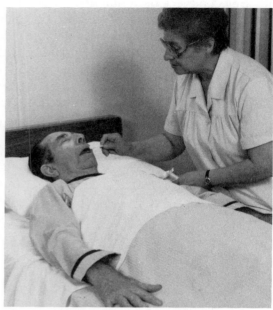

FIGURE 20–23. *Unconscious residents must be given special oral care.*

Residents who are unconscious still require oral hygiene, figure 20–23. Lemon and gycerin swabs may be used. Since the resident cannot participate, the staff must carry out this procedure for the resident.

▪▪▪ PROCEDURE: Assisting with Special Oral Hygiene ▪▪▪▪▪▪▪▪▪▪▪▪▪▪▪▪▪▪▪

1. Wash hands and assemble the following equipment:
   a. mouthwash solution in cup or mixture of glycerin in lemon juice
   b. emesis basin
   c. bath towel
   d. plastic bag
   e. applicators
   f. tissues
   g. tongue depressor
   h. lubricant for lips
2. Identify resident and explain what you plan to do. Screen unit.
3. Cover pillow with towel and turn resident's head to one side.
4. Place emesis basin under resident's chin.
5. Open mouth gently with tongue depressor.
6. Dip applicators into mouthwash solution or glycerin mixture. (In some cases, a physician may order hydrogen peroxide solution.)
7. Using moistened applicators, wipe gums, teeth, tongue and inside of mouth.
8. Discard used applicators in plastic bag.
9. Lubricate lips with cold cream or petroleum jelly.
10. Clean and replace equipment. Wash hands.
11. Report and record completion of task.

DRESSING RESIDENT ▪▪▪▪▪▪▪▪▪▪▪▪▪▪▪▪▪▪▪▪▪▪▪▪▪▪▪▪▪▪▪▪▪▪▪▪▪

Dressing in his or her own clothes contributes to the resident's sense of identity. It is for this reason that residents are encouraged to wear their own clothes and to dress after morning care every day.

Some residents will be able to dress themselves with assistance, others who are totally dependent will have to be dressed by the staff.

It is part of your responsibility to see that the clothing is clean and neat and in good repair. You should remember to:

- Select clothing that is lightweight but that will provide adequate warmth.
- Whenever possible, allow the resident to choose the clothing to be put on, figure 20–24. Do not, however, offer too many choices since it may confuse the resident.
- Encourage resident to participate, in the dressing or undressing procedure, to the extent of his or her ability.

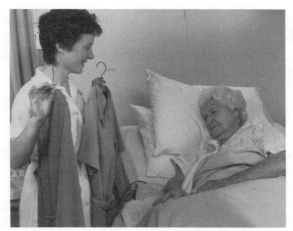

FIGURE 20–24. Whenever possible, assist the resident but allow her to make decisions.

It is easiest to dress the resident who requires complete help while he or she is in bed. Residents who can help themselves may wish to sit in a chair with clothing placed nearby. You can help by:

- Arranging the clothing in the order that they will be put on.
- Being prepared to assist with shoes and stockings even for residents who can do much themselves. Bending over to adjust shoes and stockings can result in dizziness and loss of balance.
- Always putting on or removing clothing from the affected side first if the resident has difficulty moving one side or is paralyzed.

PROCEDURE: Dressing and Undressing Resident

1. Wash hands.
2. Identify resident and explain what you plan to do.
3. Select appropriate clothing and arrange in order of application. Encourage resident to participate in selection.
4. Screen unit or draw curtains for privacy.
5. Raise bed to comfortable working height.
6. Elevate head of bed to sitting position.
7. Cover resident with bath blanket and fanfold top bedclothes to foot of bed.
8. Assist resident to comfortable sitting position.
9. Remove night clothing, keeping resident covered with bath blanket.

10. Gather undershirt and slip over the resident's head, or helps hook bra.
11. Grasp resident's hand and guide it through the arm hole by reaching into the arm hole from the outside.
12. Repeat procedure with opposite arm.
13. Assist resident to sit forward, adjusting undershirt so it is smooth and over upper body. *Note:* A similar procedure may be followed for applying a dress or pullover shirt.
14. Shirts or dresses which fasten in the front should be applied as follows:
    a. Insert your hand through sleeve of shirt or dress and grasp hand of resident, drawing sleeve over your hand and resident's.
    b. Adjust sleeve at shoulder.
    c. Assist resident to sit forward. Arrange clothing across back.
    d. Gather sleeve on opposite side by slipping your hand in from the outside.
    e. Grasp resident's wrist and pull sleeve of shirt or dress over your hand and resident's. Draw upward and adjust at shoulder.
    f. Button or secure front of shirt or dress.
15. Facing foot of bed, gather resident's underwear from waist to leg hole.
16. Slip underwear over feet and draw up the legs as high as possible.
17. Assist resident to raise his or her buttocks and draw underwear over buttocks and up around waist. (Have resident roll first to one side and then to other to adjust underwear if this appears to be the easier of the two methods of adjusting underwear.)
18. For male resident, repeat process with outer trousers. Fasten or zip trousers.
19. Put on socks by rolling socks and adjusting over toes and drawing over foot. Adjust so that socks lie flat and smooth.
20. For female residents, gather pantyhose and adjust over toes and feet. Draw up over feet and legs as high as possible.
21. Assist resident to raise hips and position pantyhose in same manner as you followed with underwear.
22. Put on shoes and secure.
23. Assist resident to comfortable position out of bed, with call bell within easy reach.
24. Wash hands and report completion of task.

VOCABULARY

axilla	dilating	pore
Century tub	dry sterile dressing (DSD)	receptor
constricting	epidermis	senile keratoses
debride	integumentary system	senile lentigines
decubiti	lesions	subcutaneous tissue
dermis	oil gland	sweat gland

SUGGESTED ACTIVITIES

1. Using a model or diagram, identify the parts of the skin and appendages.
2. Working in pairs, practice carrying out the special procedures described in this Lesson.
3. Give supervised care to residents using the procedures you have learned.

REVIEW

Brief Answer/Fill in the Blanks

1. Three functions of the integumentary system include

   a. _____

   b. _____

   c. _____

2. Name five characteristics of the aging integumentary system:

   a. _____

   b. _____

   c. _____

   d. _____

   e. _____

3. The elderly person should be bathed at least _____ each week.

4. Hair should be shampooed at least _____ each month.

5. Substances that are highly irritating to the skin and need to be removed include

   a. _____

   b. _____

   c. _____

6. Three benefits of a whirlpool bath are that it: _____ circulation, the warm water can be _____, and warm water is both _____ and _____.

7. Liver spots are more properly called _____.

8. Roughened, wart-like lesions thought to be formed from exposure to sun are called _____.

9. Pressure sores are also called _____.

10. Three things you can do to prevent decubiti from developing include

    a. _____

    b. _____

    c. _____

11. Briefly explain the three stages of decubiti development and list your actions.

    a. _____

    b. _____

    c. _____

CLINICAL SITUATION

Mary Mandell, one of your residents, is bright and charming. Her hair is long and she wears it braided around her head. She tells you that she would like to have it washed and cut but can't do it herself. What could or should you do to help?

Answer: _____

_____

_____

LESSON 21 The Cardiovascular System

OBJECTIVES

After studying this lesson, you should be able to:

- Name the parts and function of the cardiovascular system.
- Identify normal cardiovascular changes as they relate to the aging process.
- List common geriatric cardiovascular conditions.
- Give appropriate care to residents with cardiovascular dysfunction.
- Define and spell all the vocabulary words and terms.

The cardiovascular system is the body's transportation system.

The cardiocvascular system is composed of the heart, blood vessels, and the blood. The spleen, liver, and bone marrow make some of the blood cells and destroy them when they are worn out. The lymphatic vessels carry **lymph**, or tissue fluid. The cardiovascular system is the transportation system of the body, carrying substances from where they are formed to where they may be used or eliminated.

Cardiovascular conditions involve diseases of the heart, blood, and blood vessels. Cardiovascular disease is the most common cause of death in the United States, so many residents in your care will suffer from cardiovascular disabilities. Cardiovascular disease is responsible for heart attacks, strokes, and peripheral vascular changes that diminish the blood flow to the body tissues. Diminished blood flow is called **ischemia**. Ischemia leads to less oxygen delivery and, eventually, to death of the tissues (**infarction**). Changes which take place in the aging cardiovascular system are summarized in figure 21–1.

- Toughening (fibrosis) of blood vessel walls
- Narrowing of blood vessels
- Increased blood pressure
- Less blood flow to vital organs
- Heart muscle less effective

FIGURE 21–1. Cardiovascular changes associated with aging.

THE HEART

The heart is a muscular organ that pumps the blood in a continuous flow throughout the blood vessels of the body, figure 21–2.

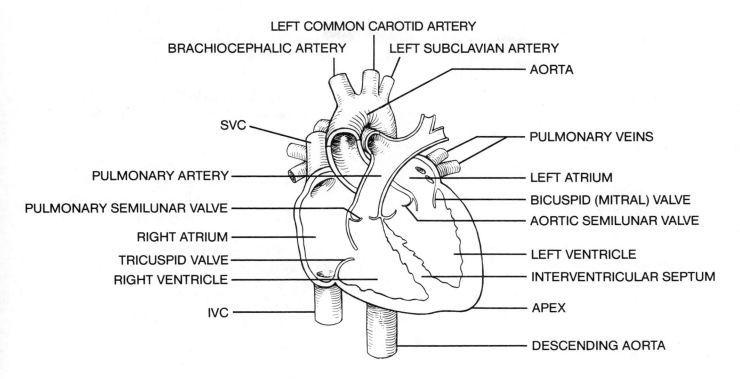

LEFT COMMON CAROTID ARTERY
BRACHIOCEPHALIC ARTERY
LEFT SUBCLAVIAN ARTERY
AORTA
SVC
PULMONARY VEINS
PULMONARY ARTERY
LEFT ATRIUM
PULMONARY SEMILUNAR VALVE
BICUSPID (MITRAL) VALVE
AORTIC SEMILUNAR VALVE
RIGHT ATRIUM
TRICUSPID VALVE
LEFT VENTRICLE
RIGHT VENTRICLE
INTERVENTRICULAR SEPTUM
IVC
APEX
DESCENDING AORTA

FIGURE 21–2. Diagram of the heart. Note the chambers and valves.

It is separated into a right and left side by a partition called the **interventricular septum**.

The *right side* of the heart receives blood from the body and sends it to the lungs to get rid of carbon dioxide and to pick up oxygen. (Both carbon dioxide and oxygen are gases.) The *left side* receives blood from the lungs by way of the pulmonary veins and sends it out to the body, where the oxygen is given up to the cells and the carbon dioxide is picked up.

Each side is further divided into upper and lower parts (chambers) by **valves**. The valves permit blood flow in one direction only. The *upper chambers* are called the right **atrium** and left atrium (plural: *atria*). The *lower chambers* are the right and left **ventricles**.

The two upper chambers contract first, forcing the blood through the open valves into the two lower chambers. The ventricles fill and the valves close. The ventricles then contract, squeezing the blood up through the large blood vessels, leaving them.

Two major blood vessels of the heart are:

- the **pulmonary artery**, which carries blood to the lungs from the right ventricle
- the **aorta** (a large artery), which carries blood to the body from the left ventricle

Valves at the base of the pulmonary artery and aorta close as the blood moves forward, preventing backflow of blood into the ventricles between contractions.

CARDIAC CYCLE ▪▪▪▪▪▪▪▪▪▪▪▪▪▪▪▪▪▪▪▪▪▪▪▪▪▪▪▪▪▪▪▪▪▪▪▪

The cardiac cycle keeps the blood moving forward.

The series of contractions and relaxations of the heart muscle is called the **cardiac cycle**, figure 21–3. The cardiac cycle is controlled by special nervous (nodal) tissues within the heart and by two sets of nerves:

1. One set of nerves carries messages to increase the heart rate.
2. The other set of nerves carries messages to slow the heart down.

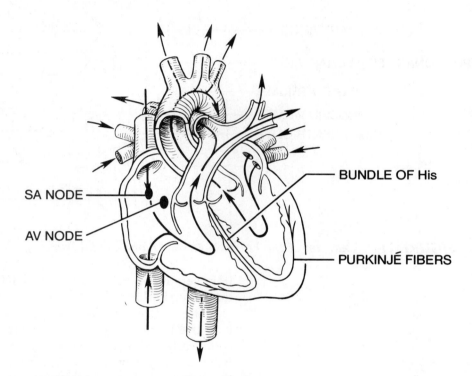

SA NODE

AV NODE

BUNDLE OF His

PURKINJÉ FIBERS

FIGURE 21–3. Messages beginning in the S-A node reach the A-V node, bundle of His, and Purkinje fibers, causing the cardiac cycle to take place.

Electrical impulses passing through the nodal tissue make the muscle contract. **Systole** (pronounced sis'tuh–lee) is the term meaning heart *contraction*. **Diastole** (pronounced dye–as'tuh–lee) is the term meaning heart *relaxation*.

For a short time, the heart rests completely in between beats. The pulse you feel at the radial artery corresponds to ventricular systole, figure 21–4. The sounds you hear when listening to the heart and when taking a blood pressure are the sounds made by the closing of the valves during the cardiac cycle.

BLOOD VESSELS ▪▪▪▪▪▪▪▪▪▪▪▪▪▪▪▪▪▪▪▪▪▪▪▪▪▪▪▪▪▪▪▪▪▪▪▪

Avoid anything that limits circulation.

There are three kinds of blood vessels:

• **arteries**
• **capillaries**
• **veins**

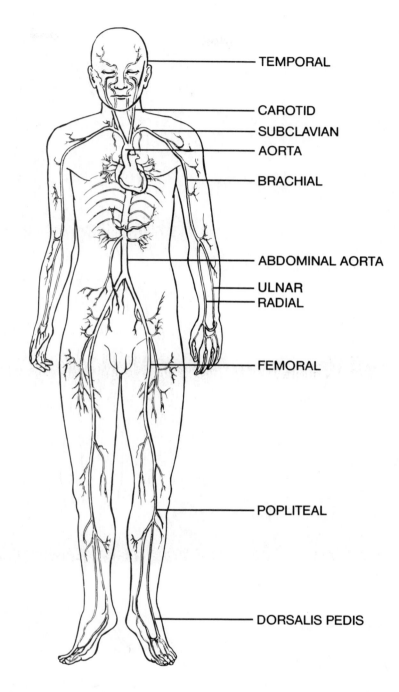

FIGURE 21–4. Pulses of the body. Pulses can be felt in any area of the body where an artery can be gently compressed.

Arteries. Arteries carry blood away from the heart, figure 21–5. The blood that arteries carry is usually high in oxygen, which is needed to keep the body cells alive and functioning. The blood is described as **oxygenated**. The arteries get smaller and finally form tiny networks of vessels called capillaries.

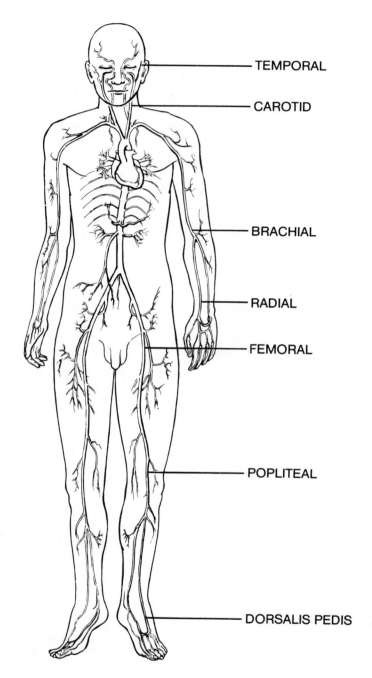

FIGURE 21–5. General plan of circulation.

Capillaries. Through the walls of the capillaries, nutrients and oxygen are exchanged for carbon dioxide and waste products. The capillaries form larger vessels called **venules** to begin the journey back to the heart.

Veins. Many venules join to eventually form larger vessels called veins. The largest veins, the **superior vena cava** and the **inferior vena cava**, return the blood to the right atrium. The blood that these veins carry has less oxygen and more carbon dioxide and is described as **deoxygenated** blood.

As you can see from figure 21–5, the cardiovascular system is a closed system with the gases and other substances passing into and out of the blood as it passes throughout the body.

Blood vessels frequently take their names from nearby bones. For example, the radial artery and radial vein are found close to the radius, which is one of the forearm bones.

Blood vessels often have the same name as a nearby bone.

LYMPH

Lymph is fluid that is drained from the tissues. It passes into lymphatic vessels through masses of cells called **lymph nodes**; and eventually it is returned to the general circulation. The lymph nodes act as filters, removing harmful substances picked up in the tissues before they can reach the general circulation.

THE BLOOD

The blood is a red body fluid that carries the nutrients, chemicals, and waste products of the body. Each person has about 4 to 6 liters (or 4 to 6 quarts) of blood in his or her body. The blood consists of two portions:

- **plasma**
- blood cells

Plasma. The liquid part of the blood, called plasma, carries water, nutrients, and wastes. Plasma also carries proteins that help blood to clot and other proteins that fight infection and help to move materials in and out of the bloodstream. **Serum** is the fluid that is left after the cells and some of the proteins have been removed.

Blood Cells. Three kinds of blood cells are (figure 21–6):

1. *Red blood cells*, or **erythrocytes**, which carry oxygen and a small amount of carbon dioxide.
2. *White blood cells*, or **leukocytes**, which protect the body by fighting infection.
3. *Platelets*, or **thrombocytes**, which are only pieces of cells but contain a chemical important to blood clotting.

DYSCRASIAS

Heart disease is a major cause of death and disability.

Blood abnormalities (**dyscrasias**) commonly seen in the elderly include:

- cancers
- **anemias**

Cancers. Cancers of the blood include some forms of **leukemia**. Excessive numbers of white blood cells are formed and too few platelets and red blood cells are produced; as a result, the person fatigues easily, is subject to infections and anemia, and is apt to bleed. Sometimes, these conditions are treated with radiation or drugs.

ERYTHROCYTES

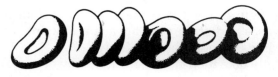

LEUKOCYTES

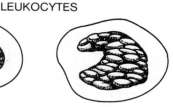

MONOCYTE   LYMPHOCYTE

THROMBOCYTES

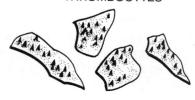

AGRANULOCYTES

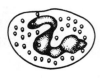 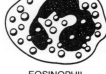 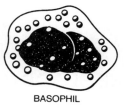

NEUTROPHIL   EOSINOPHIL   BASOPHIL

FIGURE 21–6. Types of blood cells.

Anemias. Anemias are the result of a decrease in the quantity of red blood cells and their ability to carry oxygen. People suffering from anemia have little energy. They:

- are usually pale or jaundiced (yellowish)
- complain of light-headedness
- feel cold
- experience dizziness
- have an increased respiratory rate
- suffer from poor digestion

Special Care

Residents with either cancer or anemia may need blood transfusions. You must:

1. Check vital signs.
2. Encourage rest and a good diet.
3. See that resident avoids unnecessary exertion.
4. Handle resident very gently.
5. Give special mouth care, since the mouth and tongue become rather sensitive.
6. Be sure to report any signs of bleeding such as bruises or discolorations, since further blood loss makes the condition worse.
7. Keep resident warm with sweaters and lap robes.
8. Protect resident against falls that may result from dizziness or weakness.
9. Change the resident's position often — at least every two hours.

VASCULAR DISEASE

Diseased blood vessels carry less blood to the tissues.

Vascular disease affects many older residents. Over the years, changes take place in the blood vessels; as a result, the amount of blood flowing through them is gradually decreased. The tissues served by the diseased vessels suffer from the loss of nourishment and oxygen, figure 21–7.

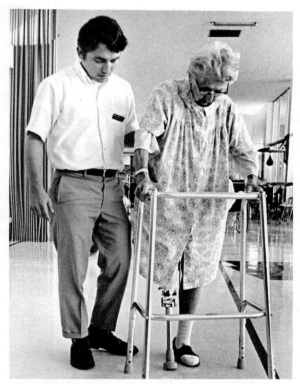

FIGURE 21–7. *Poor circulation due to disease of blood vessels may lead to death of the tissues and the need for amputation.*

The brain, heart, arms, and legs are the body parts most seriously affected. Inadequate blood flow is associated with pain and diminished function of the tissues served by the narrowed vessels.

Arteriosclerosis

The general term **arteriosclerosis** or hardening of the arteries describes several forms of vascular disease such as **atherosclerosis, arteriolosclerosis** and **arteriosclerosis obliterans**.

Atherosclerosis. Deposits of fatty materials and calcium form roughened areas (**plaques**) on the inner wall of the arteries. As the plaques get larger, the space within the vessels (the **lumen**) narrows, blocking the blood flow. The vessels of the heart, brain and deep body areas are most often involved. Blockage of these vessels cause **cerebrovascular accidents** (strokes or CVAs) and myocardial infarction (heart attacks).

The exact cause of atherosclerosis is unknown, but the lifestyle of the individual seems to play an important role. Factors that seem to contribute to atherosclerosis include:

- excess weight
- diets high in fat and sugar
- little exercise
- smoking and stress

These factors seem to promote unhealthy changes in the vascular walls.

Arteriolosclerosis. This affects the smaller arteries that carry blood to organs like the kidneys. The vessels are gradually narrowed, making it more difficult for the organs to carry on their work. Disease of the arterioles also raises the blood pressure.

Arteriosclerosis obliterans. This is complete closing of the vessels. It leads to extreme pain, breakdown of the tissues and, sometimes, amputations. It most often affects the vessels of the extremities (peripheral vascular disease).

When peripheral vascular disease is present:

1. The skin becomes dry and scaly or shiny.
2. Pigmentation deepens.
3. The skin feels cold to touch.
4. The skin is pale or cyanotic.
5. Nails become thickened and brittle.
6. The resident complains of pain, described as throbbing or gnawing, especially at night and during exercise.

Confusion and diminished brain function occur when the cerebral vessels are involved. This state is known as **chronic brain syndrome** or **cerebral arteriosclerosis**.

Special Care

Your conscientious care of the feet can make the difference between the saving or loss of a limb. You can best assist your resident with circulatory impairment by the following measures:

1. Avoid anything that would further limit the circulation, such as too-tight clothing, circular garters, shoes that are too tightly tied, or sitting with the legs crossed.
2. Give careful attention to the feet, figure 21-8:
   a. inspect feet as you carry out foot hygiene.
   b. bathe feet regularly.
   c. use a lanolin lotion if feet are dry.
   d. dry area between toes well.
   e. use light dusting of powder, but be sure not to use so much powder that it cakes, as this may prove irritating.
   f. report any signs of irritation, such as corns or calluses, so that they can be treated by a podiatrist, figure 21-9.
3. Encourage water intake to promote the elimination of wastes and to help dilute the blood.
4. Do not permit smoking. Smoking or the use of tobacco in any form is forbidden, since tobacco causes vasoconstriction.
5. Provide warmth by maintaining the room temperature at about 70°F. You can also add additional coverings and warm clothes and socks. Residents will often complain of coldness in their legs and feet. Never be tempted to provide external heat in the form of a heating pad or hot water bottle, since heat increases the need for additional circulation that cannot be met, and decreased sensitivity may result in a severe burn.

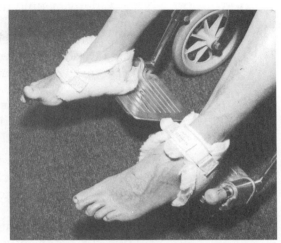

FIGURE 21–8. Protect the resident's heels from injury by using heel protectors.

- Broken skin
- Coldness
- Color change
- Cracking between toes
- Corns or callouses

FIGURE 21–9. Note and report.

6. Follow planned exercise programs. A specific exercise program will be planned for each resident and should be followed by all staff members.
7. Protect resident against injury. Always keep in mind the fact that decreased circulation predisposes the resident to tissue breakdown and ulcer formation from even a minor injury. Such ulcerations are very difficult to heal. The ulcerated tissue can become infected, further complicating the healing process. Remember, the signs and symptoms of infection include:

- redness
- heat
- swelling
- pain
- loss of function
- drainage

Hypertension

Hypertension means elevated blood pressure. Diseases of the blood vessels elevate the overall blood pressure. When blood vessels are narrowed due to disease, the heart attempts to make up for the resistance in the vessels by enlarging. Over a period of time, the heart eventually fails. Hypertension further increases the rate at which disease progresses in the vessels.

Uncontrolled hypertension leads to strokes and heart attacks.

Elderly people usually have a somewhat higher pressure than younger persons. The normal blood pressure for young adults is 120/80, but in the elderly, the norm is higher, with about 150/90 mmHg being the highest level of normal. Above this level, the incidence of stroke and heart attack is dramatically increased.

Control of Hypertension. Control of hypertension is essential. Steps can be taken to avoid the serious consequences of stroke and heart attack and to bring the hypertension under control. These include:

* drugs to lower the pressure
* weight reduction
* dietary restrictions, such as limiting salt intake

You will recognize high blood pressure as you take the vital signs. Look for other indications of an elevated blood pressure. These include:

* flushed face
* dizziness
* nose bleeds
* headaches
* changes in speech patterns
* blurred vision

Be sure to report any of these signs and symptoms to the nurse.

Cerebrovascular Accidents_____

A **cerebrovascular accident (CVA)** is also called **stroke** and **apoplexy**. It is as much a problem of the nervous system as it is of the cardiovascular system. The complete or partial loss of blood flow to the brain tissue is frequently a complication of atherosclerosis.

Transient Ischemic Attack (TIA)_____

A temporary interruption of the blood flow to the brain is known as a **transient ischemic attack** (TIA). TIAs frequently occur in the elderly and are usually due to **thrombi** (sing., *thrombus*), or blood clots that block a small vessel. They may or may not cause loss of consciousness or paralysis, figure 21–10.

A TIA is associated with signs and symptoms that are seen in varying degrees of intensity and combination. The resident may experience:

* nausea
* dizziness
* momentary loss of contact
* temporary weakness
* loss of vision
* forgetfulness
* irritability
* confusion

Sitting up suddenly may cause a resident to experience a temporary decrease in the flow of blood to the brain. The condition is usually progressive, so the resident will need close care and supervision.

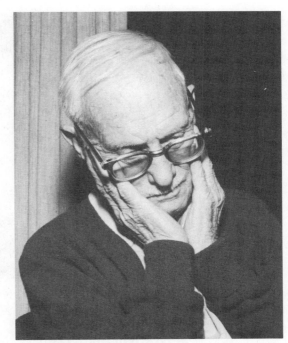

FIGURE 21-10. A temporary interruption of blood flow to the brain (TIA) can make the resident experience confusion and depression.

ACUTE CARDIOVASCULAR ATTACK

When a larger vessel in the brain is blocked, the situation becomes critical and requires acute care. To assure that proper care will be given, you must recognize the signs and symptoms of an acute CVA. The signs and symptoms are summarized in figure 21-11. If the blockage of blood vessels occurs in the right side of the brain, the left side of the body will be affected, and vice versa.

- Loss of consciousness
- Labored respirations
- Elevated blood pressure
- Unilateral paralysis
- Derangement of thought process
- Incontinence

FIGURE 21-11. Signs and symptoms of a CVA.

Paralysis of one side of the body is called **hemiplegia**, figure 21-12. Other forms of paralysis are **paraplegia** (paralysis of the lower limbs) and **quadriplegia** (paralysis of all four limbs).

Left Brain Damage. Left-sided brain damage may affect the speech and communication centers, so the resident will be **aphasic** (unable to communicate verbally).

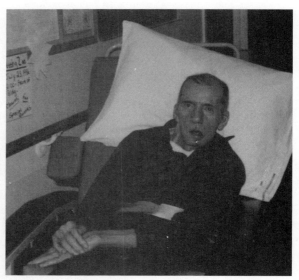

FIGURE 21–12. This resident has right brain damage. Note paralysis on left side of body.

Right Brain Damage. May affect thought processes, memory, written computation, and the ability to put time and events together properly.

The resident with an acute CVA may be transferred to an acute care hospital for immediate care. At some point later, he or she may return to your facility for continued care and rehabilitation.

Convalescence and Rehabilitation

The process of rehabilitation starts with the admission for acute care. Because this is an intense period of care, the stroke victim is referred to as a patient. Care in the early post-stroke period centers around maintaining vital functions.

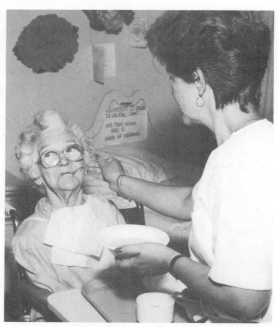

FIGURE 21–13. Assist the post-stroke resident with the activities of daily living.

Rehabilitation is an ongoing process that begins with admission.

Therapy started in the immediate care period is continued and expanded as the patient recovers, figure 21-13. Short- and long-range goals are established in a team effort which involves the patient, specialists and, when possible, the family, figure 21-14. Emotions are very unstable for a long period following a stroke, and this can be difficult to deal with for you, the resident, and the family. For example, residents may seem depressed and cry with seemingly little reason or they may become angry or irritated. They may have mood swings, seeming more hopeful in the morning and frustrated and upset an hour later. It is important that you remain calm and positive in your behavior. Being consistent and understanding is an important contribution you can make to your resident's sense of security and stability.

- Bowel/bladder retraining
- Oral hygiene
- Evaluation of disability
- Retraining in activities of daily living (ADL)
- Retraining in communication skills

FIGURE 21-14. Long-term goals for the resident suffering a CVA.

One of the most significant contributions the staff can make is to *motivate* the patient to take an active interest in his or her own progress. This early period is a very difficult phase for most people who must relearn the activities of daily living, often with the severe limitations of paralysis and faulty brain functions. Bowel and bladder retraining may be started immediately, and the frustrating experience of trying to learn to eat, dress, and communicate begins. (Bowel retraining is presented in lesson 22; bladder retraining in lesson 23.)

Trained therapists prescribe special programs to overcome each of the patient's limitations. Speech therapists help the resident learn to communicate. The physiotherapist and occupational therapists work with the resident to regain motor skills such as ambulating and carrying out the activities of daily living. Learning to balance, stand and, eventually, walk again requires a great deal of practice — practice that is tiring and frustrating and that often leads to periods of depression.

The training begins with relearning the transfer activities needed to move from bed to chair, wheelchair to toilet, and chair to tub. The patient must learn to use hand rails and ambulatory aids such as walkers, canes, and wheelchairs. Raised toilets, lap boards, and ramps are available to help in the retraining process. Step by step, the patient is brought to greater self-sufficiency.

Aphasia limits the ability to communicate.

Aphasia. Perhaps the most frustrating problem to overcome is that of the inability to form thoughts and express those thoughts so that others can understand, figure 21-15. Language impairment is known as **aphasia**. Some people have no useful language skills after a stroke. They cannot write, speak, or comprehend the written word. Other

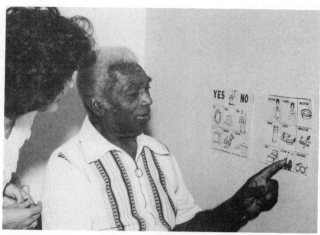

FIGURE 21–15. This stroke victim has language impairment (aphasia) and uses picture cards to help convey his thoughts.

stroke victims are not as severely damaged and, with patience and guidance, can regain some communicating skills.

Automatic Speech. In **automatic speech** words are spoken that have no relationship or meaning. This is a common occurrence spoken in the post-stroke period. During periods of automatic speech, words may be spoken that are considered profane and may be frequently repeated.

Nursing Assistant Responsibilities___

When a post-stroke resident returns to your care, you can cooperate in continuing the rehabilitation process by:

- Following the resident's care plan.
- Assisting in the activities of daily living (ADL).
- Using pillows to support the resident to maintain proper alignment whether the resident is in bed or sitting up in a wheelchair or geri-chair, figure 21–16.
- Using good communication skills, since communication may be a real challenge. Use short, precise sentences, speaking slowly, looking at the resident, and working from the non-affected side. Focus on one request or direction at a time. Even if the resident doesn't seem to comprehend you, continue to try since the resident needs examples to follow and needs to practice his or her communication skills.
- Helping resident stay aware of the surroundings, figure 21–17. Clocks, radios, calendars, and signs of the seasons and holidays are sensory stimuli that are helpful in establishing and maintaining proper orientation.
- Allowing resident to do as much as possible for himself or herself.

Success in helping the resident reach a level of independence equal to that of the pre-stroke period probably will not be realized. Rehabilitation should strive to bring each resident to the highest level that is consistent with the individual's limitations, figure 21–18.

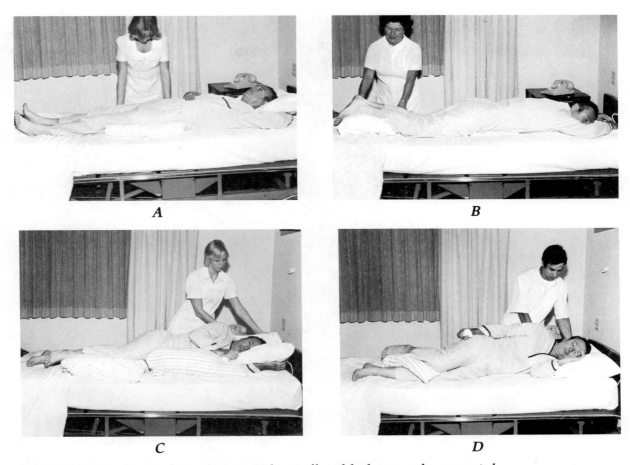

A

B

C

D

FIGURE 21–16. *The stroke patient must have affected body properly supported.*
A. *The resident's weak hand is tucked under the pillow with fingers open. Rolled sheet or bath blanket is used to maintain position of leg.*
B. *When it is not possible for the resident's toes tohang over the end of the mattress, a large pillow can be used to support the feet so that the toes do not touch the mattress.*
C. *In this side-lying poistion, a pillow is used to support the weak arm. Another pillow is used to support the weak leg.*
D. *Here is one more side-lying position. The weak arm is placed on a pillow right behind the resident. Notice the rolled towel under the hand.*

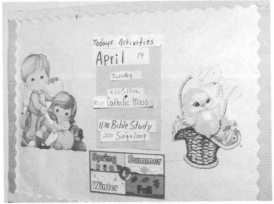

FIGURE 21–17. *Call attention to signs that will keep the resident oriented to time and place.*

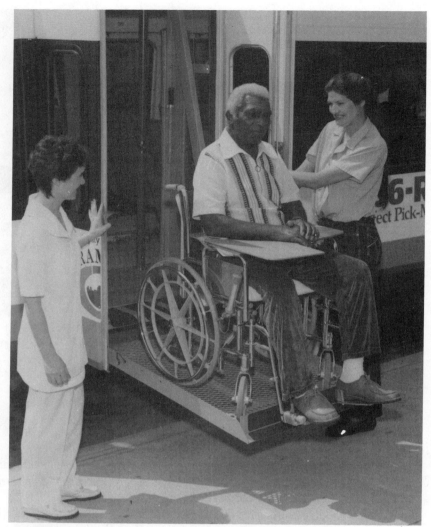

FIGURE 21–18. *This post-stroke victim makes visits to a nearby rehabilitation center twice each week for rehabilitative exercises and treatment of his left arm.*

HEART DISEASE

Many of your residents will suffer from some form of heart disease. Heart disease often makes self-care difficult, and residents become depressed and frustrated by their limitations. Heart disease may sometimes be due to an infection but the majority of heart disease develops because of changes in the blood vessels that make the space inside the vessels smaller. These changes make it harder and harder for the heart to do its job of pumping blood.

Heart Attack

In heart attack the heart fails to pump blood adequately.

A **heart attack** refers to an occurrence when the heart no longer is able to function properly, figure 21–19. There are different kinds of attacks, and some have more serious consequences than others. Every attack is serious though, and each requires some form of treatment (**therapy**).

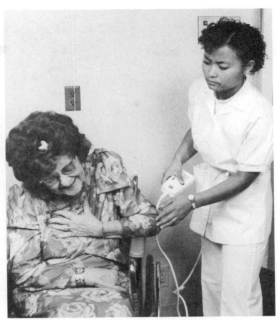

FIGURE 21-19. If you suspect the resident is having a heart attack, do not leave her but summon help.

Myocardial Ischemia

In **myocardial ischemia** the normal flow of blood to the heart is decreased. Narrowing of the coronary (heart) blood vessels that supply blood to the heart may occur so slowly over a period of years that some new circulation can develop. However, when the heart attack occurs, the flow of blood has diminished so much that not enough blood reaches the heart and the heart muscle may die. This lack of blood flow is known as ischemia.

Sometimes the flow of blood is cut off abruptly because a blood clot lodges in a coronary artery. When there is generalized narrowing of the blood vessels, the heart labors, enlarges, and gradually fails.

Angina Pectoris

Angina pectoris is a condition in which there is a temporary myocardial ischemia, figure 21-20. Signs and symptoms of an angina heart attack that you should note and immediately report include:

- Pain when exercising or under stress. The pain is described as dull, with increasing intensity. It is usually centered under the breast bone (**sternum**), spreading to the left arm and up into the neck.
- Pale or flushed face.
- Resident is freely perspiring.

Signs and symptoms may differ with individual residents, but the symptoms are usually the same each time that a resident experiences an attack. Stress causes a need for an immediate increase in the coronary circulation. You may assist the resident with angina pectoris by:

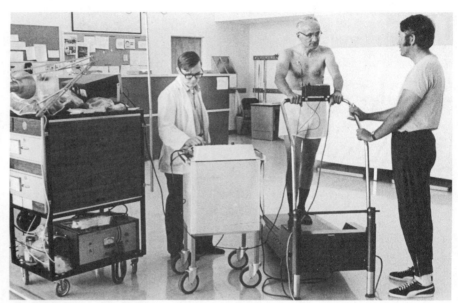

FIGURE 21–20. *The treadmill is a commonly used test for angina patients.*

- Helping the resident to avoid unnecessary emotional or physical stress.
- Encouraging the resident not to smoke.
- Reporting any signs and symptoms of an attack to the nurse at once.

Nitroglycerin tablets are sometimes kept at the bedside. This medicine, a **vasodilator,** increases the blood flow to the heart, relieving the ischemia. The effect of each tablet lasts about one half hour. Relief from pain is achieved in 2 or 3 minutes. There may be some headache but few other side effects.

Coronary Occlusion

In **coronary occlusion,** or **myocardial infarct** (MI), the coronary blood vessels that serve the heart muscle are completely blocked. The size of the blocked vessel and its location determine the seriousness of the attack.

Silent Coronary. If the narrowing has been gradual and additional circulation has had time to develop, the blockage may cause little damage and the resident may have little awareness of the situation. This type of attack is called a **silent coronary**. The damage from this type of occlusion is relatively minor and may not be recognized until it is discovered during a physical examination that includes an **electrocardiogram (ECG)**. An ECG is a special test that measures the response of the heart muscle to nervous stimulation.

Acute Myocardial Infarction

An *acute coronary heart attack*, or acute MI, is a serious medical emergency. The blood flow to the myocardium is cut off suddenly. The closure of a large vessel can result in death (infarction) of that part of the heart muscle not being supplied with blood. If too much of the heart muscle dies, the resident cannot survive.

Survival depends, to a large extent, upon how quickly proper medical help is administered. You must recognize the signs and symptoms of this type of heart attack and report to the nurse immediately.

Signs and Symptoms. These include:

- crushing chest pain, spreading down the arms and up into the neck and jaw; sometimes described as "severe indigestion"
- clammy, ashen, or pale skin
- excessive sweating (**diaphoresis**)
- nausea
- vomiting (sometimes)
- anxiety and weakness
- weak pulse
- low blood pressure
- shock

Nursing Assistant Care. You can help by:

- staying with the resident
- using the intercom or call bell to summon help
- staying calm

The resident will usually be transferred immediately to an intensive care unit of an acute care hospital. Early treatment is designed to reverse the shock, relieve the pain, and keep the heart functioning.

Cor Pulmonale

Cor pulmonale is a condition that involves both heart and lungs. The normal heart loses some of its elasticity and muscle strength as it ages. Narrowing of blood vessels adds additional stress. Disease in the lungs also causes stress on the heart by making it more difficult to send proper volumes of blood through the pulmonary artery. The right side of the heart enlarges (*hypertrophies*); this condition is called cor pulmonale. Gradually, the heart muscle tires and becomes less effective and fails, leading to **congestive heart failure**.

Congestive Heart Failure

Many residents will have hearts that are less efficient. Signs of acute failure include:

- cough
- **dyspnea** (difficulty breathing)
- **orthopnea** (difficulty in breathing unless sitting upright)
- cyanosis
- **hemoptysis** (spitting up blood)
- fluid retained in the lungs and throughout the body
- **edema** (fluid in the tissue spaces)
- **ascites** (fluid collecting in the abdomen)
- neck veins swell
- easily fatigued
- **hypoxia** (inadequate oxygen levels)
- confusion

Nursing Assistant Care. Acute failure is an urgent situation requiring expert care. You will assist in this care. Watch the resident carefully and report any increase in signs and symptoms at once.

Positioning. The resident is usually more comfortable sitting up in bed, supported by pillows, or supported in a chair (**orthopneic position**). The position must be changed frequently, but changes in position should be made slowly. Padded footboards help keep the weight of the bedding off the toes.

TED Hose. **TED hose** are elastic anti-embolism stockings. TED hose and Ace bandages help channel blood to the deeper vessels, figure 21–21. They must be checked often and reapplied every 6 to 8 hours. Check the extremities carefully for adequate circulation. The skin should be pink and warm.

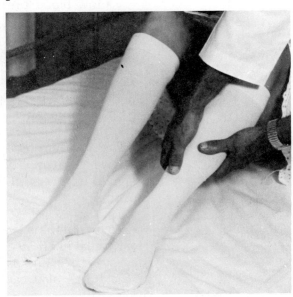

FIGURE 21–21. TED hose smoothly applied helps support the peripheral circulation.

PROCEDURE: Application of TED Hose

1. Wash hands and take elasticized stockings of proper length and size to the resident's bedside.
2. Identify resident and explain what you plan to do.
3. With resident lying down, expose one leg at a time.
4. Grasp stocking with both hands at the top and roll toward toe end.
5. Adjust over toes, positioning opening at base of toes (unless toes are to be covered). Remember that the raised seams should be on the outside.
6. Apply stocking to leg by rolling upward toward body.
7. Check to be sure stocking is applied evenly and smoothly and that there are no wrinkles.
8. Repeat procedure on opposite leg.
9. Report and chart:
   a. date and time
   b. procedure: application or reapplication of elasticized hose
   c. any unusual observations

General Hygiene. Complete bathing is fatiguing, but partial baths can stimulate circulation and provide comfort. Special attention must be given to the skin since the combination of position, edema, and poor circulation contributes to the greater likelihood of tissue breakdown.

Oxygen Therapy. Oxygen therapy may be ordered, either by face mask or nasal cannula, figure 21–22. Since cardiac residents tend to be mouth breathers, there is a tendency for the mouth to be very dry. Special mouth care may be needed.

Oxygen Safety
- NO smoking
- NO woolen blankets
- NO open flame
- DISCONNECT OXYGEN before using any electrical equipment

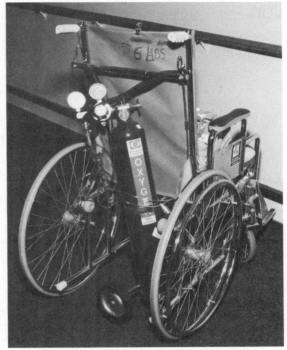

FIGURE 21–22. A portable oxygen unit attached to the wheelchair is useful for residents requiring a constant supply of oxygen.

Elimination. A bedside commode is convenient and the use of a commode is less fatiguing for the resident than using a bedpan for elimination.

Nutrition. Small meals that are easily digested should be encouraged. You may need to assist in the feeding process to prevent fatigue.

Fluid Intake. Residents with acute congestive heart failure may be given drugs that increase the output of urine and alter the heart rate. Measuring the intake and output and taking daily weights are ways of determining water retention. These procedures are part of the care you will give.

Checking Vital Signs. Sometimes the force of heart contraction, which propels the blood foward into the blood vessels, doesn't have enough strength to make the vessels expand. This is called a **pulse deficit**.

You will recall that each heart contraction is normally accompanied by an expansion of blood vessels and, when the expansion is felt, it is recorded as the pulse. To be sure that you are accurately recording heart activity and its effectiveness, an apical pulse should be taken on cardiac residents. Remember, to determine pulse deficit, you and someone else will need to record the apical and radial pulses simultaneously. Review Lesson 17 for the apical pulse procedure.

Chronic Congestive Heart Failure

Residents can live for years with some level of chronic failure. This will be the situation of many of those in your care. These people need a calm environment with planned activity that keeps them mobile but not fatigued. Visiting should be limited to one or two visitors at a time, since too many visitors at one time can be tiring.

The same basic care is required for the resident in chronic failure as that given for a resident with acute failure. This includes:

- measuring fluid intake and output
- taking apical and radial pulse
- assisting when necessary to prevent fatigue and maintain mobility

Since medications are needed for such long periods of time, there is a tendency for drug levels to accumulate. Elderly people are more sensitive to drugs and, therefore, you must be very alert to unusual responses or behavior that could indicate a drug reaction. Be sure to report anything unusual about the residents in your care.

Heart Block

Heart block is a heart condition that develops due to an interference in the normal flow of electrical current through the heart that makes the normal cardiac cycle possible.

An electronic device called a **pacemaker** is implanted under the chest muscles or in the abdomen to replace the lost control, figure 21–23. Small wires carry electrical current from the electronic device directly into the heart muscle. The electrical current signals the heart to contract. Some pacers send messages only if normal messages carried by the conduction system are delayed. This type of pacer is called a **demand pacer**. Other pacers send regular signals to keep the heart contracting. The rate of signals is pre-set.

When caring for a resident who has a pacemaker:

- Carefully take and record the pulse rate.
- Report any irregularities or changes below the present rate.
- Report any discoloration over the implant site.
- Report hiccoughing, since this may indicate problems.
- Keep resident clear of microwave ovens, since they may disrupt the function of the pacer.

Residents usually function very well with pacers so long as they are adequately monitored.

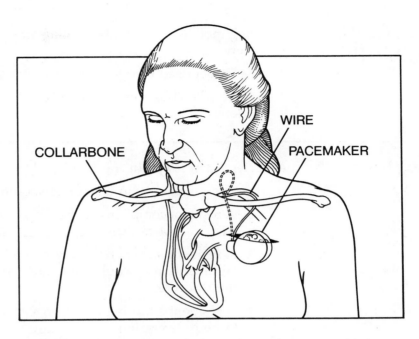

FIGURE 21–23. The electronic pacer sends electrical impulses to the heart muscle, causing it to contract.

VOCABULARY

apoplexy	deoxygenated	myocardial ischemia
aphasic	diaphoresis	nitroglycerin
atrium (plural; *atria*)	diastole	pacemaker
anemia	dyscrasia	paraplegia
angina pectoris	dyspnea	plaque
aorta	edema	plasma
artery	electrocardiogram	platelet
ascites	(ECG)	pulmonary artery
arteriosclerosis	erythrocytes	pulse deficit
arteriosclerosis	heart block	quadraplegia
obliterans	hemiplegia	serum
arteriolosclerosis	hemoptysis	sternum
atherosclerosis	hypertension	stroke
automatic speech	hypoxia	superior vena cava
capillaries	infarction	systole
cardiac cycle	inferior vena cava	TED hose
cerebral	interventricular	therapy
arteriosclerosis	septum	transient ischemic
cerebrovascular	ischemia	attack (TIA)
accident (CVA)	leukemia	thrombocyte
chronic brain	leukocytes	thrombi
syndrome	lumen	vasodilator
congestive heart	lymph	valve
failure	lymph node	veins
cor pulmonale	orthopneic position	ventricle
coronary occlusion	oxygenated	venule
demand pacer	myocardial infarct	

SUGGESTED ACTIVITIES

1. Using models, wall charts, or diagrams, learn the parts of the cardiovascular system.
2. Give supervised care to residents who suffer from cardiovascular disease.
3. Practice with classmates or a manikin the proper positioning for the post-stroke resident.

REVIEW

A. Brief Answer/Fill in the Blanks

1. The resident who is anemic should avoid unnecessary _____.

2. A resident complains of chest pain, is perspiring and anxious. You should suspect myocardial _____ and should summon _____.

3. A resident suffers from angina pectoris. She and her visitor get into an argument. You would intervene because the stress could _____ the disorder.

4. A resident suffering from congestive heart failure may be weighed daily to help determine _____.

5. When TED hose are used, they should be checked every_____ hours.

6. Residents with congestive heart failure are more comfortable in a _____ position as long as they are properly supported.

7. The resident with a pacer should have the _____ carefully checked.

8. Residents suffering from peripheral vascular disease should not _____ or use tobacco in any form.

9. A resident is 6-months post-stroke and still cannot move her left arm or leg. You know that the CVA has affected the _____ side of the brain.

10. A resident suffering from a stroke may have limited _____ skills.

B. Matching. Match the words on the left with the explanations on the right.

1. _____ upper heart chambers
2. _____ fluid in the tissue spaces
3. _____ vessels that carry blood away from the heart
4. _____ located close to the radius
5. _____ lower heart chambers
6. _____ name of heart muscle
7. _____ form of vascular disease in which plaques are formed in the walls of arteries
8. _____ diminished blood flow

a. edema
b. myocardial infarct
c. ventricles
d. ischemia
e. myocardium
f. radial artery
g. atria
h. valves
i. atherosclerosis
j. arteries

9. _____ separate upper heart chambers from
lower heart chambers

10. _____ death of heart tissue

C. **Identification.** Identify the parts of the heart and vessels indicated in the
diagram.

1. _____

2. _____

3. _____

4. _____

5. _____

6. _____

7. _____

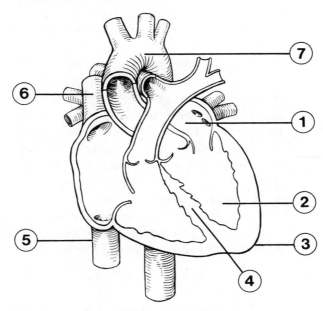

**CLINICAL
SITUATION**

Walter Rabinovitz has poor circulation in his feet. He is always complaining
that his feet are cold. When you give him morning care, he asks for a hot water
bag to put on his feet. How will you respond?

Answer: _____

_____

LESSON 22 The Gastrointestinal System

OBJECTIVES

After studying this lesson, you should be able to:

- Name the parts and function of the gastrointestinal system.
- Identify normal changes as they relate to the aging process.
- Practice safely carrying out procedures related to the gastrointestinal tract.
- Define and spell all the vocabulary words and terms.

The digestive tract processes food, transports and absorbs nutrients.

The digestive system processes the foods eaten, releasing simple nutrients that are needed by the body. You will remember that there are six nutrients: vitamins, minerals, water, fats used as fatty acid and glycerol, proteins used as amino acids, and carbohydrates. The nutrients and their role in the body are discussed in detail in Lesson 12. The nutrients in their simple forms pass through the wall of the intestinal tract, into the bloodstream and are transported to where they can be used by the body cells.

Chemicals (**enzymes**) help break down or digest the food and the non-digestible portion of what is eaten is eliminated from the body, in the bowel movement (BM), as solid waste called **feces**. Another term for bowel movement is **defecation**.

THE DIGESTIVE SYSTEM

The digestive system is also called the gastrointestinal tract (GI tract) or **alimentary canal**, figure 22–1. It is a tube about 30 feet long, stretching from the mouth to an opening called the **anus**. It consists of the true digestive organs (figure 22–2) which are the:

- mouth
- **pharynx**
- **esophagus**
- stomach
- small and large intestines

Accessory organs include the:

- liver
- pancreas
- gallbladder

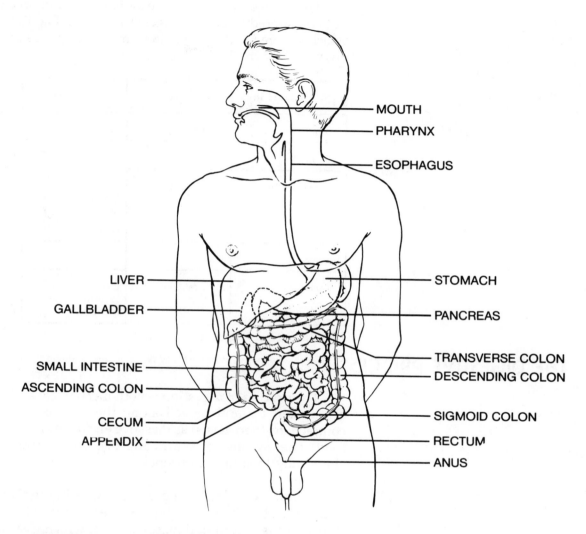

MOUTH
PHARYNX
ESOPHAGUS
LIVER
GALLBLADDER
SMALL INTESTINE
ASCENDING COLON
CECUM
APPENDIX
STOMACH
PANCREAS
TRANSVERSE COLON
DESCENDING COLON
SIGMOID COLON
RECTUM
ANUS

FIGURE 22–1. *The digestive system.*

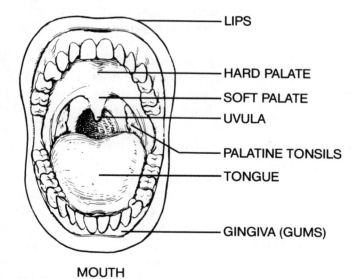

LIPS
HARD PALATE
SOFT PALATE
UVULA
PALATINE TONSILS
TONGUE
GINGIVA (GUMS)

MOUTH

FIGURE 22–2. *The mouth.*

The accessory organs contribute to the digestive process but are not considered to be true digestive organs. The liver produces bile, which is stored in the gallbladder, and the pancreas produces digestive enzymes, figure 22–3.

Produced in	Located in	Enzyme	Acts on
Mouth	Saliva	Salivary amylase	Starches
Stomach	Gastric juice	Pepsin	Protein
Small intestine	Intestinal juice	Maltase Lactase Maltase }	Sugars
		Peplidases	Protein
Liver	Bile		Fats
Pancreas	Pancreatic juice	Lipase Trypsin Amylase	Fats Protein Carbohydrates

FIGURE 22–3. Digestive enzymes.

THE DIGESTIVE PROCESS

The process of **digestion** is both mechanical and chemical. Foods are broken up and moved along the tract by rhythmic muscular contractions (**peristalsis**) as digestive enzymes and bile are mixed with food. The digestive enzymes and bile act to break the foods down chemically to simple nutrients.

The Mouth. The digestive process begins in the mouth as the teeth and tongue break the food into smaller pieces, mix it with saliva and form a **bolus** (a rounded mass) of food, which is swallowed into the pharynx and down the esophagus into the stomach. The teeth, numbering 32 in the adult, with care should last a lifetime. Many older persons, however, must rely on dentures to replace lost teeth.

The Stomach. The stomach is a hollow, muscular organ that is guarded by two circular muscles called **sphincter muscles**, one at each end. Contraction of the muscles allows food to remain in the stomach about 4 hours, where it is churned and mixed with the gastric juice to form liquid **chyme**. Protein digestion begins in the stomach and continues as the chyme moves into the small intestine.

Small Intestine. The small intestine is about 20 feet long, coiled in the abdominal cavity. It is divided into three parts: the **duodenum, jejunum,** and **ileum**. It is attached by the duodenum to the stomach and by the ileum to the large intestine.

Most absorption of nutrients takes place in the small intestines.

Bile (from the liver and gallbladder) and pancreatic juice (from the pancreas) flow from these organs into the duodenum. The bile prepares fat for further breakdown by the pancreatic enzyme **lipase**. The other digestive enzymes produced by the pancreas mix with the intestinal enzymes and the chyme and complete the digestive process. Most of the digestion and absorption of nutrients that are taken into the body in the forms shown in figure 22–4 takes place in the small intestine.

The Colon. The large intestine is called the **colon**. It extends from the end of the small intestine to the rectum, which ends in the anus. It is larger but not as long as the small intestine and, although its main purpose is to carry the unused food out of the body, some vitamins and water are absorbed through the colon walls. A sphincter muscle guards the anal opening and can be voluntarily controlled to relax and permit defecation.

Nutrient	Form Used	Function
Complex carbohydrates	Glucose	Supply blood sugar — primary energy for body
Proteins	Amino acids	Build and repair tissues
Fats	Fatty acids Glycerol	Supply stored energy; Needed to benefit from fat-soluble vitamins
Water	Water	Needed to carry on body chemistry
Vitamins	Fat-soluble — A,D K,E; Water-soluble — B,C	Act as co-enzymes in promoting body activities
Minerals	Calcium, phosphorus, potassium, sodium, and traces of others	Important in formation of body tissues and body chemistry

FIGURE 22–4. Basic nutrients and their functions.

AGING CHANGES

Aging lessens the efficiency of digestion and elimination.

As the body ages, the digestive process remains adequate but some changes do take place (figure 22–5):

- The flow of enzymes is somewhat diminished.
- The muscle walls of the tract lose some tone, so that movement along the tract is sluggish.
- The gag reflex that prevents food from slipping into the windpipe is not as active so there is greater likelihood of choking.
- Absorption of nutrients is slower.
- Constipation and **flatulence** (gas) are more common.

Some older persons find that foods they previously enjoyed are less well tolerated.

- Decreased taste buds
- Reduced digestive enzymes
- Thicker saliva
- Tongue more sensitive
- Peristalsis not as efficient
- Less effective gag reflex
- Poorer tolerance to some foods
- Slower absorption of nutrients
- Decreased chewing/poor dentures
- Weaker muscular walls

FIGURE 22–5. Digestive system changes associated with aging.

COMMON DIGESTIVE SYSTEM CONDITIONS

Hernias

A **hernia** occurs when a structure such as the intestines pushes out of its normal body position. Hernias are also known as **ruptures**. These may develop as the intestines or peritoneal membranes push through a weakened area in the abdominal wall.

There are different kinds of hernias, depending on location. Two hernias common to the elderly include:

- inguinal hernia
- hiatal hernia

Inguinal Hernia. This is a protrusion of the intestines through the wall in the groin area. It is felt as a small lump, especially when the resident strains.

Hiatal Hernia. In a hiatal hernia, the stomach protrudes upward into the thoracic cavity, through the normal opening that allows the esophagus to pass through the diaphragm to the stomach. Signs and symptoms of hiatal hernias include:

- difficulty swallowing (**dysphagia**)
- pain and pressure in the chest under the sternum, as food and gastric juice become trapped in the esophagus

The hydrochloric acid in the trapped juice can be very irritating, causing inflammation and ulceration of the esophagus.

Hiatal hernias tend to be a chronic recurrent problem. Residents feel better when they eat smaller meals and eat sitting up. They also feel more comfortable when sleeping when the head of the bed is raised. Antacids are sometimes ordered to overcome the acidity and reduce discomfort.

Inflammations

Inflammation anywhere along the gastrointestinal tract can cause distress and the possibility of tissue breakdown and the formation of ulcers. For example, inflammation of the stomach (**gastritis**) can lead to **dyspepsia** (indigestion). A combination of overeating, foods which are too spicy and natural aging changes can cause gastric distress. Also, ulcerations in the colon can cause blood in the stool and painful defecation.

Diverticulosis

Diverticuli are small, weakened areas in the wall of the colon. These areas form small pockets. Seeds and other hard food particles sometimes become trapped, causing inflammation (**diverticulitis**). When the diverticuli become inflamed, the resident complains of constipation, pain, and is more susceptible to infection.

Usually diverticuli are multiple and the condition is then called **diverticulosis**. Residents who have diverticulosis feel best when:

- eating a bland diet
- weight is controlled
- constipation is avoided

Sometimes the part of the bowel that is affected must be removed to correct the problem.

Malignancy

Malignancies, or cancers, of the digestive system occur frequently in older people. Cancers may occur anywhere along the tract, but commonly occur in the lower colon. Because the lumen of the large intestines is fairly big, cancer can grow inside the colon for a relatively long time before it becomes large enough to cause an obstruction or change the character of the feces.

OSTOMIES ▪▪▪▪▪▪▪▪▪▪▪▪▪▪▪▪▪▪▪▪▪▪▪▪▪▪▪▪▪▪▪▪▪▪▪▪▪

It may be necessary to surgically remove the section of the bowel which is cancerous and create an artificial opening in the abdominal wall for solid waste elimination. The opening is called an **ostomy**. When the colon is brought through the abdominal wall, the opening is called a **colostomy**, figure 22–6. The ostomy may be temporary or permanent.

As ostomy is an artificial opening.

Some surgical procedures bring the remaining section of the bowel through the wall after the diseased part of the bowel has been removed. This procedure forms a single colostomy. In other surgical procedures, a section of the bowel is removed and both ends of the remaining bowel are brought out of the abdominal wall, creating a "double-barreled" colostomy.

Evacuation through the ostomy or **stoma** (opening, or "mouth") cannot be voluntarily controlled in the same way that evacuation through the anus can. Proper diet can help residents have better control. The drainage that occurs may cause odor and irritation of the skin around the stoma. You can help the resident by:

- keeping the area around the stoma clean.
- assisting in irrigations as ordered.
- encouraging the resident to eat foods helpful in controlling elimination.

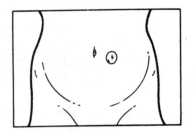

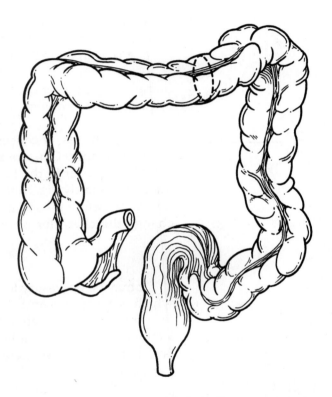

FIGURE 22–6. *Positions of colostomy stoma.*

If the colostomy is at a portion of the bowel where the stool is formed, regularity may be established and the drainage bag worn over the stoma gradually with a simple dressing. Tablets can be added in the bag to cut down on odors.

▮▮▮ PROCEDURE: Caring for a Stoma ▮▮▮▮▮▮▮▮▮▮▮▮▮▮▮▮▮▮▮▮▮▮▮▮▮▮▮

1. Wash hands and assemble the following equipment:
   a. washcloth/towel
   b. basin of warm water
   c. bath blanket
   d. bed protector
   e. bedpan
   f. disposable colostomy bag and belt

    g. disposable gloves
    h. skin lotion, as directed
    i. toilet tissue

2. Take equipment to bedside. Identify resident and explain what you plan to do.
3. Replace top bedclothes with bath blanket.
4. Place bed protector under resident's hips.
5. Put on disposable gloves.
6. Remove soiled disposable stoma bag and place in bedpan. Note amount and type of drainage.
7. Remove belt that holds stoma bag and save, if clean.
8. Gently clean area around stoma with toilet tissue to remove feces and drainage. Dispose of tissue in bedpan.
9. Wash area around stoma with soap and water.
10. Rinse thoroughly and dry.
11. If ordered, apply skin lotion lightly around the stoma; too much lotion may interfere with proper adhesion of fresh ostomy bag.
12. Position clean belt around resident. Inspect area for irritation or breakdown.
13. Place clean ostomy bag over stoma and secure to belt, (figure 22–7).
14. Remove bed protector. Check to be sure bottom bedding is not wet. Change if necessary.
15. Replace bath blanket with top bedding, making resident comfortable.
16. Gather soiled equipment and dispose of according to facility policy.
17. Clean bedpan and basin and return to unit.
18. Wash hands.
19. Report completion of task and your observations to nurse.
20. Record on resident's chart:
    a. procedure: ostomy care
    b. type and amount of drainage
    c. signs of irritation
    d. lotion applied, if any
    e. resident's reaction

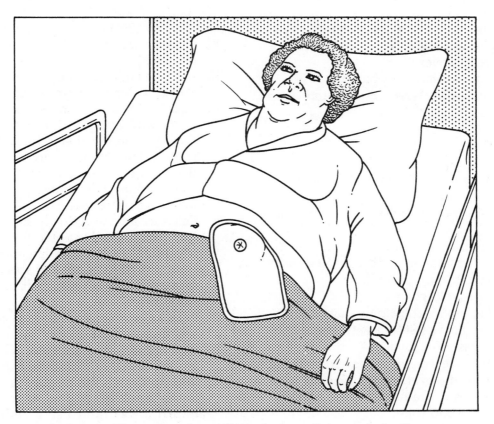

FIGURE 22–7. The ostomy bag collects drainage between irrigations.

Colostomy Irrigations_____

Nursing assistants may be assigned to irrigate permanent colostomies.

Initial colostomy irrigations are nursing responsibilities. The nurse will also teach the resident how to carry out the irrigation of the colostomy if the colostomy is to be permanent.

You will care for the stoma between irrigations, keeping it clean and dry and you may be assigned to assist in irrigating older, permanent colostomies. Protect the skin around the stoma according to facility policy. Some frequently used protectants are petroleum jelly, zinc oxide, and tincture of benzoin.

A wet colostomy is one that drains freely. A plastic solution of 10 percent Vinylite in alcohol is sometimes applied around the stoma. This acts as a coating that remains in contact with the skin for 12 to 24 hours and then is peeled away. The area is cleaned and a new film applied.

Commercially produced plastic colostomy bags can be positioned to collect the drainage and can be used for the irrigations. Whenever possible, use the resident's own equipment. Let the resident do as much as possible but lessen the resident's fatigue by preparing the solution and cleaning up the equipment after the irrigation is completed.

▆▆▆ PROCEDURE: Irrigating a Colostomy in the Bathroom ▆▆▆▆▆▆▆▆▆▆▆▆▆▆▆▆▆▆▆▆▆▆▆

1. Wash hands, check the orders, and assemble the following equipment in the resident's bathroom:
   a. irrigating can, tubing, and clamp
   b. connector and catheter
   c. disposable gloves
   d. disposable irrigating apparatus
   e. dressings for fresh ostomy bag and clean belt if needed
   f. lubricant
   g. toilet tissue
   h. washcloth and towel
   i. IV pole or other fixture to support irrigating can
2. Identify resident and explain what you plan to do.
3. Assist resident into bathroom.
4. Position resident on toilet and drape legs with towel (figure 22–8).
5. Put on disposable gloves.
6. Remove disposable colostomy bag or dressing. Cleanse area of stoma with tissue and dispose of tissue in toilet.
7. Apply disposable irrigating sleeve by placing faceplate directly over stoma. Secure with belt. Drop plastic drainage sheath between resident's legs into toilet.
8. Attach catheter to connector and then to tubing. Attach tubing to irrigating container.
9. Fill container with solution as ordered, usually 1000 to 2000 ml of warm tap water (100° to 105°F) or saline solution.
10. Place container on IV pole no more than 12 inches above colostomy site.
11. Allow a small amount of fluid to fill tubing and catheter to warm tubing and expel air.
12. Squeeze small amount of lubricant onto toilet tissue and apply to tip of catheter.
13. Gently insert catheter into stoma approximately 3 to 4 inches, using a rotating motion. If cone tip is used, press against stoma to control return flow. If resistance is met do not force, but inform nurse.
14. Release clamp and slowly allow approximately 500 ml of fluid to enter the ostomy. Flexing the tube between your fingers will allow you to control the amount and speed of flow. Stop immediately if resident complains of discomfort.
15. Remove catheter and allow return to flow into toilet. Note character of return.
16. Repeat procedure until returns are clear. This is a process that cannot be hurried and may take up to an hour. Be sure to check resident for fatigue. If resident becomes fatigued, return to bed and use a bedpan to collect returns.

16. Detach irrigating bag from belt and dispose of according to facility policy. You may flush the sleeve. Wash and dry for reuse.
17. Clean area around stoma with warm, soapy water. Rinse and dry thoroughly.
18. Apply small amount of lotion, if ordered.
19. Apply a small dressing or a clean ostomy bag and secure with belt.
20. Remove gloves and dispose of according to facility policy.
21. Assist resident back to bed.

22. Clean equipment and replace according to facility policy.
23. Wash hands.
24. Report completion of procedure and results to nurse.
25. Record on resident's chart:
    a. date and time
    b. procedure: colostomy irrigation
    c. solution used
    d. character and amount of returns
    e. resident's reaction to procedure

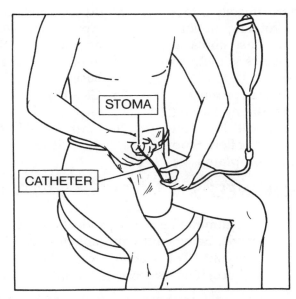

FIGURE 22–8. Irrigating the colostomy in the bathroom.

PROCEDURE: Irrigating an In-Bed Colostomy

1. Wash hands and assemble the following equipment:
   a. bed protector/bath blanket
   b. toilet tissue
   c. lubricant
   d. basin
   e. disposable gloves
   f. emesis basin lined with paper towels
   g. disposable irrigating apparatus
   h. IV pole to support irrigating can
   i. solution, as ordered
   j. washcloth and towel
   k. irrigating can, tubing, catheter, and connector
   l. dressing or fresh ostomy bag and belt

2. Identify resident and explain what you plan to do.
3. Replace top linen with bath blanket.
4. Position resident close to edge of bed, either sitting or in semi-Fowler's position.
5. Place protective bed covering in position.
6. Place bedpan on a chair beside bed.
7. Attach tubing, connector, and catheter to irrigating can. Clamp tubing.
8. Fill irrigating container with 1000 to 2000 ml of solution at 100° to 105°F.
9. Allow a small amount of fluid to flow through tubing to expel air.

10. Hang container from IV standard near bed, approximately 18 inches above stoma.
11. Place emesis basin on bed with concave surface next to resident.
12. Put on disposable gloves, remove dressing or disposable bag and place in emesis basin.
13. Clean gently around stoma with toilet tissue and dispose of tissue in emesis basin.
14. Apply disposable irrigation bag over stoma and place open end in bedpan so that return and drainage will flow into it.
15. Squeeze small amount of lubricant onto toilet tissue and apply to tip of catheter.
16. Gently insert catheter approximately 3 to 4 inches into stoma, using a rotating motion. If cone tip is used, press against stoma to control return flow. If resistance is met, do not force but inform nurse.
17. Release clamp and slowly allow approximately 500 ml of fluid to enter the ostomy. Flexing the tube between your fingers will allow you to control the amount and speed of flow. Stop immediately if resident complains of discomfort.
18. Remove catheter and allow return to flow into bedpan. Note character of return.
19. Repeat procedure until returns are clear. This process cannot be hurried and may take up to an hour. Be sure to check resident for fatigue. Stop procedure and allow resident to rest.
20. Detach irrigating bag from belt and dispose of according to facility policy. You may flush the sleeve. Wash and dry for reuse.
21. Clean area around stoma with warm, soapy water. Rinse and dry thoroughly.
22. Apply small amount of lotion if ordered.
23. Apply a small dressing or a clean ostomy bag and secure with belt.
24. Remove gloves and dispose of in emesis basin.
25. Clean equipment and replace according to facility policy.
26. Wash hands. Report completion of procedure. Record and report observations.

ASSISTING ELIMINATION NEEDS

Eliminating waste products regularly is one of the basic human needs. Being **continent** (able to control elimination) is important to everyone. The inability to predict and control elimination (**incontinence**) hinders social interaction. You should remember these terms:

- A continent resident — one who is able to control elimination.
- An incontinent resident — one who has no control over elimination.

The Continent Resident

You have specific responsibilities in helping continent residents to meet their elimination. needs. You must:

- Be aware of the resident's need to reach the proper facilities on time. Be observant so that you can be available to help the resident reach the toilet or commode, figure 22–9. Answer call bells promptly for residents who use a bedpan.
- Always note and chart the frequency and character of the excreta.

Normal feces should be brown in color; formed but soft. Record bowel movements on the health record and report anything unusual about the bowel movement. For example:

- Infections and medications such as antibiotics can cause loose or watery stools.
- Iron can make the stool black and can make the stool loose in some residents while constipating others.

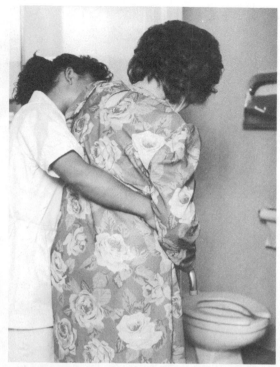

FIGURE 22–9. Be observant so that you can help the resident reach the toilet on time.

- **Hemorrhoids** (**piles**) are distended blood vessels (varicose veins) in the rectum and can sometimes bleed. The blood may show red in the stool or make the stool unusually dark.

▪▪▪ PROCEDURE: Giving and Receiving Bedpan ▪▪▪▪▪▪▪▪▪▪▪▪▪▪▪▪▪▪▪▪▪▪▪▪▪▪▪

1. Wash hands and assemble the following equipment:
   a. bedpan and cover (figure 22-10)
   b. toilet tissue
   c. basin of warm water
   d. soap
   e. washcloth and towel
2. Identify resident and explain what you plan to do.
3. Screen unit.
4. Lower head of bed.
5. Place bedpan on bedside chair. Never place it on side stand or overbed table. Put tissue on bedside stand within easy reach of resident. Place remaining articles on bedside table.
6. Place bedpan cover at foot of bed between mattress and springs. The bedpan may be warmed by running hot water into it and emptying it. In hot weather, talcum powder may be used on the bedpan to prevent the resident's skin from sticking to it. Plastic bedpans may be comfortable without warming.
7. Fold top bedclothes back at a right angle and raise resident's gown. Pad bedpan with folded towel if resident is thin or has pressure sores.
8. Ask resident to flex knees and rest weight on heels, if possible.
9. Help resident to raise buttocks by putting one hand under small of resident's back and lifting gently and slowly with one hand. With other hand, place bedpan under resident's hips. If resident is unable to raise buttocks, two assistants may be needed to lift, or pan may be placed by rolling resident to one side, positioning bedpan against buttocks, and

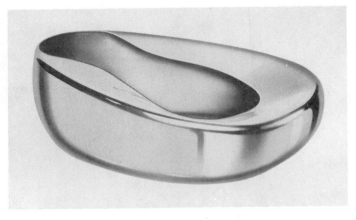

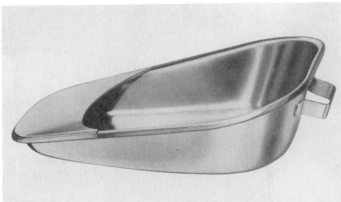

FIGURE 22–10. Regular adult bedpan (top), orthopedic bedpan (bottom).

rolling resident back on it, figure 22–11. Alternately, if a trapeze is in place over bed, you can place bedpan under the resident as he or she raises himself or herself using trapeze, figure 22–12. Resident's buttocks should rest on rounded shelf of bedpan. The narrow end should face foot of bed.

10. Replace top bedclothes. Raise head of bed to a comfortable height.

11. Make sure signal cord is within easy reach of resident. Leave resident alone unless contraindicated.

12. Answer resident's call signal immediately. Fill basin with warm water. Lower head of bed.

13. Ask resident to flex knees and rest weight on heels. Place on hand under small of back and lift gently to help raise buttocks off bedpan. Remove bedpan with other hand. Cover bedpan and place on the chair.
    a. If resident is unable to raise buttocks, two assistants may be needed to lift. Otherwise, roll resident off pan to side and remove pan. Lift and move carefully,

holding pan firmly with one hand.
    b. Many residents have difficulty cleaning adequately after using bedpan. You may need to clean and dry resident yourself.

14. Assist resident to clean area of bed. Discard tissue in bedpan unless specimen is to be collected. Cover the bedpan again and place on chair. Cleanse resident with warm water and soap.

15. Replace bedclothes. Encourage the resident to wash hands and freshen up after procedure. Change linen or protective pads as necessary.

16. Take bedpan to the bathroom or utility room and observe and note contents. Measure, if required.

17. Empty bedpan. Rinse with cold water and disinfectant; rinse, dry, and cover bedpan.

18. Put bedpan inside resident's bedside table. Clean and replace other articles.

19. Wash hands. Leave unit in order.

20. Report any unusual observations to nurse and chart according to facility policy.

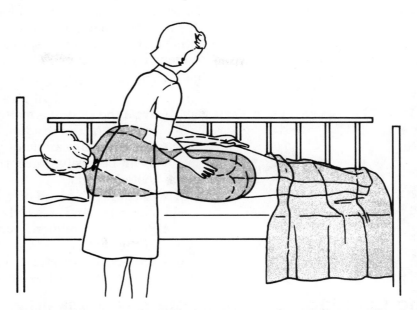

FIGURE 22–11. *The assistant rolls the patient away from her. She supports the patient with one hand on her hip and arm and places the bedpan with her other hand. Then she rolls the patient toward her and onto the bedpan.*

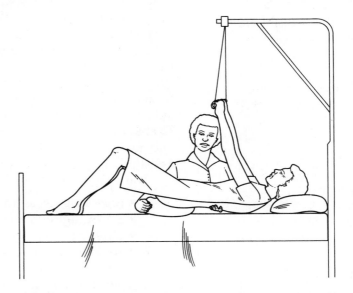

FIGURE 22–12. *The patient assists by lifting herself with the trapeze as the assistant places the bedpan under her. Note that the assistant supports the patient's back with her hand.*

The Incontinent Resident_____

Incontinence is very stressful for the resident.

Incontinence is embarrassing and uncomfortable. Feces can be very irritating to the skin and unpleasant for the resident. The stool may be soft and formed or loose and watery. The incontinence may be occasional or frequent. Bowel incontinence may be temporary or may require retraining.

Diarrhea. The elimination of loose, watery stools is called **diarrhea**. This may be caused by infection, intolerance to food or fecal impaction. You have specific responsibilities in caring for the incontinent resident with diarrhea. You must:

- Check the resident frequently for soiling.
- Clean the resident as soon as evacuation occurs.
- Treat the care in a matter-of-fact manner. Be sensitive to the feelings of the resident.
- Be especially careful of handwashing. If infection is present, it can be easily transferred to yourself or others on contaminated hands.
- Encourage a bland diet, if ordered. This kind of diet is easily digestible and has little bulk to irritate the colon.
- Report the frequency and character of the bowel movement to the nurse.
- Provide the resident with room deodorizers as needed to assure an odor-free environment.

The Constipated Resident_____

Constipation — look for
- loss of appetite
- complaints of abdominal pain
- distension

The resident with the problem of **constipation** (difficulty in evacuating bowels) may not have any appetite and may complain of abdominal discomfort. The abdomen may be distended. If **fecal impaction** — the most serious form of constipation — is present, there may be frequent, small evacuation of diarrhea.

Fecal impaction results when the fecal mass loses so much water that it becomes dehydrated and difficult to eliminate. The dried waste acts as an irritant to the bowel. Mucus tends to dissolve the outer part of the mass, which then drains from the bowel as diarrhea. Whenever there are frequent, small amounts of diarrhea, this should be reported, and the resident should be checked for impaction.

In some facilities, nursing assistants are permitted to check for fecal impaction and report their findings, so that an order for a bowel aid such as a **suppository** or **enema** can be ordered and given for relief. To check for fecal impaction, the resident must be in the Sims position and not sitting on the toilet. Be sure your facility permits nursing assistants to perform this procedure before you undertake to do so.

You may assist the constipated resident by:

- Encouraging as much activity as possible.
- Encouraging a high-roughage diet.
- Offering fluids frequently.
- Assisting the resident to the bathroom and allowing adequate time for defecation.
- Administering bowel aids as ordered.

Nursing assistants may give oil-retention enemas, soapsuds enemas and, in some facilities, are permitted to insert lubricating suppositories. Each of these procedures requires a specific order.

■■■ PROCEDURE: Checking for Fecal Impaction ■■■■■■■■■■■■■■■■■■■■■■■■■■■

Note: Check the facility policy to be sure that this is a nursing assistant function.

1. Wash hands.
2. Assemble the following equipment:

a. disposable glove
b. lubricant
c. protective pad
d. bath blanket
e. toilet tissue
f. basin of warm water
g. washcloth and towel

3. Identify resident and explain what you plan to do.
4. Draw curtains for privacy.
5. Raise bed to comfortable working height.
6. Lower side rails on side closest to you.
7. Ask resident to raise hips.
8. Place bed protector under hips.
9. Turn resident to lay on side, facing away from you.
10. Cover with bath blanket and fanfold top bedclothes to foot of bed.
11. Put disposable glove on your dominant hand.
12. Lubricate index finger of that hand.
13. Ask resident to take deep breath and bear down as you insert lubricated finger into rectum. *Note:* Rectum should feel soft and pliable. You may feel no feces or you may feel a soft stool, a large solid mass, or multiple hard formations.
14. Withdraw finger. *Note:* If a spontaneous bowel movement occurs, note amount and character.
15. Wash the resident's buttocks with warm water and dry.
16. Assist the resident onto back.
17. Ask resident to raise hips and withdraw bed protector.
18. Remove protector and glove, folding from outside to inside-out, and place on chair.
19. Pull bedding up and remove bath blanket.
20. Fold bath blanket and place in bedside table.
21. Make resident comfortable.
22. Raise side rail.
23. Leave call bell within reach.
24. Empty basin and dry. Return to bedside table.
25. Put towel and washcloth in laundry hamper.
26. Dispose of protector and glove according to facility policy.
27. Wash hands and report completion of procedure and findings to nurse.

Enemas

An enema is the introduction of fluid into the rectum, through the anal sphincter to remove feces (**stool**) or **flatus** (gas). The fluid is expelled a short time after introduction, along with the waste products. The need to empty the bowel is signaled by a feeling of urgency. Sometimes a small amount of warm oil is given to soften the stool (oil-retention enema) and then is followed by a cleansing enema of soapsuds, figure 22–13.

Pre-packaged enema solutions may be used, but since they contain sodium, which is poorly tolerated by many older people, they are not often prescribed. When possible, enemas should be given before breakfast or morning care. There must be a specific order for an enema before it is given.

▧▧▧ PROCEDURE: Giving Oil-Retention Enema ▧▧▧▧▧▧▧▧▧▧▧▧▧▧▧▧▧▧▧▧▧▧▧▧▧▧▧▧

1. Wash hands and assemble the following equipment:
   a. prepackaged oil-retention enema
   b. bedpan and cover
   c. towel, soap, and basin with water
   d. toilet tissue
   e. bath blanket
   f. bed protector
2. Identify resident and explain what you plan to do. Instruct resident that it will be necessary to hold in the solution for at least 20 minutes.
3. Place chair at foot of bed; cover with towel. Place bedpan on chair.
4. Cover resident with bath blanket and fanfold top linen to foot of bed.
5. Place bed protector under buttocks.
6. Help resident assume the Sims' position.
7. Open prepackaged oil-retention enema.

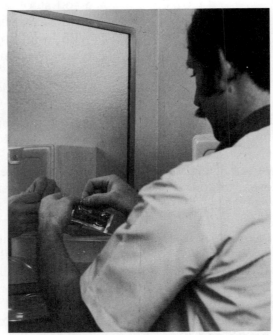

FIGURE 22–13. *Preparing to administer a soapsuds enema using a disposable kit.*

8. Expose resident's anus. Remove cap from enema container. Instruct resident to take a deep breath and insert pre-lubricated tip into anus.
9. Squeeze container until all the solution has entered the rectum.
10. Remove container and place in package box to be discarded.
11. Encourage resident to remain on side.
12. Check resident every 5 minutes until fluid has been retained for 20 minutes.
13. Position resident on bedpan or assist to bathroom.
14. If resident is on bedpan, raise head of bed to comfortable height.
15. Place toilet tissue and signal cord within easy reach of resident. If resident is in bathroom, stay nearby.
16. Dispose of expendable material per facility policy.
17. Remove bedpan or assist resident to return to bed. Observe and note contents of bedpan or toilet. Cover pan and dispose of in flush toilet.
18. Give resident basin of soap, water, and towel to wash and dry his or her hands.
19. Replace top bedclothes and remove bath blanket and bed protector. Dispose of protector according to facility policy. Fold bath blanket and return to bedside stand.
20. Report completion of task and results to nurse.
21. Wash hands and enter on chart:
    a. date and time
    b. procedure: oil-retention enema
    c. return (color, consistency, flatus, unusual characteristics)
    d. resident reaction to procedure

▪▪▪ PROCEDURE: Giving Soapsuds Enema ▪▪▪▪▪▪▪▪▪▪▪▪▪▪▪▪▪▪▪▪▪▪▪▪▪▪▪▪▪▪▪▪▪▪

1. Wash hands. Obtain disposable enema equipment, which is commercially available, consisting of a plastic container, tubing, clamp, and lubricant.
   a. Connect tubing to solution container.
   b. Adjust clamp on tubing and snap shut.
   c. Fill container with warm water (105°F) to the 1000-ml line.
   d. Open packet of liquid soap and put soap in the water.

e. Using the tip of the tubing, mix solution gently so that no suds form.

f. Run small amount of solution through tube to get rid of air and to warm tube.

2. If disposable equipment is not available, you will need:
   a. a funnel
   b. tubing and clamp
   c. graduated pitcher with warm, soapy water (105°F)
   d. connecting tube
   e. rectal tube

3. Take the following equipment to bedside:
   a. disposable enema unit as in step #1 or items listed in step #2.
   b. lubricant
   c. toilet tissue, bedpan and cover
   d. towel, soap, and water-filled basin
   e. bath blanket
   f. bed protector (Chux)
   g. IV pole

4. Identify resident and explain what you plan to do. Screen unit.

5. Place chair at foot of bed and cover with towel. Place bedpan on chair.

6. Cover resident with bath blanket and fanfold top linen to foot of bed.

7. Place bed protector under buttocks.

8. Help resident to turn on left side and flex knees (Sims' position).

9. Place container of solution on chair so tubing can reach resident. Lubricate tip.

10. Adjust bath blanket to expose anal area.

11. Expose anus by raising upper buttock.

12. Insert tube. Never force tube. If tube cannot be inserted easily, get help. There may be an impaction.

13. Open the clamp, raise container 12 inches above anus and hang it on the IV pole so that the fluid flows in slowly, figure 22–14. Ask resident to take deep breaths to relax the abdomen. If the resident complains of cramping, clamp tube and wait until resident is comfortable. Then open the tubing to continue fluid flow.

14. When enough solution has been given, clamp the tubing.

15. Instruct resident to hold breath while upper buttock is raised and tube is gently withdrawn.

16. Wrap tubing in paper towel. Put in disposable container.

17. Place resident on bedpan or assist to bathroom.

18. Raise head of bed to comfortable height if resident is on bedpan.

19. Place toilet tissue and signal cord within reach of resident. If in bathroom, stay nearby.

20. Take tray with used equipment to utility room. Rinse enema equipment thoroughly in cool water and then wash in warm soapy water. Return it to bedside or discard according to facility policy.

21. Remove bedpan or assist resident back to bed and observe contents.

22. Give resident soap, water and towel to wash hands.

23. Replace top bedding and remove bath blanket. Air room. Leave room in order.

24. Clean and replace all other equipment used, according to facility policy. Wash hands.

25. Report completion of procedure and results to nurse.

26. Chart:
    a. date and time
    b. procedure: enema (type, amount, and temperature of solution)
    c. return (color, consistency, unusual materials, flatus)
    d. resident reaction to procedure

PROCEDURE: Inserting Lubricating Suppository

1. Wash hands and assemble the following equipment:
   a. suppository, as ordered
   b. lubricant
   c. toilet tissue
   d. gloves
   e. bedpan and cover if ordered

2. Identify resident and explain what you plan to do.

3. Draw curtains for privacy. Help person assume left Sims' position.

4. Expose buttocks only.

5. Put on gloves and unwrap suppository.

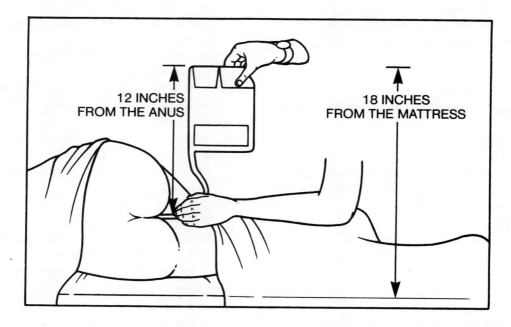

12 INCHES
FROM THE ANUS

18 INCHES
FROM THE MATTRESS

FIGURE 22–14. Container of soapsuds should not be higher than 12 inches from the anus.

6. With left hand, separate buttocks, exposing anus.
7. Apply small amount of lubricant to anus and insert suppository. It must be inserted deeply enough to enter the rectum beyond the sphincter (approximately 2 inches), figure 22–15.
8. Encourage resident to take deep breaths and relax until the need to defecate is experienced, approximately 5 to 15 minutes.
9. Remove gloves and dispose of according to facility policy.
10. Adjust the bedclothes and help resident assume a comfortable position.
11. Place call bell near resident's hand.
12. Check resident every 5 minutes.
13. After 15 minutes, assist resident to bathroom or on bedpan.
14. Report completion of procedure and results to nurse.
15. Record time of insertion, type of suppository, and results on chart.

Collecting a Stool Specimen

There may be occasions when it will be necessary to collect a stool specimen, figure 22–16. This is usually the case when infection or bleeding in the colon are suspected. When carrying out this task:

- Make sure to collect the specimen in a bedpan or commode.
- Do not allow the specimen to touch the outside of collection container.
- Use throatsticks to handle the specimen.
- Make sure that the specimen is properly labeled and promptly transported.

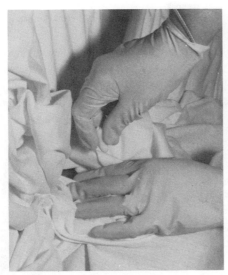

FIGURE 22–15. Expose the anus and insert the suppository approximately two inches.

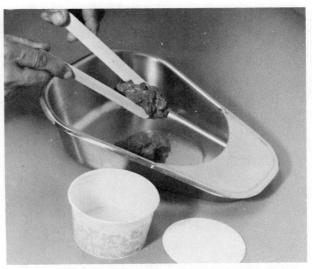

FIGURE 22–16. Use tongue blades to transfer the stool specimen from the bedpan to the specimen container.

▧▧▧ PROCEDURE: Collecting Stool Specimen ▪▪▪▪▪▪▪▪▪▪▪▪▪▪▪▪▪▪▪▪▪▪▪▪▪▪▪

1. Make out label including: resident's full name, room number, date and time of collection, doctor's name, examination to be performed, and other information as requested.
2. Wash hands and assemble the following equipment:
   a. specimen container and cover
   b. tongue blades
3. Follow the procedure for giving and receiving the bedpan, through step 15.
4. Take the covered bedpan containing the specimen to the utility room.
5. Use tongue blades to remove specimen from bedpan and place in specimen container. Discard tongue blade.
6. Wash hands. Do not contaminate outside of container.
7. Cover container and attach completed label. Make sure that cover is on container tightly.
8. Clean and replace equipment, according to facility policy.
9. Take or send specimen promptly to laboratory.
10. Wash hands. Report completion of task to nurse.
11. Record procedure on resident's chart.

Bowel Retraining___

When bowel incontinence is a problem, a retraining program may be undertaken. There are several steps in this process:

- Assess bowel pattern.
- Check for fecal impaction.
- Clear the colon.
- Establish regularity.
- Administer bowel aids, when necessary.
- Assist the defecation process.

Assessment. The retraining process is planned after the nurse has made an assessment of the resident's bowel pattern and emotional and physical status, figure 22-17. Your observations regarding the resident can be very helpful to the nurse in this evaluation:

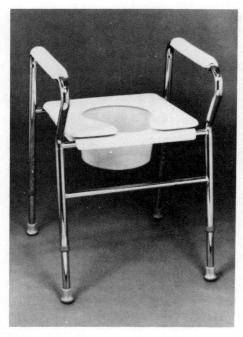
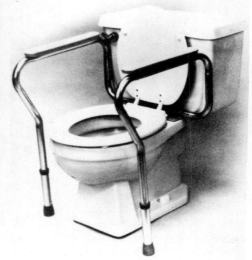
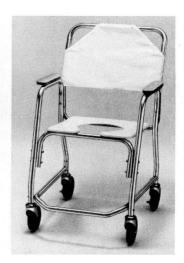

FIGURE 22–17. Proper facilities help the resident during the retraining period. (Courtesy of Invacare Corporation).

Bowel retraining takes time, patience, and consistency.

- Keep a record of the time of each bowel movement.
- Note the character of each bowel movement.

Check for Fecal Impaction. The next step is to make sure that there is no fecal impaction. This can be done by examining the rectum with a lubricated, gloved finger.

Clear the Colon. To clear the colon, it may be necessary to give an oil enema, followed by a soapsuds enema.

Establish Regularity. The key to all bowel training is regularity. During the retraining program, you will learn when the resident usually has an evacuation and you will plan to help him or her to the bathroom or commode at the appropriate time.

Administer Bowel Aids. You may be instructed to administer bowel aids such as rectal suppositories or contact laxatives. Be sure to be available when the resident needs help. You must place the suppository or contact laxative high against the bowel wall, about 2 inches beyond the anus and not into a fecal mass.

Assist the Defecation Process. If the resident has difficulty defecating:

1. Instruct him or her to take a deep breath and bear down with the abdominal muscles while you massage the abdomen with a downward, or circular motion.
2. Make sure that the resident is seated properly with feet flat on the floor, or on the bedpan, comfortably supported. Guard rails add a sense of security.

3. Provide privacy and maintain an unhurried attitude.
4. Offer resident something warm to drink since warm drinks may stimulate peristalsis.
5. Be patient and available.

During the bowel retraining period, you will need to encourage the resident to be as active as possible and to eat a well-balanced, roughage-containing diet. Offer water frequently. Regaining continence raises the resident's self-esteem and is an important step in rehabilitation. Your positive attitude is an important factor in helping a resident to successfully manage elimination needs.

VOCABULARY

alimentary canal	dysphagia	incontinence
anus	dyspepsia	inguinal hernia
bolus	enema	jejunum
chyme	enzymes	lipase
colon	esophagus	ostomy
colostomy	excreta	peristalsis
constipation	fecal impaction	pharynx
continent	feces	piles
defecation	flatulence	rupture
diarrhea	flatus	sphincter muscle
digestion	gastritis	stoma
diverticuli	hemorrhoids	stool
diverticulitis	hernia	suppository
diverticulosis	hiatal hernia	urgency
duodenum	ileum	

SUGGESTED ACTIVITIES

1. Review the parts of the gastrointestinal system, using diagrams or wall charts.

2. Review Lesson 12, "Special Needs of the Geriatric Person."

3. With a partner or manikin, practice procedures designed to promote elimination.

4. Under supervision, carry out procedures that you have practiced with selected residents.

REVIEW

A. Brief Answer/Fill in the Blanks

1. Name the six nutrients needed by the body.

a. _____

b. _____

c. _____

d. _____

e. _____

f. _____

2. Name the true digestive organs.

   a. _____

   b. _____

   c. _____

   d. _____

   e. _____

3. In the elderly, peristalsis is _____, absorption is _____, and the gag reflex is _____.

4. Gastrointestinal conditions common to the elderly include _____ hernia, _____, inflammations, diverticulosis, and _____.

5. When a resident has a colostomy, the opening, called the _____, must be kept _____ and _____.

6. When giving a colostomy irrigation the irrigating tip should be inserted approximately _____ inches into the stoma, using a _____ motion.

7. When the resident experiences urgency following an enema, it means that _____.

8. The best position for the resident receiving an enema is on the _____ with the knees flexed.

9. The resident should be encouraged to retain an oil enema approximately _____ minutes.

10. When collecting a stool specimen, use _____ to transfer the sample from the bedpan to the specimen container.

B. **Identification.** In the diagram shown, label the digestive system:

   1. _____
   2. _____
   3. _____
   4. _____
   5. _____
   6. _____
   7. _____
   8. _____
   9. _____

CLINICAL SITUATION

Jessica Beebe, 79, is assigned to your care. She seems rather listless, complaining of an upset stomach and cramps. She refuses breakfast and you note some fecal soiling on the bedding. When you ask her about her last bowel movement, she can't remember. You report the situation to the charge nurse, who examines the resident for fecal impaction. You are told to give a soapsuds enema. List the equipment and fluid you will assemble.

Answer: _____

_____

_____

_____

SECTION V Achievement Review, Part A

A. **Multiple Choice.** Select the one best answer to each of the following:

1. The organ that pumps blood around the body is the
   a. liver
   b. spleen
   c. brain
   d. heart
   e. capillaries

2. Blood vessels that carry oxygenated blood are called
   a. arteries
   b. venules
   c. veins
   d. capillaries
   e. lymphatics

3. The artery that is close to the femur is called
   a. posterior
   b. femoral
   c. radial
   d. sternal
   e. brachial

4. The disease that causes a decrease in the number or quality of erythrocytes is called
   a. leukemia
   b. cerebrovascular accident
   c. anemia
   d. hemophilia
   e. atherosclerosis

5. Excessively high blood pressure is known as
   a. hypertension
   b. TIA
   c. CVA
   d. hypotension
   e. aphasia

6. Which of the following is a true digestive organ?
   a. gallbladder
   b. stomach
   c. liver
   d. spleen
   e. heart

7. Most of the digestion and absorption take place in the
   a. colon
   b. mouth
   c. stomach
   d. pancreas
   e. small intestine

8. Solid waste excreted through the digestive tract is known as
   a. feces
   b. stool
   c. BM
   d. all of the above
   e. none of the above

9. Rhythmic waves that move food along the digestive tract are known as
   a. micturition
   b. defecation
   c. peristalsis
   d. cardiac cycle
   e. voiding

10. The number of adult teeth is normally
    a. 20 teeth
    b. 32 teeth
    c. 45 teeth
    d. 50 teeth
    e. 60 teeth

11. A resident has anemia. You know that
    a. he may suffer from dizziness
    b. his pulse rate will probably be low
    c. his skin will be rosy
    d. he will feel clear-headed
    e. none of the above

12. A resident with arteriosclerosis obliterans is sitting with her legs crossed. You had best
    a. rub her feet
    b. suggest that she sit with her legs uncrossed
    c. allow her to wear circular garters
    d. suggest that she sit with her ankles crossed
    e. tie her shoes tighter so they won't fall off

13. A resident is 87 years old. What would be considered a high but normal blood pressure for a person her age?
    a. 90/50
    b. 100/66
    c. 120/80
    d. 150/90
    e. 190/100

14. A resident has a history of TIA. You should report to the nurse that he
    a. seems talkative
    b. has a momentary loss of consciousness
    c. has an improved appetite
    d. is playing cards
    e. has a visitor

15. The resident has had a stroke. Something helpful you can do is to
    a. be consistently calm and positive
    b. let the resident know when you are depressed
    c. tease the resident when she can't find the right words to say
    d. do everything for the resident
    e. keep the resident in bed as long as possible

16. The resident with a stroke has aphasia. He repeatedly says a swear word. You know
    a. he is frustrated and swearing at you
    b. he is angry about the care he is getting
    c. this is called automatic speech and you should be insulted
    d. this is the only word he remembers
    e. this is called automatic speech and means nothing

17. If a resident is nicked while you are shaving him, you had best
    a. use light, long strokes for the remaining areas
    b. let the area bleed until it stops
    c. apply pressure directly over the area
    d. forget the matter, since it isn't serious
    e. tell another nursing assistant

18. Because the skin changes with age, you will
    a. rarely wash the resident
    b. give a total bath two or three times a week
    c. only give showers
    d. give a bath every day
    e. give a bath both morning and night

19. Routine foot care includes
    a. bathing the feet
    b. massaging the feet
    c. trimming toenails
    d. applying lotion
    e. all of the above

20. A resident's position should be changed at least every
    a. 2 hours   c. 4 hours   e. 8 hours
    b. 3 hours   d. 6 hours

21. When dressing a resident, you should
    a. offer many choices
    b. choose only dark colors
    c. arrange the clothes in the order to be donned
    d. always put clothes on the unaffected side first
    e. none of the above

22. The resident is to have a Sitz bath. You understand that you will
    a. soak the hands in warm water
    b. have the resident sit in warm water
    c. apply an icepack
    d. apply an Aqua-K pad
    e. give a cooling sponge bath

23. The temperature of a continuous heat unit, such as an Aqua-K pad, should be about
    a. 60–65°F   c. 95–100°F   e. 115–125°F
    b. 80–85°F   d. 105–115°F

24. When using a heat lamp, the distance from the resident
    a. is not important
    b. need not be measured
    c. can be easily measured with your eye
    d. must be at least 18 inches
    e. should be at least 25 inches away

25. After soaking a body part you
    a. pat gently to dry
    b. rub vigorously
    c. leave the area wet
    d. allow the area to air dry
    e. wrap in a towel to dry

B. **Brief Answer/Fill in the Blanks.** Write or orally present brief answers to the following:

1. List four ways you can help the resident with poor circulation to the legs:

    a. _____

    b. _____

    c. _____

    d. _____

2. List five nursing assistant responsibilities while caring for the resident who has had a CVA:

a. _____

b. _____

c. _____

d. _____

e. _____

3. List three special nursing assistant responsibilities while caring for a resident suffering from congestive heart failure:

a. _____

b. _____

c. _____

4. List three observations about the resident with a pacemaker that you should report to the nurse:

a. _____

b. _____

c. _____

5. List four functions of the skin:

a. _____

b. _____

c. _____

d. _____

6. Your resident uses an ambulatory aid. List four ways you can improve the resident's safety:

a. _____

b. _____

c. _____

d. _____

7. Name two ways of supporting a fracture and explain the nursing care:

a. _____

_____

b. _____

_____

8. Describe four actions you should take when applying a hot water bag:

a. _____

b. _____

c. _____

d. _____

9. Describe three observations that should be reported, if noted, during the application of cold treatments:

   a. _____

   b. _____

   c. _____

10. List four things you should know before giving a hot or cold temperature application:

   a. _____

   b. _____

   c. _____

   d. _____

C. **Matching.** Match the words on the right with the explanations on the left.

   1. _____ hardening of the arteries

   2. _____ difference between apical heart rate and radial pulse rate

   3. _____ excessive perspiration

   4. _____ food that has been broken down into a liquid

   5. _____ permanent shortening of a muscle

   6. _____ removal of dead tissue

   7. _____ fluid in the abdomen

   8. _____ artificial opening in abdominal wall

   9. _____ decubitus ulcer

   10. _____ unable to voluntarily control elimination

   a. diaphoresis
   b. incontinent
   c. contracture
   d. atherosclerosis
   e. debridement
   f. acities
   g. chyme
   h. alignment
   i. ostomy
   j. pressure sore
   k. gait belt
   l. pulse deficit
   m. ambulatory aid

D. **Word Search.** Place a circle around the word in the diagram that is described in the list below. Identify by horizontal line number or vertical line letter.

   1. _____ making a blood vessel smaller

   2. _____ death of a tissue

   3. _____ another name for a cerebrovascular accident

   4. _____ eliminating solid wastes

   5. _____ the act of processing and absorbing nutrients

   6. _____ solid wastes

7. _____ yellow discoloration of the skin

8. _____ treatment that decreases body temperature

9. _____ break in a bone

10. _____ the second layer of skin

	a	b	c	d	e	f	g	h	i	j	k	l	m	n
1	A	D	O	F	G	T	V	C	I	J	Q	R	B	Z
2	N	B	P	D	M	K	A	B	E	A	T	D	Q	R
3	L	D	C	N	Q	B	S	T	R	O	K	E	S	T
4	U	W	J	K	V	A	O	C	M	Z	B	F	X	A
5	A	O	A	T	R	O	C	K	F	E	C	E	S	L
6	B	D	U	P	Q	E	O	A	N	M	X	C	Y	T
7	R	C	N	A	D	M	N	Q	P	T	Z	A	A	F
8	F	T	D	O	R	N	S	E	I	O	R	T	C	B
9	A	D	I	G	E	S	T	I	O	N	E	I	O	N
10	Q	B	C	T	O	M	R	N	T	E	Q	O	A	D
11	V	O	E	X	T	E	I	O	N	B	C	N	D	F
12	A	N	M	F	R	A	C	T	U	R	E	O	E	T
13	I	N	F	A	R	C	T	I	O	N	A	D	R	C
14	R	Y	Z	K	L	E	I	X	W	T	I	E	M	S
15	F	Q	C	H	Y	P	O	T	H	E	R	M	I	A
16	C	N	O	P	R	A	N	D	F	A	N	O	S	P
17	R	X	T	A	D	P	B	M	B	T	I	N	W	V

E. **Demonstrations.** Your teacher may wish to have you demonstrate or role play some of the following. Select a partner, select equipment, and follow the instructions that follow.

1. Demonstrate ROM exercises for the upper extremities.

2. Demonstrate ROM exercises for the neck.

3. Demonstrate ROM exercises for the lower extremities.

4. Explain your understanding of decubitus ulcer care; include stages and interventions.

5. Demonstrate the proper techniques for assisting a resident from bed into a wheelchair.

6. Show the technique of using a mechanical lift to assist a resident from a wheelchair into bed.

7. Show the proper body mechanics for both the resident and yourself where lifting or turning is required.

8. Tell the proper procedure for admitting a patient.

9. Explain how you would handle a resident who insists on crossing his or her legs when it is contraindicated.

10. Demonstrate the proper technique for determining an apical pulse.

LESSON 23 The Urinary System

After studying this lesson, you should be able to:

- Name the parts and function of the urinary system.
- Identify normal changes as they relate to the aging process.
- Give proper care to residents with conditions which involve the urinary system.
- Define and spell all the vocabulary words and terms.

The urinary system is composed of the kidneys which filter blood and form urine and the tubes which carry the urine to the outside, figure 23–1.

THE KIDNEYS

The kidneys are two bean-shaped organs about 6 inches long found on either side of the spinal column in the lumbar area. They are made up of the:

The urinary system
- forms urine
- stores urine
- excretes urine

- **Cortex** — the dark reddish brown outer part that contains the urine-producing unit called the **nephron**.
- **Medulla** — the lighter colored middle part made up of tubules that receive the formed urine.
- **Renal pelvis** — the central basin-like area into which the formed urine passes. The pelvis directs the urine out of the kidney and into the ureters.

THE URETERS

The **ureters** are tubes about 12 inches long that lead, one from each kidney, down to the urinary bladder.

THE URINARY BLADDER

The **bladder** is a hollow muscular organ found in the pelvis. It receives the urine from the ureters and stores it until it can be eliminated from the body. The normal bladder holds about 1 cup (250 ml) of urine. A small circular muscle (sphincter) guards the opening so that urine will not escape involuntarily.

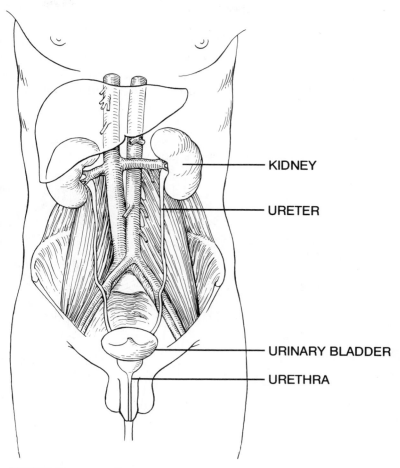

FIGURE 23–1. The urinary system.

THE URETHRA

The **urethra** is a small tube that carries the urine out of the body. The opening to the outside is called the **meatus**. In women, the urethra is about 1½ inches long. In men, it is about 8 to 10 inches long. As the male urethra passes from the urinary bladder it is surrounded by a gland called the **prostate gland**. The male urethra functions both in the excretion of urine and carries the male reproductive fluids to the outside. These two activities cannot take place at the same time.

As you can see, the doughnut-shaped prostate gland would close off the urethra were it to enlarge. This often happens in elderly men, making urine elimination more difficult.

URINE FORMATION

The nephron is a filtering system of tubules and blood vessels that produces the urine. There are one million nephrons in each kidney.

Blood is brought to the kidneys, carrying waste products such as acids and salts that need to be eliminated from the body. The first process in urine production is to filter these waste products through the capillary walls of the **glomerulus** into the filtrate of **Bowman's capsule**, figure 23–2. A great deal of water also passes into the liquid filtrate with the waste products, along with some non-waste products such as sugar. As the fluid filtrate moves slowly through the convoluted tubules, water and helpful substances like sugar are reabsorbed. The liquid left is called urine and drains into the collecting tubes of the medulla and eventually reaches the kidney pelvis.

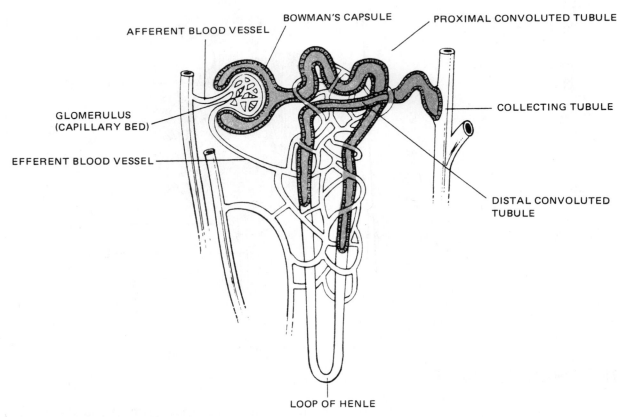

FIGURE 23–2. The glomerulus.

Urine is a liquid waste solution. It contains water and dissolved substances.

Note color, amount, character of all urine.

- *Normal* urine is acid in reaction and pale to deep yellow in color.
- *Dilute* urine has more water and fewer dissolved substances, so it will be white to pale yellow.
- *Concentrated* urine has less water and more dissolved substances, so it will be darker in color and have a stronger odor.

Because the substances in the urine provide good information about the chemistry of the body, tests are frequently performed in the urine (**urinalysis**). You should note the amount, color, odor of the urine and the presence of any sediment. So as not to introduce foreign substances, the specimen of urine to be studied is collected carefully.

▪▪▪ PROCEDURE: Giving and Receiving the Urinal ▪▪▪▪▪▪▪▪▪▪▪▪▪▪▪▪▪▪▪▪▪▪▪▪▪▪

1. Wash hands and assemble the following equipment:
   a. urinal and cover
   b. basin of warm water
   c. soap
   d. washcloth and towel
2. Identify resident and explain what you plan to do.
3. Screen unit.
4. Lift top bedclothes and place the urinal under the covers so the resident may grasp the handle.
5. Make sure the signal cord is within easy reach of resident. Leave resident alone if possible.
6. Answer the resident's signal immediately. Fill a basin with warm water and lay out soap, washcloth, and towel so resident can wash and dry hands.
7. Ask resident to hand the urinal to you. Cover it and rearrange bedclothes if necessary.
8. Take urinal to bathroom or utility room and observe contents. Measure, if required. Do not empty urinal if anything unusual (such as blood) is observed. Rather, save contents of urinal for your supervisor's inspection.
9. Empty urinal. Rinse with cold water and clean with warm soapy water. Rinse, dry, and cover urinal.
10. Place urinal in resident's bedside table. Clean and replace other articles. Leave resident comfortable and unit tidy.
11. Wash hands.
12. Report any unusual observations to nurse, and chart according to facility policy.

▪▪▪ PROCEDURE: Collecting Routine Urine Specimen ▪▪▪▪▪▪▪▪▪▪▪▪▪▪▪▪▪▪▪▪▪▪▪▪

1. Fill out label, including resident's full name, room number, facility number, date and time of collection, doctor's name, examination to be done, and other information as requested.
2. Wash hands and assemble the following equipment:
   a. bedpan or urinal and cover
   b. container and cover for specimen, figure 23–3
   c. graduate
   d. laboratory requisition slip, properly filled out
   e. soap and basin of water
3. Identify resident and explain what you plan to do. Tell resident not to discard toilet tissue in the pan with urine. Provide paper towels or a small plastic sack in which to place soiled tissue.
4. Screen unit. Offer bedpan or urinal.
5. After resident has voided, take pan to utility room. Offer wash water to resident.
6. Pour specimen from bedpan into graduate. Note the amount if resident's intake and output are to be recorded.
7. Pour about 120 ml into specimen container, figure 23–4. *Note:* Some facilities require only 10 to 20 ml.
8. Wash hands. Do not contaminate outside of container.
9. Cover container. Attach completed label and requisition slip to container.
10. Clean and replace equipment according to facility policy.
11. Take or send specimen to laboratory.
12. Record procedure on resident's chart.

▪▪▪ PROCEDURE: Collecting Midstream Urine Specimen (Clean Catch) ▪▪▪▪▪▪▪▪▪▪▪▪▪▪▪▪▪▪▪▪▪

1. Fill out label for container, with resident's full name, room number, date and time of collection, physician's name, type of specimen/test to be performed, and any other information requested.

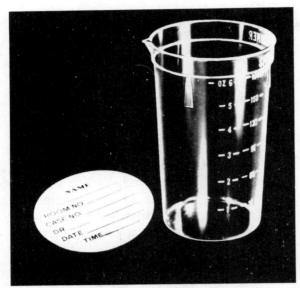

FIGURE 23–3. Urine specimen container.

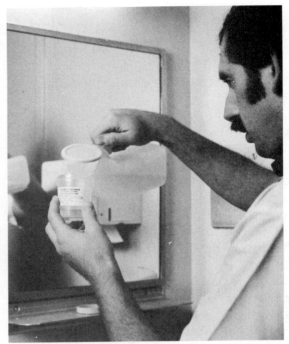

FIGURE 23–4. Carefully pour a sample of urine from the urinal into the specimen container. Do not spill onto your hands or the container.

2. Wash hands and assemble the following equipment (figure 23–5):
   a. sterile urine specimen container
   b. gauze squares or cotton
   c. soap and basin of water
   d. antiseptic solution
   e. laboratory requisition slip, properly filled out
3. Identify resident and explain what you plan to do. Screens unit.
4. Wash resident's genital area or have resident do so. For female resident:
   a. Using gauze or cotton and antiseptic solution, cleanse outer folds of vulva (the folds are also called labia or lips) with a front-to-back motion.
   b. Discard gauze or cotton.
   c. Cleanse inner folds of vulva with another piece of gauze and antiseptic solution, again with a front-to-back motion and discard gauze or cotton.
   d. Finally, cleanse the middle, innermost area (meatus or urinary opening) in the same manner. Discard gauze or cotton.
   For male resident:
   a. Using gauze or cotton and antiseptic solution, cleanse the tip of the penis from the urinary meatus (opening) down, using a circular motion.
   b. Discard gauze or cotton.
5. Instruct resident to void, allowing first part of urine stream to escape. Then, catch urine stream that follows in sterile specimen container. Allow last portion of urine stream to escape. *Note:* If intake and output are being monitored or if the amount of urine passed must be measured, catch first and last part of urine in a bedpan or urinal.
6. Place sterile cap on urine container immediately to avoid contamination of urine specimen.
7. Allow resident to wash hands.
8. With cap securely tightened, wash outside of the specimen container.
9. Wash hands.
10. Label container as instructed and attach requisition slip for appropriate test.
11. Clean and replace all equipment according to facility policy.
12. Take or send specimen to appropriate area immediately.
13. Report completion of task to nurse.
14. Record procedure on chart.

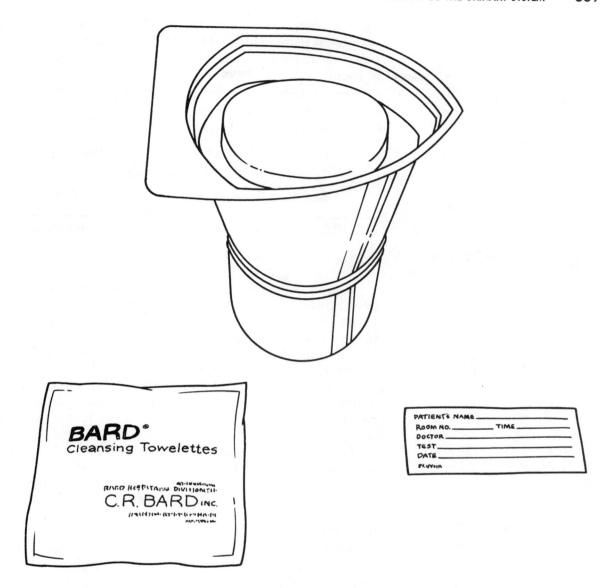

FIGURE 23–5. Equipment needed for obtaining a clean-catch specimen. From Brooks, The Nurse Assistant, *copyright 1978 by Delmar Publishers Inc.)*

AGING CHANGES IN THE URINARY SYSTEM ▪▪▪▪▪▪▪▪▪▪▪▪▪▪▪▪▪▪

As a person ages, the kidneys decrease somewhat in size and some renal cells are lost and replaced by scar tissue, figure 23–6. Though adequate, unless diseased, the kidneys are less efficient filters. Blood vessels carrying the blood to the kidneys for filtration undergo changes that diminish the delivery of blood. The lower blood flow decreases urine production.

Loss of pelvic muscular tone and strength makes bladder emptying less efficient and urine may be retained in the bladder (**retention**). Urine production influences acid-base and fluid balances of the body so these mechanisms will be affected.

Remember, urine is continually being produced and, in younger persons, is more concentrated during the night. Older people lose some concentrating ability and experience more need to empty their bladder at night. This problem is called **nocturia**. Make sure the call bell is available and that there is adequate light for safe ambulation at night.

- Kidneys decrease in size
- Scars replace renal cells
- Poorer renal concentration, with nocturia
- Less efficient bladder emptying
- Reduced filtration ability

FIGURE 23–6. Aging changes in the urinary system.

ELIMINATION

The act of eliminating urine from the bladder is called **micturation, urination,** or **voiding**. Voiding or urinating are the most frequent terms used to describe emptying the bladder. Some residents may prefer to say "passing my water."

Voiding can occur involuntarily when the bladder fills to about 250 ml as the sphincter which guards the bladder exit relaxes and the bladder walls contract. With training, the signals that the bladder is filling is brought to the level of conscious thought and voiding becomes voluntarily controlled. Remember, loss of voluntary control of elimination is called **incontinence**.

A **catheter** is a tube placed into the bladder to drain the urine. Continuous catheter drainage of the bladder causes the bladder wall to lose responsiveness, so that when the catheter is removed, it is difficult to achieve voluntary control again. Catheters are also a potential source of infection. The use of catheters should be avoided if at all possible.

Proper positioning makes it easier for the resident to void. Sitting upright with the feet flat on the floor is preferred for females but men may prefer to stand. Guard rails offer support in both positions.

Bed residents who can be placed on a bedside commode will probably be more comfortable than when using a bedpan but there will be times when a bedpan will be needed. The bedpan can be placed on the bed edge and the resident's feet rest on a chair. The bedpan can be padded and the resident supported by pillows. Always make sure the resident is safely and comfortably supported.

Bedpans are not comfortable in any position when left in place for prolonged periods. Orthopedic bedpans (fracture pan) with their flatter troughs are used when movement is most difficult and should be considered more often for use with the bed-bound resident.

PROCEDURE: Assisting with Bedside Commode

1. Wash hands and assemble the following equipment:
   a. portable commode containing removable receptacle
   b. basin of warm water
   c. towel

d. washcloth and soap

e. toilet tissue

2. Identify resident and explain what you plan to do.
3. Draw curtains for privacy.
4. Place tissue on bedside table within reach.
5. Position commode beside bed, facing head. Lock wheels and remove cover. Be sure receptacle is in place under seat.
6. Lower side rails and lower bed to lowest horizontal position.
7. Assist resident to sitting position. Swing legs over edge of bed.
8. Put slippers on and assist resident to stand.
9. Have resident place hands on your shoulders.
10. Supporting resident under the arms, pivot resident to the right, and lower to commode.
11. Leave call bell and tissue within reach.
12. When signaled, return promptly. Draw warm water in basin and bring to bedside along with soap, towel, and washcloth.
13. Assist resident to stand.
14. Cleanse anus or perineum if resident is unable.
15. Allow resident to wash and dry hands.
16. Help resident return to bed. Adjust bedding and pillows for comfort.
17. Put cover on commode.
18. Remove receptacle from commode. Cover with bedpan cover.
19. Take to bathroom. Note contents and measure if required.
20. Empty and clean according to facility policy. Return commode. Clean remainder of articles and return to their place.
21. Put commode in proper place.
22. Wash hands.
23. Report completion of task. Indicate any unusual observations. Record on resident's chart.

URINARY RETENTION AND INCONTINENCE ▪▪▪▪▪▪▪▪▪▪▪▪▪▪▪▪▪

Elderly residents face two major problems related to the urinary system. The problems are retention and incontinence.

Urinary retention is most often due to poor bladder tone or incomplete emptying because of an obstruction. Poor tone may be related to the aging process or prolonged catheter drainage. Obstruction may be due to tumor growths and most often due to enlargement in men of the prostate gland.

Retention is an inability to urinate. Incontinence is involuntary elimination.

Urinary incontinence may be due to one or a combination of factors. For example, some common problems are:

- emotional withdrawal
- lack of awareness of need
- physical changes

Urinary incontinence may occur simply because the resident cannot reach the toilet or commode on time. Infections, fecal impaction, and stroke and other brain damage can all be causes of incontinence.

When the incontenence is prolonged, tests to determine the cause may be undertaken and, if needed, a urinary retraining program will be started.

Retraining

Adult diapers or incontinence pads may be used until the training program is complete. Treat the use of the protective pads in a very matter-of-fact way, stressing the added comfort they will give the resident, figure 23–7.

The retraining program begins by determining the frequency and timing of elimination. A record is kept of each time that the resident voids or defecates, the use of any bowel aids, and the resident's

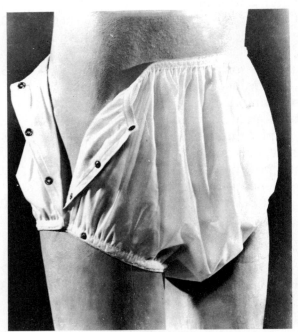

FIGURE 23–7. *Treat the use of incontinence pants as routine nursing care.*

Successful retraining requires great understanding and support.

response. Your observations and those of other staff members are added to the record along with information obtained from the family.

A retraining program is then planned by the nurse, but success requires the cooperation of all staff members and of the resident. Remember, not all residents will be able to participate in the retraining program to the same degree. Retraining is a long-term project, requiring 6 to 8 weeks of effort. You may assist in the retraining program by:

- Helping to keep the record and reporting your observations.
- Seeing that the resident gets to the bathroom or has a bedpan or urinal in place one hour before the established incontinence time. The incontinence time will be determined by studying the record. This care must be consistently and patiently done, day or night.
- Keeping a record of fluid intake. Fluid levels need to be monitored and facility policy regarding forcing or limiting fluids at specific times followed.
- Providing understanding and support.

One of the most important contributions that the staff can make to the retraining process is to provide the essential support needed to help the resident through this difficult period. Each successful elimination should be encouraged and any lapses accepted as a natural occurrence.

Intractable (Uncontrolled) Incontinence

When retraining is not successful or not possible, other steps must be taken so that the resident will not be exposed to the effects of urine against the skin. Constant wetness will cause skin breakdown very quickly.

External Drainage___

Male incontinence can be controlled by applying external drainage using a condom or **urosheath** on the penis. The condom or sheath is attached to a drainage tubing and collection bag. The sheath is removed every 24 hours, and the penis is washed and dried. A thin film of tincture of benzoin is applied to the penis before replacing the condom or sheath.

▪▪▪ PROCEDURE: Replacing Urinary Condom ▪▪▪▪▪▪▪▪▪▪▪▪▪▪▪▪▪▪▪▪▪▪▪▪▪▪▪▪▪▪

1. Wash hands and assemble the following equipment:
   a. basin of warm water
   b. washcloth and towel
   c. bed protector and bath blanket
   d. condom with drainage tip
   e. gloves
   f. plastic bag
   g. tincture of benzoin
   h. paper towels
2. Identify resident and explain what you plan to do.
3. Screen unit and elevate bed to comfortable working height. Arrange equipment on overbed table.
4. Lower side rail closest to you.
5. Cover resident with bath blanket and fanfold bedding to foot of bed. Place bed protector under resident's hips.
6. Adjust bath blanket to expose genitals only.
7. Put on gloves.
8. Remove present sheath by rolling toward tip of penis. Place in plastic bag if disposable, or place on paper towels to be washed and dried if reusable.
9. Wash and dry penis carefully. Observe for signs of irritation.
10. Check to see if condom has "ready-stick" surfaces. If not, a thin spray of tincture of benzoin may be applied to the penis. Do not spray on head of penis.
11. Apply fresh condom and drainage tip to penis by rolling it toward base of penis. If the resident is uncircumcised, be sure that the foreskin remains in good position.
12. Reconnect drainage system.
13. Remove gloves and discard in plastic bag.
14. Adjust bedding and remove bath blanket. Fold bath blanket and place in bedside stand.
15. Lower bed and raise side rail. Make resident comfortable, with call bell at hand. Leave unit tidy.
16. Clean and replace equipment and disposables according to facility policy.
17. Wash hands.
18. Report completion of task to nurse. Record on resident's chart the date and time, procedure (urinary condom replaced), and any observations you have made.

Internal Drainage___

The indwelling catheter permits continuous drainage.

Because external drainage is difficult for women and some men, internal drainage may be ordered.

Using sterile technique, a slender rubber or plastic tube (Foley catheter) is inserted into the bladder to drain the urine, figure 23–8. A balloon around the neck of the catheter is inflated once the catheter is in place. The inflated balloon keeps the catheter in place so that it will not easily slip out. The other end of the catheter is connected to a drainage tube and collection bag. This type of catheter is known as an **indwelling catheter**. The catheter is attached to a closed drainage system. The insertion of a sterile catheter is the responsibility of the nurse.

Catheter Care. Care of the resident with a catheter and urinary drainage is the nursing assistant's responsibility. The catheter is cared for daily. You should:

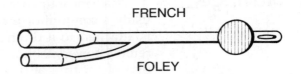

FIGURE 23–8. A sterile Foley catheter is inserted into the bladder. The balloon is then inflated to maintain the catheter in the bladder.

- Keep the urinary meatus clean.
- Check regularly for signs of irritation or urinary discomfort.
- Secure the tubing in such a way that there is no strain on the catheter or tubing.
- Always maintain the drainage bag below the level of the bladder.
- If the catheter is to be clamped at specific intervals, it is absolutely essential that you follow the times of clamping and unclamping exactly. The clamping allows the bladder to fill, stimulating muscular tone.
- Never permit the collection bag to touch the floor.
- Measure the drainage at the end of each shift, noting the character of the urine, and report and record the information.
- Check the entire drainage set-up each time care is given and at the beginning and end of your shift.

PROCEDURE: Routine Drainage Check

1. Wash hands.
2. Identify resident and explain what you plan to do. Screen unit.
3. Raise bedding to observe tubing.
4. Check position of catheter and meatus.
5. Keep drainage tube coiled smoothly on bed so there is a direct drop to collection bag, figure 23–9.
6. Adjust collection bag level below resident's hips.
7. Keep end of drainage tube above urine level in bag.
8. Attach drainage tube to bed frame.
9. Note color and character and flow of urine.
10. Measure urine using proper technique.
11. Wash hands.
12. Report and record findings.

PROCEDURE: Giving Indwelling Catheter Care

1. Wash hands and collect the following equipment:
   a. disposable gloves
   b. bed protector
   c. bath blanket
   d. plastic bag for disposables
   e. daily catheter care kit
   f. antiseptic solution
   g. sterile applicators
   h. tape
2. Identify resident and explain what you plan to do. Screen unit.
3. Raise bed to working height and lower side rail closest to you. Be sure opposite side rail is up and secure. Position resident on back, legs separated, and knees bent, if permitted.
4. Cover resident with bath blanket and fanfold top bedclothes to foot of bed.

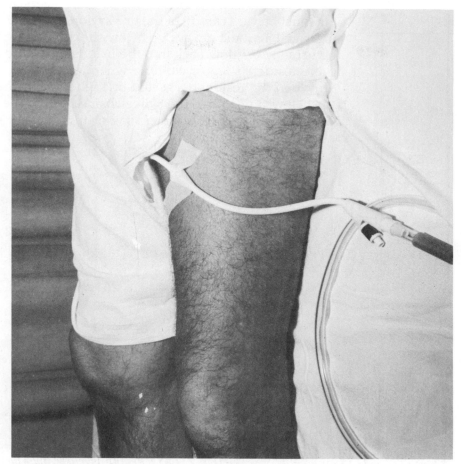

FIGURE 23–9. The tube must be coiled on the bed so there is a straight drop to the collection bag.

5. Position bath blanket so that only genitals are exposed.
6. Ask resident to raise hips and place bed protector underneath.
7. Arrange catheter care kit and plastic bag on overbed table. Open kit.
8. Put on gloves and draw drape back.
9. For male resident:
   a. Gently grasp penis and draw foreskin back.
   b. Dipping a fresh applicator in antiseptic solution for each stroke, cleanse glans from meatus toward shaft for approximately 4 inches.
   c. Place each applicator into disposable plastic bag after use.
   For female resident:
   a. Separate labia.
   b. Using a fresh applicator dipped in antiseptic solution for each stroke, clean from front to back.

   c. Dispose of used applicators in plastic bag.
10. Remove gloves and place in plastic bag.
11. Check catheter to be sure it is taped properly. Retape and adjust for slack, if needed.
12. Check to be sure tubing is coiled on bed and hangs straight down into drainage container. Check level of urine in container. End of tubing should not be below urine level. Empty bag and measure if necessary.
13. Replace bedding and remove bath blanket.
14. Fold bath blanket and place in bedside stand.
15. Help resident to assume a comfortable position, with call bell within easy reach.
16. Lower bed and raise and secure side rail. Leave unit tidy.
17. Dispose of equipment according to facility policy.
18. Wash hands and report completion of task. Record on resident's chart the date and time, procedure, antiseptic solution used, and any observations you have made.

Ambulating with a Catheter_____

When residents are ambulatory or using a geri-chair or wheelchair, you must be very careful of the urinary drainage. Remember that the drainage bag must always be below the level of the bladder so that the urine won't flow back into the bladder. The bag may be secured to the resident's leg or clothing when ambulating.

When the resident is seated in a wheelchair, the tubing should run below and under the wheelchair so it can be secured to the wheelchair back. The drainage bag or tubing must never touch the floor, figure 23–10.

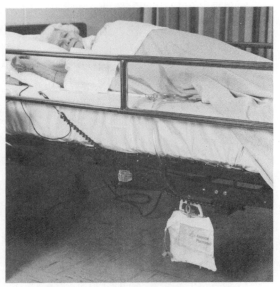

FIGURE 23–10. *The drainage bag must never touch the floor.*

▪▪▪ PROCEDURE: Disconnecting Catheter ▪▪▪▪▪▪▪▪▪▪▪▪▪▪▪▪▪▪▪▪▪▪

Note: It is preferable never to disconnect the drainage set-up, but it may be necessary. If sterile caps and plugs are available, they should be used. If not, the disconnected ends must be protected with sterile gauze sponges.
1. Wash hands.
2. Identify resident and explain what you plan to do. Screen unit.
3. Clamp catheter.
4. Disinfect area where catheter is connected to tubing.
5. Disconnect catheter and drainage tubing. Do not put them down or allow them to touch anything.
6. Insert sterile plug in end of catheter, figure 23–11. Place sterile cap over exposed end of drainage tube.
7. Secure drainage tube to bed in such a way that it will not touch floor. Wash hands.
8. Reverse procedure to reconnect catheter. If you find an unprotected, disconnected tube in bed or on floor, do not reconnect it but report it at once.

There is always the danger of infection when an indwelling catheter is used.

At times, the catheter may be disconnected to make ambulation easier, but when this is done, there is always the danger of contamination. You must follow the procedure for disconnecting the

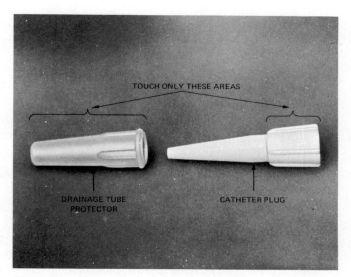

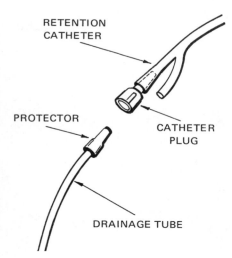

FIGURE 23–11. Left: Sterile catheter plug and protector; right: plug and protector in place.

catheter very carefully. The resident who has an indwelling catheter is at risk for infection. There are several sites where infection can enter the drainage system, figure 23–12. They are:

- urinary meatus, where the catheter is inserted
- connection between the catheter and drainage tube
- connection between the drainage bag and drainage tubing
- opening used to empty the drainage bag

INTAKE AND OUTPUT (I&O)

The amount of fluid taken into the body and the amount of fluid lost should be just about equal. The intake and output (I&O) is frequently measured and recorded. Imbalances in intake and output can result in severe fluid imbalances such as **edema** (water retention) and **dehydration** (excessive water loss).

Intake. Intake includes everything taken in that is liquid at room temperature. For example, included in the intake would be fluids such as:

Intake and output are recorded in metric measurements.

- water or tea
- jello, junket, or pudding
- fluids given directly into a vein (IV)

Output. The output includes all fluids lost. This includes:

- the amount of urine eliminated
- perspiration
- blood
- diarrhea
- vomiting

If the resident is incontinent, indicate the number of times on the output record. Do not forget to check the resident often and to change the linen each time it is wet.

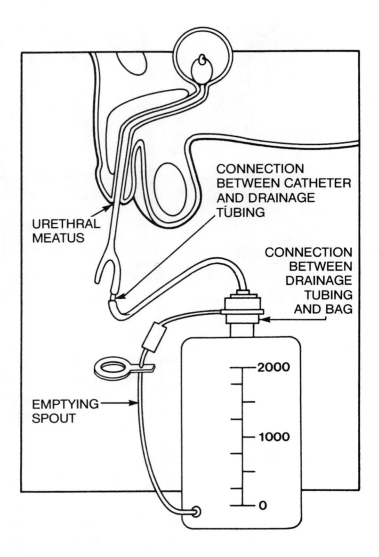

FIGURE 23–12. Special care must be taken to protect possible sites of contamination.

Measuring Intake and Output_____

The **metric system** of measurements is generally used to measure I&O. Most of the containers for fluids used in the facility are marked in metric measurements. Urine drainage bags, intravenous fluids, and enema solution containers are routinely marked with this system in milliliters (ml) or **cubic centimeters** (cc).

You must learn the metric unit equivalents of commonly used U.S. customary units. One ml is approximately the same as 1 cc. See figure 23–13 for a listing of those you will need to learn.

A special form for recording I&O may be kept at the bedside to be used each day. A summary of fluids taken in and lost is made on the I&O sheet in the resident's health record.

Your facility will also use standardized cups, bowls, and glasses. Familiarize yourself with the values of each (figure 23–14). It will make your job of computing intake easier.

U.S. Customary Units		Metric Units
16 minims	=	1 ml (1 cc)*
1 ounce (oz)	=	30 ml (30 cc)
1 pint (pt)	=	500 ml (500 cc)
1 quart (qt)	=	1000 ml (1000 cc)
1 inch (in)	=	2.5 centimeters (cm)
1 foot (ft)	=	30 cm
* cc = cubic centimeters		

FIGURE 23–13. Metric and U.S. Customary Units.

Drinking glass = 6 oz = 180 cc   Jello = 4 oz = 120 cc
Styrofoam cup = 6 oz = 180 cc   Ice cream cup = 5 oz = 150 cc
Juice glass (small) = 4 oz = 120 cc   Creamer = 1 oz = 30 cc
Juice glass (large) = 8 oz = 240 cc
Full water pitcher (1 qt) = 32 oz = 960 cc   **Abbreviations**
Coffee or tea pot = 10 oz = 300 cc
Coffee cup = 5 oz = 150 cc   oz = ounce = 30 cc
Milk carton = 8 oz = 240 cc   pt = pint = 16 oz = 480/500 cc
Soup bowl (small) = 6 oz = 180 cc   qt = quart = 32 oz = 960/1000 cc
Soup bowl (large) = 10 oz = 300 cc   gal = gallon = 128 oz = 3840/4000 cc

Residents may not finish all fluids furnished to them. Estimate how much fluid has actually been taken and record the amount. For instance, the resident is given 8 ounces of milk but drinks only 4 ounces. Therefore, record intake of 120 cc.

FIGURE 23–14. Average container amounts.

▮▮▮ PROCEDURE: Emptying Urinary Drainage Unit ▬▬▬▬▬▬▬▬▬▬▬▬▬▬▬▬▬▬

1. Wash hands.
2. Identify resident and explain what you plan to do.
3. If drainage bag has an opening in bottom, place graduate under it and allow urine to drain, figure 23–15.
4. If there is no opening, tube must be removed before emptying. Protect end of drainage tube with sterile cup or sterile gauze sponge.
5. Empty urine and measure it.
6. Remove protective cover from end of tube and reinsert it in bag. Be careful not to hit sides of bag.
7. Wash hands.
8. Record I&O on proper resident chart.

▮▮▮ PROCEDURE: Measuring and Recording Fluid Output ▬▬▬▬▬▬▬▬▬▬▬▬▬▬▬▬

1. Save urine specimen and take to utility room or resident's bathroom. You will need:
   a. graduate pitcher
   b. pen for recording, I&O record
2. Pour urine from bedpan or urinal into graduate. Measure amount, figure 23–16.
3. Record amounts immediately under output column on bedside I&O record. All liquid

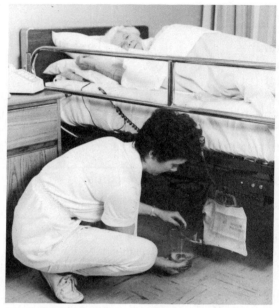

FIGURE 23–15. *Carefully open the tubing in the drainage bag and measure the urine with a graduate.*

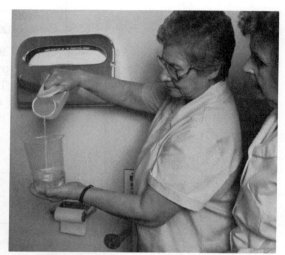

FIGURE 23–16. *Take the urinal and measure the urine in the bathroom. Do not forget to record the amount.*

output should be recorded. Output includes urine, vomitus (also called emesis), drainage from wound or stomach, liquid stool, blood loss, and perspiration. Fluids used to irrigate bladder or for enema are not included in calculating output.

4. Empty urine into bedpan hopper. If specimen is accidentally lost, estimate amount and make notation that it is an estimate. *Note:* In some cases, the physician will request that the totally incontinent resident's diapers be weighed to determine output.

5. Rinse graduate with cold water. Clean according to facility policy.
6. Clean bedpan or urinal and return to proper place according to facility policy.
7. Wash hands.
8. Copy information on chart from I&O record, according to facility policy. Perspiration and blood loss may be described as little, moderate, or excessive. Also record on chart instances in which linens or dressings have been changed or reinforced because of fluid losses.

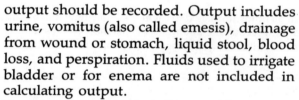

PROCEDURE: Measuring and Recording Fluid Intake

1. Wash hands and assemble the following equipment:
   a. I&O record at bedside (figure 23–17)
   b. pen
   c. graduated pitcher
2. Identify resident and explain what you plan to do. Ask resident to help by recording the amount of fluid taken by mouth.
3. Record intake on the I&O record at bedside. Intake includes:
   a. Amount of liquid resident takes with meals. This includes anything liquid at room temperature such as ice cream or jello.
   b. Amount of water and other liquids taken between meals.
   c. All other intake including fluids given by mouth, intravenously, or by tube feeding. How it is taken should also be reported.
4. Copy information on resident's chart from the bedside I&O record, according to facility policy. Remember, intake and output are recorded in millimeters (ml), which are the same as cubic centimeters (cc). The total is recorded at the end of each shift and at the end of 24 hours.

INTAKE AND OUTPUT

Room: *103 B*   Name: *Simon, Grace*   Date:

Instructions: *Record all I and O*

11-7		7-3		3-11	
Intake	Output	Intake	Output	Intake	Output
Total		Total		Total	

Drinking Glass......200cc   Full Water Pitcher..950cc   Milk Carton.........236cc   Jello...........90cc
Styrofoam Cup.......200cc   Coffee or Teapot....300cc   Soup Bowl...........250cc   Ice Cream Cup...90cc
Juice Glass (small).100cc   Coffee Cup..........150cc   Soup Bowl (small)...100cc   Creamer.........50cc
Juice Glass (large).250cc

FOLEY CATHETER DRAINAGE: (Circle the following when applicable)

Color: Yellow   Amber   Brown   Red

Appearance: Cloudy   Clear   Sediment   Mucous   Bloody   24 hour INTAKE_____

Abdomen Distended   Catheter Irrigated   Catheter Changed   24 hour OUTPUT_____

FIGURE 23-17. An intake and output chart becomes part of the resident's record.

OTHER COMMON CONDITIONS ■■■■■■■■■■■■■■■■■■■■■■■■■■■■■■

Rectocele and Cystocele_____

The urinary bladder, part of the ureters and urethra are found in the pelvic cavity. Some of the female reproductive organs are also in the pelvis. Each group of organs can be affected by disease or stress in the other group.

Frequent pregnancies and general loss of muscle tone due to the aging process results in the development of the bladder protruding into the vagina (**cystocele**) and the rectum into the vagina (**rectocele**).

The weakness of the bladder wall can cause urinary incontinence, especially when there is extra stress such as laughing or coughing. The weakened rectal wall can lead to constipation and hemorrhoids. Surgery can be helpful in repairing the cystocele and rectocele.

Renal Calculi

Renal calculi or kidney stones form as various salts and compounds settle out of the forming urine. Starting as tiny grains of sediment, they become larger and larger until they block part of the drainage system, often a ureter. When blockage occurs the resident experiences extreme pain. Pain associated with urine elimination is known as **dysuria**. Most kidney stones are passed when fluids are forced, but surgery may be required to relieve the obstruction.

The urine may have to be strained through gauze or filter paper before being measured and discarded to determine when the stone is passed. Blood may cause the urine to become pink to deep red in color. Blood in the urine is called **hematuria**.

Renal Failure

Renal failure (**uremia**) may occur suddenly but usually is a chronic situation that develops gradually over a period of years due to changes in the blood vessels that serve the kidneys, to hypertension, or to the aging process.

The resident in chronic renal failure doesn't eliminate effectively, so water and wastes accumulate in the body. Urine output is diminished (**oliguria**) and in terminal stages, ceases altogether (**anuria**). The blood pressure increases and edema and chemical imbalance develop throughout the body. The resident may complain of headache, nausea, and a bad taste in the mouth. The perspiration glands begin to eliminate uric acid. The uric acid accumulates as white crystals on the skin. This accumulation is called **uremic frost**. The perspiration has an unpleasant odor. Careful attention is needed to keep the skin clean and free from breakdown.

Renal failure can only be helped by hemodialysis which uses a machine to filter the blood or surgical replacement with a compatible kidney transplant.

VOCABULARY

anuria	incontinence	prostate gland
bladder	indwelling catheter	rectocele
Bowman's capsule	I&O (intake and output)	renal calculi
catheter	intake	renal pelvis
cortex	meatus	retention
cubic centimeter (cc)	metric system	uremia
cystocele	medulla	uremic frost
dehydration	micturation	ureter
dysuria	milliliter (ml)	urethra
edema	nephron	urinalysis
frequency	nocturia	urination
glomerulus	oliguria	urosheath
hematuria	output	voiding

SUGGESTED ACTIVITIES

1. Review the parts of the urinary system by drawing and labeling a simple diagram.

2. Practice giving catheter care using a manikin.

3. Using different size containers, practice measuring fluids accurately.

4. Under supervision, give proper care to residents with urinary problems.

REVIEW

A. Brief Answer/Fill in the Blanks

1. List the organs of the urinary system: _____

_____

2. In what other system does the urethra function in men?

3. One normal effect of aging is a loss of pelvic tone and muscular bladder strength, which can lead to _____ of urine.

4. When using adult diapers, you should stress the _____ they will provide.

5. The best position to encourage voiding in a female resident is to have her _____.

6. A person who is unable to voluntarily control urine output is said to be _____.

7. During continence retraining, the resident should be assisted to void _____ prior to the time of the incontinence pattern.

8. Intake includes everything taken in that is _____ at _____ temperature.

9. Fluid output includes the amount of fluid lost in urine, perspiration, blood, and in _____ or _____.

10. Intake and output is added and recorded at the_____.

B. **Matching.** Match the metric amounts on the right with their equivalents on the left.

1. _____ 1 minim   a. 500 ml

2. _____ 1 quart   b. 0.06 ml

                        c. 30 ml

3. _____ 2.2 pounds   d. 1 kg

4. _____ 1 pint   e. 1000 ml

5. _____ 1 ounce

C. **Identification.** Label the anatomic parts indicated on the diagram of urinary system:

1. _____

2. _____

3. _____

4. _____

D. On the chart provided below, make a record of the resident's intake and output for an 8-hour period.

7:30 a.m.	urine	300 ml
8:00 a.m.	orange juice	90 ml
	coffee	120 ml
9:30 a.m.	water	60 ml
11:30 a.m.	tea	120 ml
	soup	120 ml
1:00 p.m.	urine	400 ml
1:15 p.m.	water	80 ml
3:00 p.m.	cranberry juice	100 ml
3:15 p.m.	vomitus	120 ml
4:20 p.m.	tea	120 ml
	sherbert	120 ml
5:30 p.m.	urine	300 ml
6:00 p.m.	water	150 ml
9:00 p.m.	ginger ale	100 ml
9:30 p.m.	urine	300 ml
10:00 p.m.	water	90 ml

BAYSIDE CONVALESCENT HOME
FLUID INTAKE AND OUTPUT

Name _____ Room _____

Date	Time	Method of Adm.	INTAKE			OUTPUT		
			Solution	Amounts Rec'd	Time	Urine Amount	Others Kind	Amount

CLINICAL SITUATION

Alicia Eidi, 82, has an indwelling catheter because she is incontinent. She spends most of her day in a geri-chair. What procedures will you follow related to care of her catheter and intake and output?

Answer: _____

_____

_____

_____

LESSON 24 The Respiratory System

OBJECTIVES

After studying this lesson, you should be able to:

- Name the parts and function of the respiratory system.
- Identify changes in the respiratory system as they relate to the aging process.
- Name six common respiratory conditions.
- Give proper care to residents in respiratory distress and receiving respiratory therapy.
- Define and spell all the vocabulary words and terms.

The respiratory system carries on the vital functions of exchanging gases to meet the body's metabolic needs. The two gases are:

- **oxygen** (O_2)
- **carbon dioxide** (CO_2)

Energy for cell activity is derived from cellular respiration.

Oxygen. Oxygen is brought into the lungs and carried to the cells to produce energy. Energy production in the cells is called **cellular respiration.** It can be expressed in the following equation:

$$\text{Glucose} + \text{oxygen} \xrightarrow[\text{metabolism}]{\text{cellular}} \text{carbon dioxide} + \text{water} + \text{energy}$$

Carbon Dioxide. Carbon dioxide is carried to the lungs for excretion. Carbon dioxide is a waste product.

There is an intimate connection between the respiratory and circulatory systems, since the body cells are dependent upon the bloodstream to deliver the gases back and forth between them and the lungs.

THE RESPIRATORY ORGANS

The respiratory organs include the:

- upper respiratory tract
- lower respiratory tract
- lungs

The Upper Respiratory Tract. This part of the respiratory tract is made up of the nose, **pharynx, larynx, trachea** (windpipe), and **bronchi,** figure 24–1.

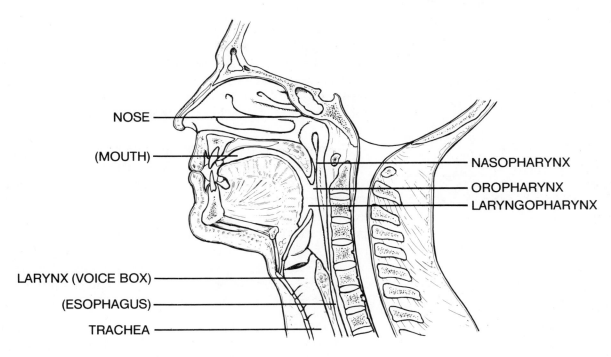

NOSE

(MOUTH)

NASOPHARYNX

OROPHARYNX

LARYNGOPHARYNX

LARYNX (VOICE BOX)

(ESOPHAGUS)

TRACHEA

FIGURE 24–1. *The upper respiratory tract — lateral view.*

The Lower Respiratory Tract. This includes the extensions of the bronchi, which branch into smaller and smaller divisions called **bronchioles.** These finally lead to the tiny air sacs called the **alveoli,** figure 24–2. The alveoli, these tiny branches leading to them, and the important pulmonary blood vessels form the lungs.

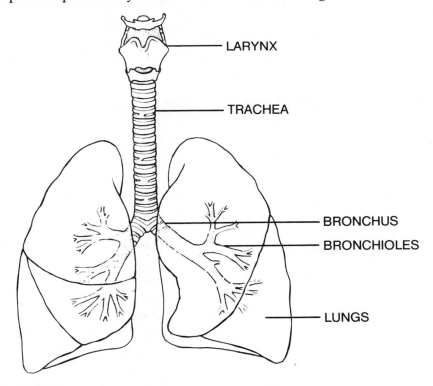

LARYNX

TRACHEA

BRONCHUS

BRONCHIOLES

LUNGS

FIGURE 24–2. *Ventral view of the lower respiratory tract.*

The Lungs. There are two lungs, each surrounded by a double-walled, serous membrane called the **pleura.** Between the two pleural layers is a small amount of serous fluid that reduces friction as the lungs alternately expand and recoil, filling with and then expelling air. The air is warmed, filtered and moistened as it passes over the vascular mucous membrane that lines the respiratory tract, from nose to alveoli.

The Act of Respiration

Respiration is the act of drawing air into the lungs (**inspiration**) and expelling the air outward (**expiration**) as the lungs expand or enlarge and recoil or become smaller. This is known as **ventilation**.

The lungs are situated in the **thorax** and follow the chest wall as it expands and decreases in size. The size of the thorax is dependent upon contraction of the diaphragm and intercostal muscles. As the muscles contract, they cause the thorax to enlarge, expanding the lungs. Air carrying oxygen rushes into the lungs. When the muscles relax, the thorax resumes its normal size and the lungs inside recoil. The air carrying carbon dioxide rushes outside. Remember:

- *Inspiration* is the act of drawing air into the lungs.
- *Expiration* is the act of expelling air.
- *Ventilation* is the combination of these two actions.

VOICE PRODUCTION

The larnyx, or voice box, is part of the respiratory tract and is important in voice production, figure 24–3. Two membranes, called the **vocal cords**, stretch across the inside of the larynx. As air passes upward through the larynx, it moves through an opening in the vocal cords called the **glottis**. Changes in the shape of the vocal cords and the size of the glottis permit controlled amounts of air to reach the mouth, nasal cavities, and sinuses, where — formed by the teeth, lips, and tongue — specific speech sounds are made.

AGING CHANGES IN THE RESPIRATORY SYSTEM

The aged lungs are less efficient in exchanging gases.

With aging, breathing capacity drops by one-half, figure 24–4. The little air sacs enlarge and lose elasticity, making recoil less effective. The respiratory rate increases. The diaphragm and intercostal muscles lose strength, so gaseous exchange is less efficient. Changes in the larynx make the voice higher pitched and weaker.

MALIGNANCIES

As with other systems, cancerous tumors can develop in any part of the respiratory tract. Although the exact causes of malignancy are not fully understood, cigarette smoking and exposure to other cancer-producing agents in the environment are known to be contributing causes. Lung cancers are treated by surgery, radiation, and chemotherapy or a combination of all three therapies. For special care related to residents receiving these therapies, see Lesson 16. You may want to review these principles now.

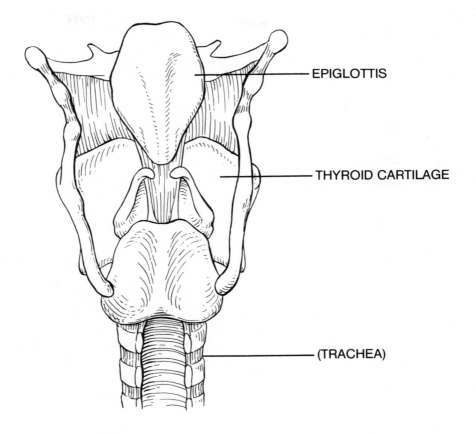

EPIGLOTTIS

THYROID CARTILAGE

(TRACHEA)

A

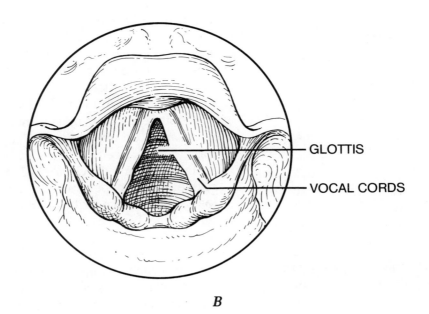

GLOTTIS

VOCAL CORDS

B

FIGURE 24–3. *Anterior view of the larynx, or voice box. Inside the cartilage, two membranes called the vocal cords are stretched.*

- Lung tissue loses elasticity
- Slower rate of gas exchange
- Breathing capacity diminished
- Diaphragm less efficient
- Rate of breathing increases
- Larynx changes make voice weaker and higher pitched

FIGURE 24–4. Aging changes in the respiratory system.

Cancer of the Larynx_____

Cancer of the larynx may make removal of that organ necessary, with the subsequent loss of voice. A **tracheostomy** is an artificial air passage made in the neck and trachea. A permanent stoma (opening) is formed through the neck, through which the resident breathes.

Loss of voice is a major catastrophy for anyone. Just think for a moment of how frustrated you would feel if you could no longer use your voice to communicate your thoughts and feelings, wants and needs to others.

Immediate care for the laryngectomy patient is given in the acute care hospital. Writing is a major form of communication available to patients during this phase of their rehabilitation. Later, the patient may be taught new ways to speak, either through esophageal speech or electronic speech.

Esophageal Speech

Esophageal speech is performed by learning to swallow air and then bring it back up (**regurgitating**) through the esophagus. This form of speech production is difficult to learn, but well-motivated patients do succeed.

Electronic Speech

Those who cannot master the technique of esophageal speech may find the use of an electronic type of artificial larynx a more satisfying method, figure 24–5. Some patients may use a combination of both techniques.

Residents who have had laryngectomies will need patience and understanding from all staff members. Even though communication is possible, do not expect the voice to sound normal and realize that more time is needed by the resident to formulate the voice sounds. A tremendous psychological adjustment must be made by the resident. Expect periods of depression, anger, and even hostility. The loss of one's voice requires an adjustment similar to that experienced when grieving for the loss of a loved one.

Stoma Care

The stoma must be protected against foreign materials.

The tracheostomy stoma (opening) (figure 24–6) must be kept clean, clear, and protected from trauma and from accidentally drawing foreign materials into the trachea (**aspiration**).

Suctioning the trachea is a licensed nursing function. As a nursing assistant, you will have responsibilities as well for the care of the resident with a tracheostomy.

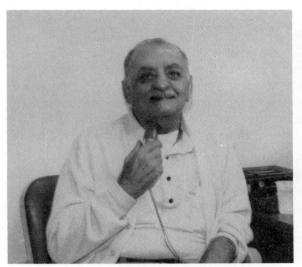

FIGURE 24–5. Electronic devices aid the laryngectomy resident to communicate. (From Huber, Homemaker—Home Health Aide, 2nd edition, copyright 1985 by Delmar Publishers Inc.)

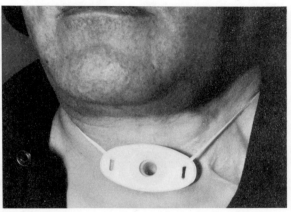

FIGURE 24–6. The tracheostomy creates a permanent opening in the trachea. (From Huber, Homemaker—Home Health Aide, 2nd edition, copyright 1985 by Delmar Publishers Inc.)

- Protect the stoma by using only lint-free cloth near it and by being sure that shaving cream and food do not find their way into the trachea. A wire cage with gauze can be used to protect the opening, figure 24–7.
- Special mouth care and frequent toothbrushing and rinsing of the mouth can help to reduce **halitosis** (bad breath) and the crusts that sometimes form in the mouth.
- Report nasal congestion. The resident will not be able to blow the nose to clear the passageway. If there seems to be nasal congestion, report to the nurse so that the nose can be suctioned.

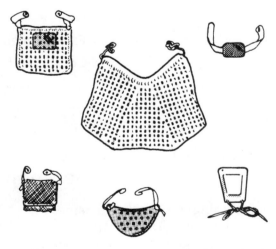

FIGURE 24–7. Stoma guards keep foreign material out of the tracheostomy opening.

INFECTIONS ▪▪▪

The respiratory tract is exposed to many germs in the environment. In the elderly, whose resistance is generally lowered, respiratory infection is very common and can be life-threatening.

Influenza and pneumonia are common complications of the aging process. Older persons' bodies do not always respond as strongly to infections as those of younger persons, so signs and symptoms of infection may not be as pronounced. Be sure to report (figure 24–8):

Common respiratory conditions
- Pneumonia
- Influenza
- Tuberculosis

- the presence of cough
- an elevated temperature
- unusual fatigue
- rapid, shallow, or noisy breathing (**tachypnea**)
- confusion
- restlessness
- complaints of chest pain

These signs and symptoms may indicate a hidden infection. Infections need to be treated vigorously with:

- rest
- antibiotics
- oxygen therapy
- drugs to keep air passageways clear
- supportive care

You may need to collect a **sputum** specimen from the resident for culture to learn the cause of the infection. *Sputum* is the matter that is brought up from deep in the lungs. You must be sure that the specimen you collect comes from the lungs and is not just saliva from the mouth, and that you handle the specimen in a proper manner.

- Respiratory distress (dyspnea)
- Easy fatigue
- Cyanosis
- Fast, labored breathing
- Confusion
- Restlessness

FIGURE 24–8. Note and report.

▪▪▪ PROCEDURE: Collecting A Sputum Specimen ▪▪▪▪▪▪▪▪▪▪▪▪▪▪▪▪▪▪▪▪▪▪▪▪

1. Fill out label including: resident's full name, room number, hospital number, date and time of collection, doctor's name, examination to be done, and other information as requested.

2. Wash hands and assemble the following equipment:
   a. container and cover for specimen
   b. glass of water
   c. tissues

d. emesis basin

e. completely filled out requisition slip

3. Identify resident and explain what you plan to do. Screen unit.

4. Have resident rinse mouth. Use emesis basin for waste.

5. Ask resident to cough deeply to bring up sputum and **expectorate** (spit) into the container. Have resident cover mouth with tissue to prevent spread of infection. Collect 1 to 2 tablespoonfuls of sputum unless otherwise ordered.

6. Wash hands. Do not contaminate outside of container.

7. Cover container tightly and attach completed label.

8. Clean and replace equipment according to facility policy.

9. Take or send specimen to laboratory promptly.

10. Record procedure on resident's chart. Be sure to include a description of specimen, such as odor and color. *Note:* If a 24-hour specimen is being collected, leave the container at the resident's bedside.

Vaccines are available for the prevention of some forms of pneumonia and influenza. Older persons can benefit from receiving them.

TUBERCULOSIS

Tuberculosis Infection_____

Tuberculosis infection can develop into tuberculosis disease.

Tuberculosis infection occurs when tuberculosis germs enter the body. The lungs are the most common site of involvement. The body responds to the invasion of the germs in a special way that usually walls off the organism from the rest of the body and prevents spread of the organisms to other body areas. The walled-off area is called a **tubercle**. As long as the tubercle remains intact and no new organisms enter the body, the condition is said to be **arrested**, or controlled.

Tuberculosis Disease_____

If the tubercle breaks down or additional organisms enter the body, more tissue damage is done and the condition is known as **tuberculosis disease**. Signs and symptoms of tubercolusis disease include:

- loss of appetite and weight
- weakness
- elevated temperature in the afternoon and evening
- sweating at night
- spitting up blood (**hemoptysis**)

Tuberculosis can be treated with a combination of drugs that can once more control the disease process and prevent spread to others.

Extra precautions must be taken when caring for the resident who has tuberculosis. This disease is transmitted primarily through respiratory secretions. In addition to the usual infections control technique, masks may be needed to prevent transmission. Also, you should turn your head so that the resident doesn't breath directly in your face as you give care and be sure to dispose of any respiratory secretions such as soiled tissues in the proper manner.

Today, with the use of drug therapy, residents can become noncommunicable within two weeks.

CHRONIC OBSTRUCTIVE PULMONARY DISEASE (COPD) ■■■■■■■■■■

Chronic obstructive pulmonary disease (COPD) is also called COLD (*chronic obstructive lung disease*). This term refers to conditions resulting from a prolonged blocking of the air passageways. The long-term obstruction causes loss of alveoli and a poor delivery of blood to the lungs. Several conditions can lead to COPD. They include infections like tuberculosis, and frequent pneumonias, **asthma**, **bronchitis**, and **emphysema.**

Asthma_____

Asthma is a disorder of respiration characterized by labored breathing and coughing. Respiratory distress is signalled by:

- constriction of the muscles of the bronchioles
- swelling of the mucous membranes
- the production of large amounts of mucus, which fill the narrowed passageways

People who suffer from asthma may experience an attack when they come in contact with the allergen or when they are under emotional stress. Common allergens are:

- pollen
- medications
- dust
- feathers
- foods such as chicken, eggs, or chocolate

If a resident has known allergies, they should be posted in the resident's health record.

Chronic Bronchitis_____

This condition stems from inflammation in the bronchi due to infection or irritants. Signs and symptoms include:

- The bronchial tissues become swollen and red, narrowing the bronchial passageways.
- There is a persistent cough, which may or may not produce sputum.
- There may be signs of respiratory distress.

Emphysema_____

Emphysema is a disease condition that develops after there has been chronic obstruction of the air flow to the alveoli. The air sacs:

- become distended
- lose their elasticity and recoil ability
- are finally completely inactivated or nonfuctional

Although it is possible to bring air into the lungs, it becomes increasingly difficult to expel the air from the lungs, and therefore there is less and less room for fresh air to reenter, figure 24–9.

There seems to be several factors that can contribute to emphysema. These factors include:

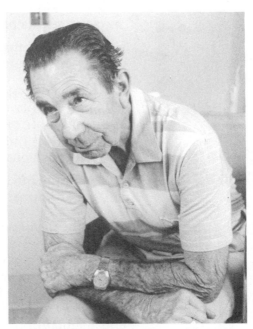

FIGURE 24–9. The resident with emphysema brings more air into and out of his lungs by pursing his lips on expiration and leaning forward.

- air pollutants such as cigarette smoke, auto exhaust fumes and insecticides
- a genetic predisposition to emphysema
- recurrent infections such as pneumonia and bronchitis
- chronic asthma

People with emphysema are at greater risk for infections such as pneumonia. They suffer from:

- chronic oxygen inadequacy and fatigue
- breathing that requires a greater and greater effort
- coughing that may bring up large amounts of heavy mucus secretions called **phlegm** or coughing that may be dry and non-productive
- feelings of dizziness and restlessness as carbon dioxide levels rise in the bloodstream
- loss of appetite and weight loss

TREATMENT AND CARE OF RESIDENTS WITH COPD ▪▪▪▪▪▪▪▪▪▪▪▪

Treatment of the resident suffering from any form of COPD is designed to:

- improve ventilation
- improve gaseous exchange

Special techniques are used to loosen the phlegm and make it easier to bring up. Just ridding the passageways of phlegm makes breathing easier. Some of these procedures will be carried out by the nurse or respiratory therapist. Procedures that you may assist in are:

- positioning for better ventilation
- positioning for improved drainage

Positioning the resident to improve ventilation and drainage activities are two major nursing activities in providing care for the resident with COPD.

Positioning for Better Ventilation____

Supported high Fowler's or orthopneic positions improve ventilation.

Two positions used are:

- **high Fowler's position**
- **orthopneic position**

In the *high Fowler's position*, the resident is sitting almost upright with the knees flexed, figure 24–10. In the *orthopneic position*, an overbed table is positioned in front of the resident, figure 24–11. The resident leans forward with arms on the table. A pillow on the overbed table supports the head. The arms may be positioned on or around the pillow. Additional pillows are used to support the resident's body and maintain proper alignment.

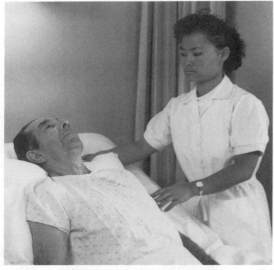

FIGURE 24–10. Position the resident in the high Fowler's position with head tilted slightly back to straighten out airway.

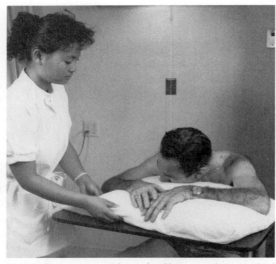

FIGURE 24–11. Place a pillow on the overbed table in front the resident so he may be supported as he leans forward.

Most out-of-bed residents with COPD breathe best when sitting forward in a chair with the body supported with the elbows on the arms of the chair or on their legs.

Positioning for Improved Drainage____

Rotary or *postural drainage* is a technique in which the position of the resident is changed so that gravity can assist in draining different areas of the chest, figure 24–12. Drugs called **mucolytics**, which loosen the sputum and dilate the bronchi, are given before each series of position changes are carried out. Position changes should be made slowly — not abruptly — and residents must be supervised during the entire activity. It is important to:

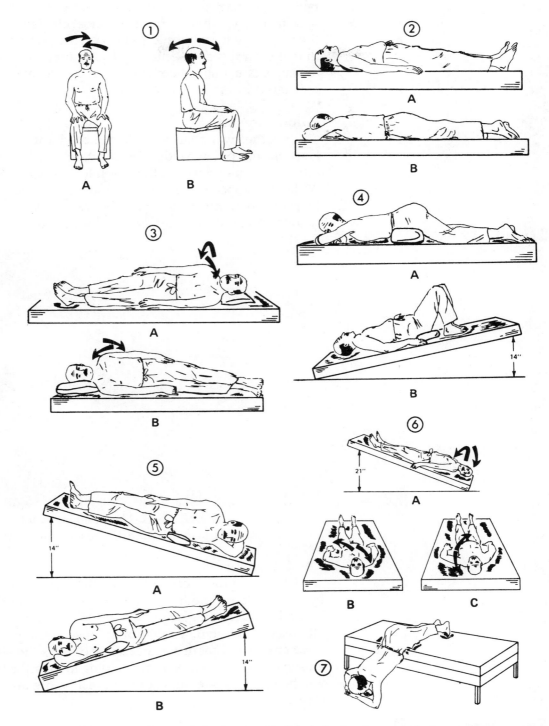

FIGURE 24–12. *Postural drainage exercises help to clear respiratory passages.*

Drainage is improved through position changes, chest tapping, mucolytic drugs.

- watch for signs of fatigue
- provide support and protection in each position

Tilt Table

The resident may be strapped to a **tilt table** during position changes. Several different positions can be maintained while on a tilt table. The exact positions chosen are determined by the resident's specific needs. This is one of the most efficient ways to carry out the therapy since it requires less effort on the part of the resident. Be sure that the straps are secure and alignment is maintained. Postural drainage is usually the responsibility of a respiratory therapist or a registered nurse.

Pillow Support

Another way that position can be changed to promote drainage is to place a pillow under the resident's abdomen, then under one hip, and then under the other, each for a specific length of time, figure 24–13. It is important that you understand the specific orders relating to postural drainage so that you can assist in the most effective manner. You must constantly guard the resident against falls or injury.

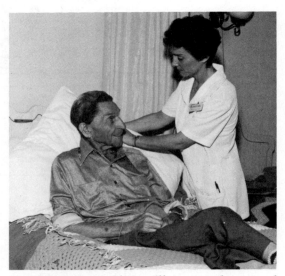

FIGURE 24–13. Three pillows may be crossed and placed behind the resident for support.

Chest Tapping

Chest tapping is carried out by the nurse, therapist or personally by the resident. The fingers are cupped and the chest wall is gently tapped with the fingertips, working in a systematic manner so that all areas are treated. The tapping loosens the phlegm, figure 24–14.

Remember that drugs that dilate or relax the air passageways and loosen and thin the mucus are helping to clear the tubes. They usually will be given by the nurse or therapist before tapping or positioning for drainage.

Exercises_____

Breathing exercises improve expiration.

Residents can be taught breathing exercises that improve respiration and that increase general respiratory muscle tone. Breathing exercises place stress on the expiration phase of respiration. The resident is first taught the basic breathing pattern, which is to breathe in through the nose to the count of "one," allowing the abdomen to rise. Air is then forced out of the lungs through pursed lips to the count of "two" and "three" as the abdominal wall is contracted.

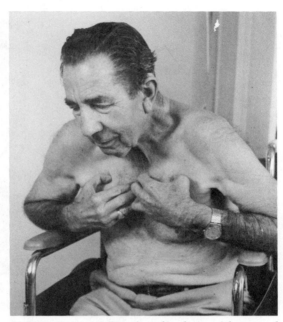

FIGURE 24–14. *Tapping the chest with cupped fingers loosens the phlegm.*

Therapy that encourages the resident to improve ventilation through the use of devices and exercise is called incentive therapy, figure 24–15. Examples include:

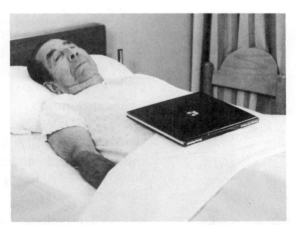

FIGURE 24–15. *Books of varying weights on the abdomen are used during ventilatory exercise periods.*

- blowing a candle out at various distances
- blowing against water resistance into a bottle
- blowing a feather or Ping Pong ball across a table

The same breathing exercises can be practiced with a weight on the abdomen, figure 24–16. The weight adds resistance to the effort and improves overall muscle tone. Ambulation, moving to music, and

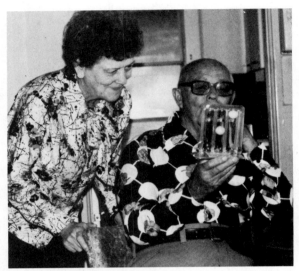

FIGURE 24–16. *Incentive spirometer improves alveolar ventilation and prevents atelectasis.*

doing bed exercises, including ROM activities, increase circulation and respiration and should be encouraged and routinely carried out.

Oxygen Therapy

Residents with COPD can benefit from low levels of oxygen. Oxygen therapy may be administered by:

- small tubes (**cannulas**) placed at the entrance of the resident's nose and held in place by straps, figure 24–17.
- **mask**, which is placed over the resident's nose and mouth and secured in place
- catheter — a small plastic or rubber tube that is inserted into the nose

The nurse will start the oxygen but you must watch the resident and equipment carefully to see that the procedure continues to be done properly. Every time you observe the resident, check the following points:

Oxygen is usually given by cannula, catheter or mask.

- The catheter, cannula, or mask are in proper position and the elastic band is snug but not constricting.
- There are no areas of irritation from straps, catheter, cannula, or mask.
- The flow meter is registering the volume properly in liters (figures 24–18 and 24–19).
- There are no kinks in the tubing. A pin tunnel around the tubing allows the resident to move without obstructing the flow of oxygen.
- The oxygen is properly moisturized.
- The resident's face is kept free of secretions.
- Safety precautions are being followed.

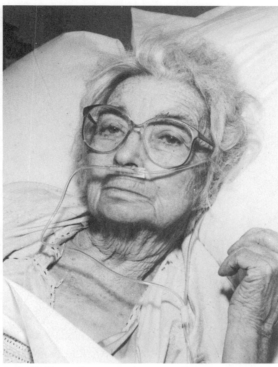

FIGURE 24–17. This resident is receiving oxygen through nipple-shaped cannulas.

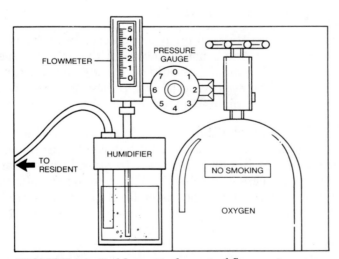

FIGURE 24–18. Note attachment of flow meter gauge to oxygen tank.

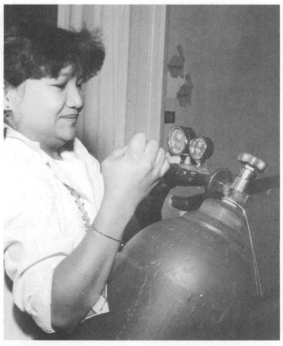

FIGURE 24–19. The gauge must be firmly attached to the tank and tightened with a wrench.

Source of Oxygen. The source of oxygen may be piped into the resident's room, but in long term care facilities tanks of oxygen may be used, figure 24–20. If a tank is used, be sure that:

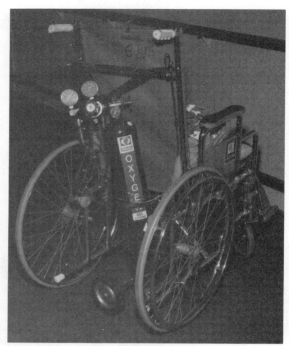

FIGURE 24–20. Resident needing continuous oxygen may transport tanks of oxygen on the back of the wheelchair.

- No smoking signs are in place.
- There is sufficient oxygen in the tank. Check the gauge each time you visit the resident.
- An additional tank is available.
- Empty tanks are marked and stored according to facility policy.
- The tank is secure on the carrier or in the stand.
- The oxygen is moisturized.

Oxygen doesn't explode, but when it is present, burning is more intense and rapid. Everyone must be aware of the safety measures and follow them carefully. If a fire should occur, sound the alarm and get the resident to safety, following facility policy. You may want to review the safety rules explained in Lesson 7.

Special Mouth Care_

Mouth breathing and inhalation of oxygen are drying. The resident may complain sputum has a bad taste. It is essential to make sure that the resident rinses his or her mouth frequently and that you provide special mouth care, figure 24–21. This nursing attention adds greatly to the resident's comfort. Encourage fluid intake since adequate fluids help decrease the thickness of secretions, figure 24–22.

PROCEDURE: Assisting with Special Oral Hygiene

1. Wash hands and assemble the following equipment:
   a. emesis basin
   b. bath towel
   c. plastic bag
   d. applicators
   e. mouthwash or solution in cup

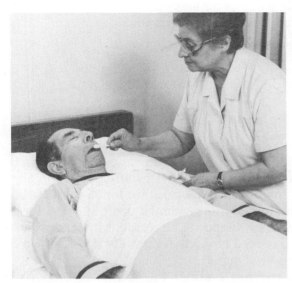

FIGURE 24–21. *Since residents with respiratory handicaps often are mouth breathers, special care is needed.*

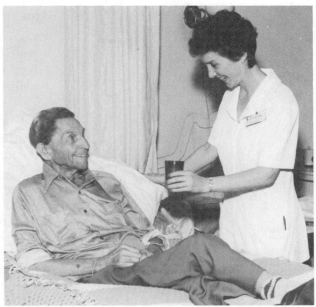

FIGURE 24–22. *Encouraging fluids helps keep respiratory secretions dilute and easier to expel.*

f. tongue depressor
g. water-based lubricant for lips
2. Identify resident and explain what you plan to do. Screen unit.
3. Cover pillow with towel and turn resident's head to one side. Place emesis basin under resident's chin.
4. Open mouth gently with tongue depressor.
5. Dip applicators into mouthwash solution. (In some cases, a physician may order hydrogen peroxide solution.)
6. Using moistened applicators, wipe gums, teeth, tongue, and inside of mouth.
7. Discard used applicators in plastic bag.
8. Lubricate lips.
9. Clean and replace equipment. Wash hands.
10. Report and record procedure on chart.

Ineffective Cough

If cough is ineffective, the resident may need to be intubated and suctioned and oxygenated through an **endotracheal tube.** The endotracheal tube is placed directly into the trachea through an opening (tracheostoma) for the delivery of oxygen and for the purpose of suctioning.

A machine that delivers oxygen under pressure at a preset rate may be needed to assist ventilation. This technique is known as **intermittent positive pressure breathing (IPPB).** The machine may be directly attached to the endotracheal tube. When a resident is receiving IPPB, you must monitor him or her very carefully for:

- change of color
- signs of congestion
- changes in vital signs
- any indications of respiratory distress

Carbon Dioxide Narcosis

The resident suffering with advanced COPD experiences increasing respiratory difficulty, eventually leading to ventilatory failure, carbon dioxide narcosis, and eventual coma and death.

Poor ventilation and exchange leads to carbon dioxide narcosis.

Carbon dioxide narcosis develops as blood levels of carbon dioxide rise. Signs of carbon dioxide narcosis include:

- poor response and lethargy
- psychotic behavior
- confusion
- belligerence

You can help by:

- Elevating the head of the bed to 30° or 40°.
- Positioning the pillow behind the shoulders so that the head is tilted slightly back. This helps straighten the airway.
- Lowering the bed to a flat position for 15 minutes every 2 to 3 hours to change the resident's position. Position changes help promote ventilation. The resident's total position should be changed every 2 hours to reduce the possibility of decubiti.
- Monitoring vital signs.
- Informing the nurse about the resident's response or any change in the resident's condition.

VOCABULARY

allergen	emphysema	pleura
alveoli	endotracheal tube	postural drainage
arrested	expectorate	regurgitating
aspiration	expiration	respiration
asthma	glottis	sputum
bronchi	halitosis	tachypnea
bronchioles	hemoptysis	thorax
bronchitis	high Fowler's position	tilt table
cannula	inspiration	trachea
carbon dioxide	intermittent positive	tracheotomy
carbon dioxide narcosis	breathing (IPPB)	tubercle
cellular respiration	larynx	tuberculosis disease
chronic obstructive lung disease	mucolytic	tuberculosis infection
chronic obstructive pulmonary disease (COPD)	orthopneic position	ventilation
	oxygen	vocal cords
	oxygen mask	
	pharynx	
	phlegm	

SUGGESTED ACTIVITIES

1. Learn the parts of the respiratory system by studying diagrams or models.
2. Observe a demonstration of oxygen administration.
3. Give supervised care to selected residents who have conditions involving the respiratory tract.
4. Review specific facility policy relating to fire safety.

REVIEW

A. Brief Answer/Fill in the Blanks

1. Cellular respiration is a process in which glucose and oxygen are combined to produce:

    a. _____

    b. _____

    c. _____

2. Another name for the windpipe is the _____.

3. As a person ages, breathing capacity diminishes by _____.

4. Changes in the larynx make the voice _____ and
_____.

5. A resident recovering from a laryngectomy needs a great deal of
_____.

6. The tracheotomy stoma must be protected against _____ and
_____.

7. Rapid, shallow breathing is known as _____.

8. Tuberculosis that is contained by a tubercle is said to be _____.

9. Three conditions leading to COPD are:

    a. _____

    b. _____

    c. _____

10. Three techniques which improve ventilation, drainage, and comfort for
the resident with COPD include:

    a. _____

    b. _____

    c. _____

B. Identification. On this diagram of the respiratory tract, label numbers 1 through
5.

    1. _____

    2. _____

    3. _____

    4. _____

    5. _____

CLINICAL SITUATION

Mary Calcetas is 72 and has been a cigarette smoker for many years. Emphysema has taken its toll and now the very act of breathing is an effort, and walking the length of the corridor to the day room requires two rest periods along the way. Smoking is only permitted under supervision in the day room so, difficult as it is, she slowly makes her way there early each morning. When an infection occurs, she requires nasal oxygen and orthopneic positioning. The nurse assigns you to collect a sputum specimen. Describe the equipment you would need.

Answer: _____

_____

_____

_____

LESSON 25 The Endocrine System and Disorders Related to Endocrine Imbalance

OBJECTIVES

After studying this lesson, you should be able to:

- Name the endocrine glands and some of their hormones.
- State the general function of the hormones.
- Define the term electrolyte.
- Explain the importance of electrolyte balance.
- Recognize reportable signs and symptoms of diabetes mellitus.
- Recognize reportable signs and symptoms of hypokalemia and hypernatremia.
- Select the proper equipment and carry out urine testing for glucose using Clinitest tablets or Tes-Tape strips, and for ketone bodies (acetone) using Acetest tablets or Ketostix.
- Report and record the findings of urine testing properly.
- Define and spell all the vocabulary words and terms.

INTRODUCTION

Hormones are chemical regulators.

The endocrine system consists of glands that are made of special tissues found in widely separated areas of the body, as you can see from figure 25-1. These glands produce chemical messengers called hormones (figure 25–2), which enter the bloodstream directly and are quickly carried to all parts of the body. The hormones are important regulators of body activities and body chemistry.

There are seven distinct endocrine glands (some of which are in pairs).

Hormones are secreted directly into the bloodstream.

Some endocrine glands secrete several hormones (see figure 25–2). In addition to the glands discussed in this lesson, glandular cells scattered throughout the body secrete minute but important regulatory hormones. The endocrine glands and cells deliver their secretions directly into the bloodstream to be carried throughout the body. These are the:

- **pituitary gland**
- **pineal body**
- **parathyroid glands**
- **thyroid gland**
- **adrenal glands**
- **islets of Langerhans (pancreas)**
- **gonads — ovaries** (in women); **testes** (in men)

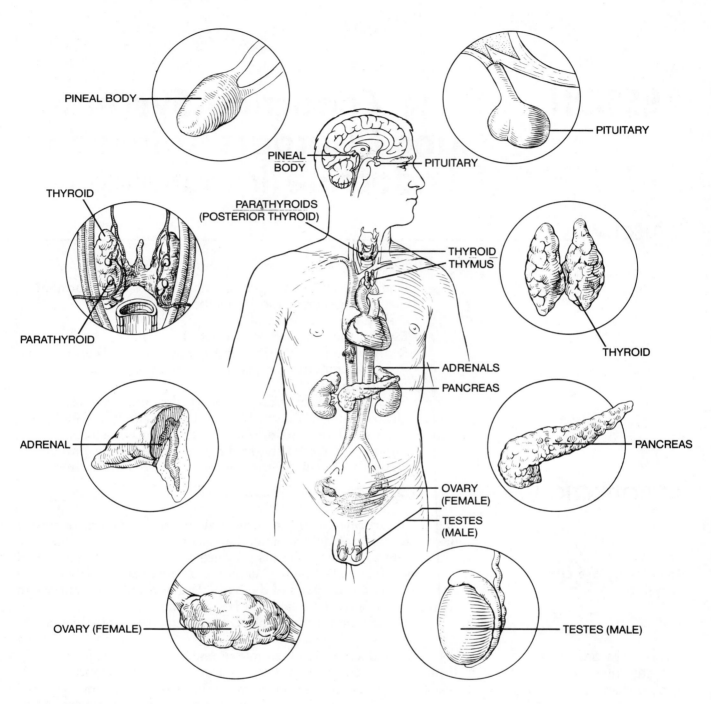

FIGURE 25-1. The endocrine glands.

Pituitary Gland_____

The pituitary is found under the brain and secretes more than one hormone. It is sometimes called the "master gland." The hormones secreted by this gland control:

- growth
- urine production
- contractions of involuntary muscles
- the activity of most of the other glands

Gland	Hormone(s)
Pituitary	Adrenocorticotropic hormone (ACTH)
	Antidiuretic hormone (ADH)
	Follicle-stimulating hormone (FSH)
	Lactogenic hormone (LTH)
	Luteinizing hormone (LH)
	Somatotropic hormone (STH)
Thyroid	Triiodothyronine (T_3)
	Thyroxine (T_4)
Parathyroid	Parathormone — also called parathyroid hormone (PTH)
Gonads	
Ovaries (female)	Estrogen
	Progesterone
Testes (male)	Testosterone
Adrenals	Androgenici hormone
	Adrenalin
	Glucocorticoids (cortisone)
	Mineralocorticoids
Islets of Langerhans (pancreas)	Insulin
	Glucagon
	Somatostatin

FIGURE 25-2. Major endocrine gland and hormone secretions.

Pineal Body

The pineal body is a small gland that is also located in the skull beneath the brain. Very little is known about this gland. It is thought to be somehow related to sexual development. It grows smaller as we age.

Adrenal Glands

There are two adrenal glands. They are located on top of each of the two kidneys. Each gland has two distinct portions, which secrete separate hormones. Two of these hormones, **adrenaline** (epinephrine) and **cortisone**, are widely used in medicine. In general, the adrenal hormones:

- control the release of energy to meet emergencies
- control water and electrolyte balance in the body
- secrete small amounts of male and female sex hormones

Gonads

The term "gonads" refers to the sex glands. In women, these are the ovaries. In men they are the testes.

Ovaries. The paired ovaries are located within the pelvis on either side of the uterus. When stimulated by the pituitary gland, they produce the hormones **progesterone** and **estrogen**.

Progesterone is the hormone that helps to maintain pregnancy. Estrogen is responsible for the development of female characteristics such as:

- enlargement of the female reproductive organs
- appearance of pubic and axillary hair
- enlargement of the breasts
- onset and regulation of menstruation

Testes. The testes, the male sex glands, are also paired and are located outside of the body in a pouch called the **scrotum**. They produce the hormone testosterone, which is responsible for secondary male characteristics. These include:

- muscular development
- deepening voice
- growth of hair on body and face
- growth and maturity of the reproductive organs

The male and female gonads also produce the special cells, the female ovum and the male sperm, that unite to form a new person during conception.

Thyroid Gland

The thyroid gland is located in the neck, just in front of the larynx. **Thyroxine**, a major hormone secreted by this gland, helps to regulate the metabolic rate of all the cells of the body.

Metabolism is the production of heat and energy by the cells. Energy production is related to the ability of the cells to take up and use oxygen to produce energy. You may remember that this process is called cellular respiration.

Parathyroids

The parathyroids are several tiny glands embedded in the back of the thyroid gland. **Parathormone**, a hormone that they manufacture, controls the use of calcium and phosphorus by the body. Calcium and phosphorus are two electrolyte minerals. (Electrolyte Balance is discussed in the next section of this lesson.)

The Islets of Langerhans

The islets of Langerhans are small groups of cells found within the pancreas. Two very important hormones produced by these cells are:

- **insulin**
- **glucagon**

Glucose is blood sugar.

Glucagon and insulin help to regulate the level of sugar in the bloodstream — this sugar is called **glucose**. Glucose is the form of energy needed for *all* body work. Glucose metabolism and the disorder of glucose metabolism called diabetes mellitus, which is often seen in residents, are discussed in detail later in this lesson.

ELECTROLYTE BALANCE

Much of the body chemistry depends on balancing certain substances called electrolytes that are found in the body fluids. You may be familiar with them as solid compounds such as sodium chloride (table salt) and sodium bicarbonate, an antacid used to relieve indigestion.

In the body fluids the electrolyte compounds break apart to form ions which influence the body's chemical reactions. Some important electrolyte compounds contain the ions of:

- sodium (Na)
- potassium (K)
- chloride (Cl)
- bicarbonate (HCO_3)

The **homeostasis** of the body functions (staying the same — balanced) is a complex process that depends on many body activities. The endocrine system plays an important part in this process.

When there is an electrolyte imbalance in the body, many problems — sometimes serious — can occur. Two problems are:

- hypernatremia — increased sodium levels in the blood
- hypokalemia — decreased levels of potassium in the bloodstream

Hypernatremia. This means that there are increased levels of sodium in the blood. These levels are controlled in a large part by the hormone vasopressin, also called antidiuretic hormone (ADH). ADH is produced in the hypothalamus and stored in the pituitary gland. When hypernatremia occurs, the sodium tends to hold excess fluid in the body, resulting in swelling, or **edema**, which is often seen in the extremities of elderly residents.

Hypokalemia. In this condition there are decreased levels of potassium in the blood. Hypokalemia is usually seen at the same time as hypernatremia, because sodium and potassium levels in extra-cellular fluids are very closely related. The hormone aldosterone, produced by the adrenal glands, is extremely important in adjusting sodium and potassium balance. In hypokalemia, the heart rate slows because of the low levels of potassium. A resident with this condition will feel weak and apathetic.

Hyponatremia (low levels of sodium in the blood) and **hyperkalemia** (increased levels of potassium in the blood) are two other conditions that may occur when there is an electrolyte imbalance. Again, various hormones are important in preventing these conditions.

GLUCOSE METABOLISM ■■■■■■■■■■■■■■■■■■■■■■■■■■■■■■■■■■■■

Remember, glucose is used as the primary energy source for all of the work done by the body. Just the right level of glucose is needed for proper functioning. Various hormones and enzymes play a part in maintaining this level and in helping the body to use (metabolize) glucose for energy, but the hormones glucagon and insulin are especially important.

Glucagon causes the plasma glucose (blood sugar) level to *rise* by converting stored sugar (glycogen) to glucose. Insulin causes the plasma glucose level to *fall* by promoting the movement of glucose from the bloodstream into the cells. It also helps in the conversion of glycogen (stored sugar) to glucose.

Abnormal plasma glucose, or blood sugar, levels are called:

- hyperglycemia — meaning that the blood sugar level is too high
- hypoglycemia — meaning that the blood sugar level is too low

A major disorder due to a breakdown in glucose homeostasis, and usually caused by insufficient insulin in the body, is **diabetes mellitus**, discussed in the following section.

DIABETES MELLITUS

In diabetes mellitus, the body is unable to use glucose in the proper manner to meet the energy needs of the body. It is a disease that is particularly common in older age groups. In fact, 1 out of every 20 persons over 65 years of age require treatment for diabetes.

There are two forms of diabetes:

- insulin-dependent diabetes mellitus (IDDM)
- non–insulin-dependent diabetes mellitus (NIDDM)

Although both forms may be seen in older persons, it is more common to see the non-insulin dependent form (NIDDM).

Insulin-Dependent Diabetes Mellitus (IDDM). IDDM is more often seen in younger persons and is associated with typical classical signs and symptoms. These include:

- abrupt onset
- excess thirst (**polydipsia**)
- excess urine elimination (**polyuria**)
- excessive hunger (**polyphagia**)

This is a more difficult form of the diabetes to control and diabetic persons may experience periods of hypoglycemia (**insulin shock**) or hyperglycemia (**diabetic coma**). These people require:

Some diabetics require insulin; in others, the disease can be controlled by diet alone.

- regular injections of insulin in order to balance their blood sugar
- regulation of food intake
- planned exercise (which uses sugar for energy) as part of the treatment program

Non-Insulin Dependent Diabetes Mellitus (NIDDM). Non–insulin-dependent diabetes mellitus (NIDDM), known as old-age diabetes or ketosis-resistant diabetes, usually begins in older age. The older the person, the more likely that the condition will develop. It is ten times more common than the insulin-dependent form. However it is more stable, with less incidents of diabetic coma or insulin shock.

Signs and Symptoms

Very often only one or two symptoms are apparent in the elderly person. The person is usually overweight and may complain of constant fatigue or have a sore or infection that takes an unusually long time to heal. About half those with diabetes show the obvious signs, figure 25–3. The others have less well-defined symptoms such as:

- easily fatigued
- skin infections
- slow healing
- itching
- burning on urination
- pain in fingers and toes and vision changes

- Polyuria
- Polydipsia
- Polyphagia
- Weight loss
- Blurring of vision
- Complaints of itching
- Burning on urination
- Redness or tenderness at injection site
- Uneaten food
- Medications not taken
- Infections or injuries

FIGURE 25–3. Note and report on diabetic residents.

Complications of Diabetes

Complications can be severe and intractable (non-reversible) in the elderly. They include:

- vision changes
- cardiovascular damage
- hyperglycemia
- hypoglycemia

Vision Changes. This is particularly common in long-term diabetes. Serious vision changes may be thought to be due to general aging and may really be related to a diabetic condition. Glaucoma, cataracts, and retinitis proliferans are common eye involvements. Blindness is also a complication of long-term diabetes.

Cardiovascular Damage. The consequences of insulin shock or diabetic coma can be very severe in the elderly patient and can include heart attacks and strokes. Because injuries heal poorly, an ingrown toenail or improperly cut nails can lead to serious consequences. Vascular changes can so interfere with the normal circulation that the tissues of toes, feet, and even legs may die and need to be removed (amputated).

Diabetic coma may develop over a 24-hour period.

Hyperglycemia. This condition (diabetic coma) occurs when there is insufficient insulin for metabolic needs and sugar and ketone compounds (e.g., **acetones**) build up in the blood (**ketosis**) and spill over into the urine (**glycosuria**). It is less apt to occur in the NIDDM, which is why this form of the disease is also known as *ketosis-resistant* diabetes. Sudden, unexpected need for insulin brought about by stress, illness, or injury or curtailed activity may bring on a state of ketosis. It usually develops slowly, sometimes over a 24-hour period. Perhaps the first symptoms noted will be headache, drowsiness, and confusion. The resident seems less responsive, irritable, confused, and drowsy and may slip slowly into unconsciousness (coma).

Signs and symptoms of hyperglycemia include:

- thirst
- blurred vision
- nausea and vomiting
- a sweet odor to the breath
- dry, flushed skin

It is important to note these indications early so that the condition can be treated right away. Carefully study and learn the signs and symptoms of diabetic coma, figure 25–4, and, if noted in a resident, report the situation immediately. The immediate treatment for hyperglycemia is insulin, which will be given by the nurse.

Diabetic Coma (Hyperglycemia)	Insulin Shock (Hypoglycemia)
Gradual onset	Sudden onset
Drowsiness	Nervousness
Deep, difficult breathing	Shallow breathing
Nausea	Hunger
Sweet odor to breath	
Hot, flushed, dry skin	Moist, pale skin
Mental confusion	Mental confusion Vision disturbance
Loss of consciousness	Loss of consciousness

FIGURE 25–4. Note and report the signs and symptoms of diabetic coma and insulin shock.

Hypoglycemia can develop very rapidly.

Hypoglycemia. Hypoglycemia or low blood sugar occurs far less commonly when oral antidiabetic agents are given than when insulin is by injection. When hypoglycemia results from an overdose of insulin, it is referred to as *insulin reaction* or **insulin shock**. Hypoglycemia can be brought on by:

- neglecting planned snacks or taking less food (e.g., when the resident has a generally diminished appetite)
- unusual activity
- stress

- vomiting
- diarrhea
- interaction of oral drugs with other medications being taken

In contrast to ketosis, which develops slowly, hypoglycemia reactions are apt to occur rapidly.

Signs and symptoms of hypoglycemia include:

- hunger
- sweating
- dizziness
- drowsiness
- blurred vision
- erratic behavior
- staggering gait
- mental confusion
- disorientation
- pale and moist skin

Make sure that you learn the signs and symptoms of hypoglycemia (see figure 25–4) and report immediately to the nurse if you observe them in a resident.

The hypoglycemic resident is treated with sugar in some form. A food containing sugar is given orally if the resident is conscious. If the resident is unconscious, glucagon may be given by injection. Orange juice or other easily absorbed sources of sugar are usually kept on the unit where they are easily accessible for emergency use. Every staff member should be aware of the storage location.

Treatment of Diabetes_____

Diet, exercise, and insulin as hypoglycemic drugs must be balanced.

For diabetics living independently, the control of the disease centers on self-care. When the diabetic person becomes a resident, the self-care is assisted. Residents should be encouraged to participate in their own care to the maximum extent possible. Whether at home or in a care setting, the goals remain the same: to maintain a proper metabolic balance and to prevent complications.

Although it is not common, it is possible for the less stable form of diabetes (IDDM) to first appear in later years. Therefore, if you notice any of the acute signs, they should be reported at once. A few elderly diabetics are insulin dependent. The treatment is then the same for any insulin-dependent person. Some people who have been diabetics since their youth will continue to require a regular routine of insulin injections.

There are three factors in each diabetic's life that need to be balanced. They are:

- diet
- exercise
- drugs

Diet. Most diabetics receive a specially planned diabetic diet tray. A large part of your responsibility will include serving the trays, assisting in feeding, and returning trays after meals. Be sure to:

- check trays carefully to be sure the correct diet is given
- notice and record how much food was eaten
- inform the nurse if food is not eaten
- give supplemental foods as ordered

If concentrated sugars such as jellies or jams are on the tray, be sure to check with the nurse before feeding the resident, since concentrated sugars are never permitted on a diabetic tray. There is not full agreement by physicians as to the rigidity of the diet that must be followed, but you must know what is allowed for each resident in your care.

Exercise. The more a person exercises, the more sugar is needed for energy. The increased need for sugar usage increases the need for insulin. Less exercise decreases the need. A resident's activity will influence the need for both food and insulin. Be sure to report either unusual activity or unusual inactivity.

Drugs. Drugs used in the treatment of diabetes are called antidiabetic drugs. Some of these may be taken by mouth (oral hypoglycemics) but insulin must be injected. The nurse will administer the drugs, but you also have some responsibilities. In the case of oral hypoglycemics, if the drugs are not taken, be sure to report this observation — for example, if a pill is given to the resident and then is spit out after the nurse leaves the room, report this to the nurse immediately.

If the resident is receiving insulin, check the injection site for:

- redness
- pain
- itching

Report any of these observations. Remember also that not all diabetics receive drugs to control their sugar levels.

URINE TESTING OF DIABETIC RESIDENTS ▪▪▪▪▪▪▪▪▪▪▪▪▪▪▪▪▪▪▪▪▪▪

Nursing measures
- urine testing
- foot care
- careful observing

Since hypoglycemic drugs and insulin are prescribed according to how well the body is using sugar for energy, blood tests and urine tests for sugar and ketone bodies (acetone) are performed regularly. Blood tests are usually done by a laboratory but routine urine testing is done in the resident's unit by the long-term care assistant, figure 25–5.

The amount of sugar and acetone that are being spilled in the urine gives valuable information about how well the metabolism is being balanced. Urine testing for sugar and acetone are important procedures which are routinely carried out.

Elderly diabetics with fairly stable conditions usually have their urine tested once each day. Those who are insulin dependent will have their urine tested four times each day: before each meal and at bedtime. The urine should be tested both for sugar and ketone bodies (acetone).

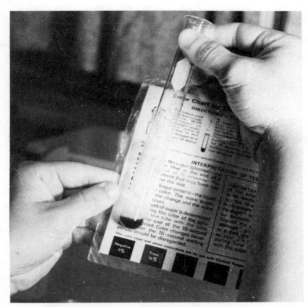

FIGURE 25–5. Compare the color of the test tube solution with the color chart.

Follow the procedures for urine testing carefully. Be sure to:

- Test freshly voided urine.
- Have the resident empty the bladder about one hour before the test. Collect the specimen for testing immediately before the test is to be done. When the morning specimen is being tested, the bladder should be emptied and the test made on the second specimen taken within the hour.
- Report to the nurse if the resident cannot void.
- Record the results on the appropriate record and report the results to the medication nurse when the test is completed.

If the resident is able to carry out the testing procedure, it is usually permitted, but you should observe the procedure and record and report the results.

Materials_____

Several materials of different types are available for conducting these tests:

- tablets such as Clinitest
- paper tapes such as Tes-Tape

Errors can occur if any of the tests are improperly timed or if the wrong chart is used for comparison. For safety, one type of test should be used routinely and the comparison chart kept posted in good light for accurate comparison.

▪▪▪ PROCEDURE: Urine Testing for Glucose Using Tes-Tape Strips ▪▪▪▪▪▪▪▪▪▪▪▪▪▪▪▪▪▪▪

1. Wash hands and assemble the following equipment:

   a. freshly voided specimen of urine
   b. Tes-Tape strips in container

c. watch with second hand

2. Open Tes-Tape container and withdraw approximately 1½ inches of Tes-Tape from container. Touch only the tip closest to your fingers.

3. Dip approximately ¼ inch of the strip into the urine sample. Withdraw, holding tip downward over urine container.

4. Time reaction for 60 seconds.

5. Check darkest area of wet strip against Tes-Tape color chart on back of Tes-Tape container, figure 25–6.

6. Read the figures above the color match. This is the value to record and report.

7. Discard tape and urine sample.

8. Clean equipment. Return to proper place.

9. Wash hands.

10. Report findings to nurse and record properly.

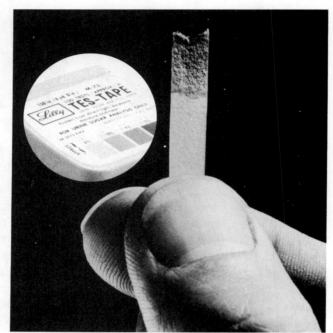

FIGURE 25–6. *The color of the Tes-Tape, which has been dipped in the specimen, is compared with a color chart.* (Courtesy of Eli Lilly and Company).

PROCEDURE: Urine Testing for Ketone Bodies Using Reagent Strips

1. Wash hands and assemble the following equipment:
   a. freshly voided sample of urine (same sample to be used for test which follows)
   b. reagent strips
   c. watch with second hand

2. Open container and remove one dipstick. Touch only one end.

3. Dip other end of dipstick into urine sample, figure 25–7A.

4. Remove and hold dipstick horizontally.

5. Wait 15 seconds. Compare color of dipstick with color code on bottle, figure 25–7B.

6. Dispose of urine sample if not to be saved.

7. Clean equipment according to facility policy.

8. Wash hands.

9. Report and record results properly.

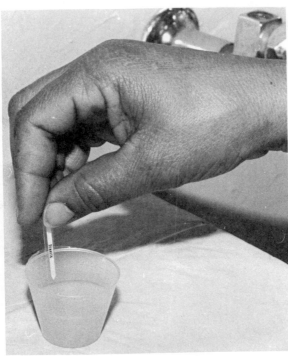

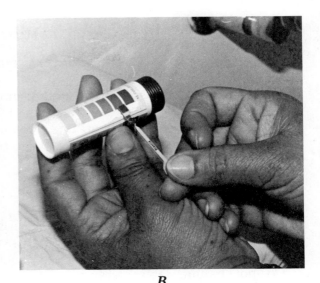

FIGURE 25–7. (A) Immerse the test area of the dipstick in the urine specimen. (B) Compare the test square on the dipstick with the color chart on the label.

▪▪▪ PROCEDURE: Urine Testing for Glucose Using Clinitest Tablets ▪▪▪▪▪▪▪▪▪▪▪▪▪▪▪▪▪▪▪▪▪

1. Wash hands and assemble the following equipment:
   a. freshly voided sample of urine
   b. Clinitest color chart
   c. medicine dropper
   d. watch with second hand
   e. Clinitest tablet
   f. test tube
   g. water
2. Read manufacturer's directions carefully.
3. Using medicine dropper, place 5 drops of urine in clean, dry test tube. Hold medicine dropper upright so urine does not touch sides of tube.
4. Rinse medicine dropper in cold water.
5. Add 10 drops of fresh water to test tube with dropper. If you miscount, empty tube and begin again.
6. Remove Clinitest tablet from wrapper. Do not touch it with the fingers. Drop tablet into test tube. If bottle of tablets is used, drop tablet into test tube from cover of bottle. Re-cover bottle at once.
7. Watch reaction carefully. (Do not handle tube during reaction since tube gets hot.) Fifteen seconds after the reaction has stopped, gently shake test tube. Compare resulting color with Clinitest color chart.
8. Discard unused portion of urine sample and contents of test tube.
9. Clean and replace equipment according to facility policy.
10. Wash hands.
11. Report and record results.

▦▦▦ PROCEDURE: Urine Testing for Ketone Bodies Using Acetest Tablets ▪▪▪▪▪▪▪▪▪▪▪▪▪▪▪▪

1. Wash hands and assemble the following equipment:
   a. freshly voided sample of urine (same sample that was used with previous procedure)
   b. medicine dropper
   c. watch with second hand
   d. Acetest tablet and color chart
   e. plain white paper
2. Read manufacturer's directions carefully.
3. Place one Acetest tablet on the white paper. Do not handle tablet with your fingers. Transfer it from the bottle to the cover, then drop it from the cover to the paper, figure 25–8.
4. Using medicine dropper, place one drop of urine on Acetest tablet.
5. Wait 30 seconds. Compare resulting color with Acetest color chart.
6. Discard tablet, paper, and urine sample.
7. Clean and replace equipment according to facility policy.
8. Wash hands.
9. Report and record results.

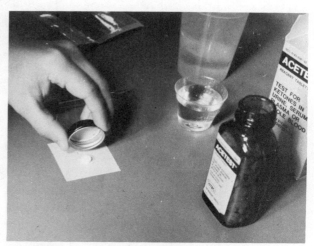

FIGURE 25–8. Place one Acetest tablet on a piece of white paper. Do not touch the tablet.

FOOT CARE OF DIABETIC RESIDENTS ▪▪▪▪▪▪▪▪▪▪▪▪▪▪▪▪▪▪▪▪▪▪▪▪▪▪▪

Since persons with diabetes do not heal as well as others, even a small injury can cause serious consequences. Circulation to the feet is especially poor, so healing of an injured toe or foot is particularly difficult. Great care must be taken of the diabetic resident's feet, including the following measures:

- Wash resident's feet daily.
- Carefully dry between toes. Do not allow moisture to collect between the toes.
- Inspect feet closely for any breaks or signs of irritation.
- Report any abnormalities to the nurse.
- Apply lanolin to dry feet.
- Massage feet daily.
- When toenails need cutting, report this to nurse. Cutting the toenails of diabetic resident should be performed only by a podiatrist.
- Be sure that shoes and stockings fit properly.
- Avoid anything that might injure the feet or interfere with circulation.

Gangrene (death of tissue), followed by amputation, is a common problem for the older diabetic, figure 25–9. Careful observations and care can help avoid this serious situation. Be sure to report any signs of infection or injury anywhere in the diabetic resident, so that proper steps can be taken quickly to prevent serious complications.

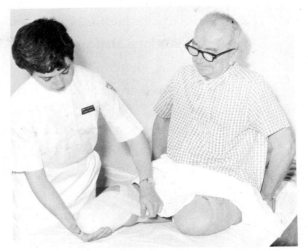

FIGURE 25–9. *Amputation is serious complication for the person who has diabetes mellitus.*

VOCABULARY

acetone	gonad	ovaries
adrenal glands	homeostasis	pancreas
adrenalin	hormone	parathormone
cortisone	hyperglycemia	parathyroid glands
diabetes mellitus	hyperkalemia	pineal body
diabetic coma	hypernatremia	pituitary gland
edema	hypoglycemia	polydipsia
electrolytes	hypokalemia	polyphagia
endocrine gland	hyponatremia	polyuria
estrogen	insulin	progesterone
extracellular	insulin shock	scrotum
gangrene	islet of Langerhans	testes
glucagon	ketone bodies	thyroid
glucose	ketosis	thyroxine
glycosuria		

SUGGESTED ACTIVITIES

1. Using a diagram or model, locate the seven endocrine glands.

2. Collect a sample of your own urine and carry out tests for sugar and ketone bodies using the Clinitest and Acetest tablets and Ketostix strips as outlined in the performance guide.

3. Practice recording urine test information on sample records.

4. Role play with classmates reporting urine testing findings to the charge nurse.

5. Carry out urine testing procedures in the clinical setting.

REVIEW

A. Brief Answer/Fill in the Blanks

1. A word meaning having low blood potassium is _____.

2. A word meaning having a high blood sugar is _____.

3. A condition that makes using sugar difficult is _____.

4. A gland that produces hormones is an _____ gland.

5. The glands that produce the reproductive cells are the _____.

6. Three areas of living to be balanced for the diabetic are diet, insulin or hypoglycemic agent, and _____.

7. Diabetic coma occurs when there is too high a level of _____ in the bloodstream.

8. The endocrine gland that secretes insulin is called the _____.

9. The endocrine gland that secretes parathormone is the _____.

10. Electrolyte compounds break apart in fluid to form _____.

11. The classical signs of diabetes mellitus are:

    a. _____

    b. _____

    c. _____

    d. _____

B. Matching. Match the word on the right with the correct term on the left.

1. _____ excessive hunger   a. polydipsia

2. _____ blood sugar   b. polyuria

3. _____ excessive thirst   c. polyphagia

                                               d. glycosuria

4. _____ increased urine output   e. glucose

5. _____ sugar in the urine

CLINICAL SITUATION

Mr. MacFarland is a diabetic and assigned to your care. You notice he seems very restless and less responsive than he usually is with you. As the morning passes, he grows increasingly confused. His 11 A.M. urine testing showed a moderate amount of acetone and a 3+ sugar. What action should you take?

Answer: _____

_____

_____

LESSON 26 The Reproductive System

OBJECTIVES

OBJECTIVES

After studying this lesson, you should be able to:

- Name the parts and functions of both male and female reproductive systems.
- Identify normal changes as they relate to the aging process.
- Describe major geriatric problems that are associated with the reproductive system.
- Properly carry out procedures related to the reproductive system.
- Define and spell all the vocabulary words and terms.

The reproductive system in men and women share some features in common but are different in other ways.

Both systems:

- consist of gonads, tubes, and accessory structures
- contribute to the reproductive process
- provide the sex hormones
- bring pleasure

Human **sexuality** is a complex interaction between the physical and emotional needs of an individual. Sexuality is intimately involved with the individual's sense of identity.

THE MALE REPRODUCTIVE SYSTEM

The male reproductive system consists of the primary organs (genitalia) and the accessory glands.

The primary organs are the:

- **penis**
- **testes**
- **epididymis**
- **vas deferens**
- **ejaculatory duct**

The accessory glands include the:

- **seminal vesicles**
- **prostate**
- **bulbourethral glands** (Cowper's glands)

The Penis

The male penis is the organ used for sexual intercourse (**coitus; copulation**) (figure 26–1). When the special tissues which the penis is made of become **engorged** (filled) with blood, the penis becomes enlarged and firm. The outer portion of the penis is covered by a loose skin fold called the **foreskin** or **prepuce**.

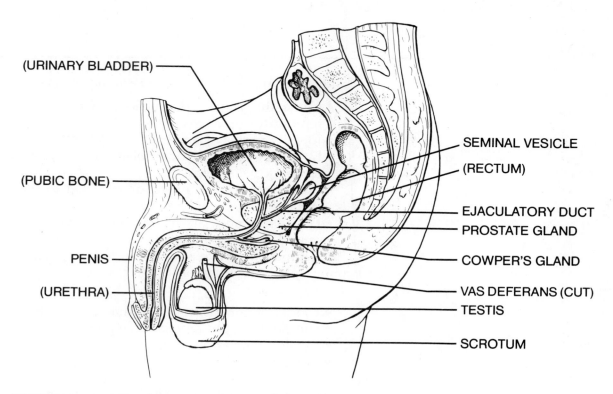

(URINARY BLADDER)

(PUBIC BONE)

PENIS

(URETHRA)

SEMINAL VESICLE

(RECTUM)

EJACULATORY DUCT

PROSTATE GLAND

COWPER'S GLAND

VAS DEFERANS (CUT)

TESTIS

SCROTUM

FIGURE 26–1. Lateral view of the male reproductive organs.

The male urethra serves two purposes. It carries:

1. reproductive fluid during intercourse
2. urine during voiding

The genitals give physical sexual identity.

The two activities cannot occur at the same time because they are under different nervous control systems.

The Testes

The testes (**testicles**) are found in a pouch-like structure called the **scrotum**, which is located outside the body. The testes produce the male sex cells (**sperm**) throughout life and the male hormone **testosterone**. You will remember that testosterone is responsible for the male characteristics.

Epididymis

The epididymis is a tube 20 feet long coiled on the back of each testis, which stores the sperm. The epididymis is the beginning of a tube system that moves the sperm upward and out of the body. The vas deferens, the ejaculatory duct, and the urethra are part of this pathway.

Vas Deferens_____

The vas deferens passes behind the urinary bladder, joining with the ejaculatory duct and entering the urethra.

Ejaculatory Duct_____

The ejaculatory duct carries the fluid produced in the seminal vesicles. This fluid contains nutrients and other substances needed to sustain the sperm. Surrounding the neck of the bladder is the prostate gland, which also contributes to the fluid.

Accessory Glands_____

As the sperm moves from the testes into the tube system, fluids from the seminal vesicles and prostate gland are added to form the seminal fluid or **ejaculate**. The ejaculate is released as a rhythmic series of muscular contractions which force the fluid through the urethra to the outside. The process is called **ejaculation** and occurs during sexual intercourse and may spontaneously occur at other times. The Cowper's glands, or the bubourethral glands, are two small glands located behind the urethra.

THE FEMALE REPRODUCTIVE SYSTEM ▦▦▦▦▦▦▦▦▦▦▦▦▦▦▦▦▦

The female reproductive system (figure 26–2) consists of the external genitalia (the vulva) and the internal organs (figure 26–3). These are the:

- **ovaries**
- **fallopian (uterine) tubes**
- **uterus**
- **vagina**

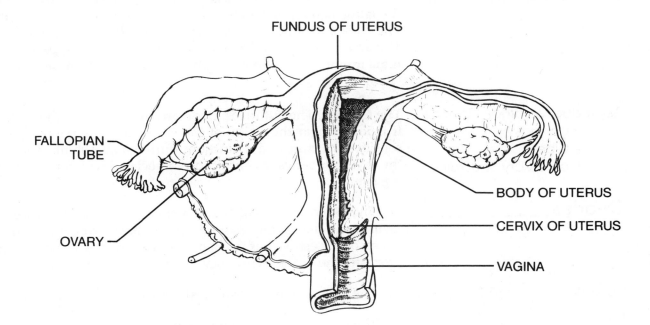

FIGURE 26–2. Internal female organs, ventral view.

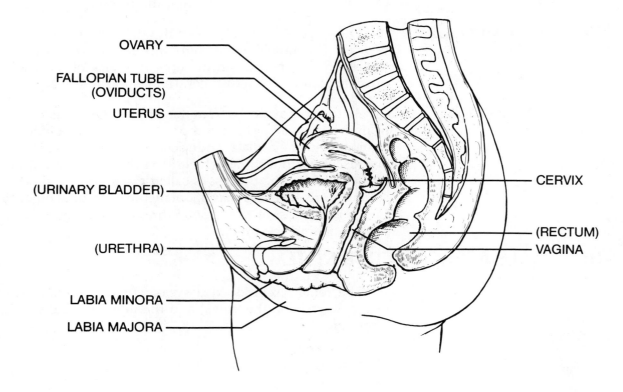

OVARY

FALLOPIAN TUBE (OVIDUCTS)

UTERUS

(URINARY BLADDER)

(URETHRA)

LABIA MINORA

LABIA MAJORA

CERVIX

(RECTUM)

VAGINA

FIGURE 26–3. Lateral view of the female reproductive organs.

The Vulva

The outside of the vulva is made up of two lip-like structures called the **labia majora**, figure 26–4. The labia majora are covered with hair. The labia surround the openings of the female urethra and vagina. The area between the vagina and anus is called the **perineum**. The **labia minora** are found inside the labia majora. They are two hairless "lips."

Reproductive organs include
• gonads
• tubes
• accessory structures

The Clitoris. The **clitoris** is an organ very similar to the male penis. It is found near the union of the labia. Like the penis, it is a very sensitive structure and it functions during sexual stimulation to begin the rhythmic series of contractions associated with female **climax**, or **orgasm**.

Ovaries

The two ovaries, which are the female gonads, produce the egg (**ovum**) and the hormones **progesterone** and **estrogen**. As discussed in Lesson 25, estrogen is needed to develop female characteristics and progesterone is the pregnancy-maintaining hormone.

Fallopian Tubes

The fallopian tubes (**oviducts**) carry the ovum toward the uterus.

Uterus

The uterus (**womb**) is a hollow muscular organ about three inches long. It is lined with a special membrane, the **endometrium**, which is periodically shed unless pregnancy exists. In pregnancy the endometrium nourishes the growing **fetus** (unborn infant in the womb).

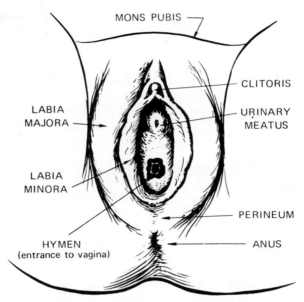

MONS PUBIS

CLITORIS

LABIA MAJORA

URINARY MEATUS

LABIA MINORA

PERINEUM

HYMEN
(entrance to vagina)

ANUS

FIGURE 26–4. External female genitalia.

Vagina_____

The vagina is a muscular tube which serves as the excretory duct for the menstrual flow and is the receptor of the penis during copulation.

MENSTRUAL CYCLE

During each menstrual cycle the uterus is prepared for pregnancy.

At **puberty** (between 9 and 17 years of age), the menstrual cycle, or female sexual cycle, begins. The cycle varies in length, usually between 25 and 30 days. The average is 28 days, which is why it is considered a monthly cycle.

During the menstrual cycle, a mature egg, or ovum (plural, *ova*), is released from one of the ovaries and travels from the ovary to one of the fallopian tubes, where it may be fertilized by a male sperm. At the same time that the ovum is being matured and expelled from the ovary (**ovulation**), the lining of the uterus (endometrium) is being built up and made ready to receive the fertilized ovum. If pregnancy does not occur, the endometrium is no longer needed and is carried out of the body as the menstrual flow. This process is known as **menstruation**.

It is interesting that, unlike the sperm cells, all the special cells that will become the ova exist at the time that a woman is born. When the last ova are released, the menstrual cycle ceases and menopause begins.

MENOPAUSE

As women age, the menstrual cycle becomes irregular and gradually ceases altogether. This is called the menopause, or **climacteric**. It usually occurs around the age of 55 and involves a natural series of changes that stops the menstrual cycle (**amenorrhea**). These changes are not abrupt but usually take place over a period of years. Because the ova are no longer being matured and released, pregnancy can no longer occur.

Some women may undergo a "surgical" menopause earlier in life after surgical removal of the uterus.

AGING CHANGES IN THE REPRODUCTIVE SYSTEM

Changes occur in both male and female reproductive organs with aging, but the need for sexual pleasure and sensual satisfaction does not stop.

Changes in the Male Reproductive System_____

Because of aging, in men there will be:

- slower sexual response
- delayed ejaculation
- decrease in the number of sperm (but number is still adequate for reproduction)
- gradual decrease in testosterone levels

Changes in the Female Reproductive System_____

These changes, which occur during menopause, include:

- decrease in estrogen levels
- thinning of tissue of vulva and vaginal walls and decrease in lubrication of vagina (because of this, elderly women are more prone to vaginal infections)
- weakening of breast tissues and muscles (sagging of breasts)

SEXUAL INTERCOURSE

Sexual intercourse is possible and is desired by many older couples (figure 26–5) even though pregnancy is no longer possible. Before sexual intercourse actually occurs, there is an excitement phase, which is induced by sexual thoughts or physical caressing. **Erection** occurs as the tissues of the penis fill with blood and the penis becomes erect (firm and enlarged). During this phase, the vagina becomes moist and receptive. The excitement reaches a plateau of arousal and is then followed by orgasm (climax) and a release of sexual tension.

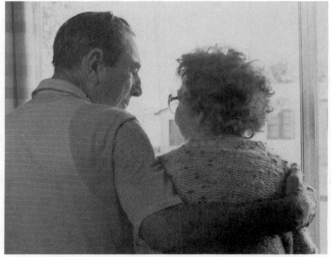

FIGURE 26–5. Elderly adults should not be denied the sexual pleasure they find in one another.

Sexual intercourse offers physical and emotional pleasure.

- In the female, the sexual sensations are centered in the vagina, uterus, and rectum.
- In the male they are associated with **ejaculation**.

Orgasm for both men and women is a series of pleasurable muscular contractions that are strong initially and gradually slow and stop. Both men and women feel satisfied and relaxed after coitus.

Men must wait awhile before repeating the act but women do not have to wait. They may experience another orgasm very soon if stimulated adequately.

Sexual intercourse has psychological and physical benefits since it meets sensual needs and is good physical exercise. Even those with severe physical limitations can have successful sexual experiences if those who give care can be open, mature, and understanding of human sexual needs.

SELF-STIMULATION

Remember that **masturbation** is the act of stimulating oneself sexually. Many people — both men and women — find this sexual outlet satisfying. It is a common way of gaining comfort when stressed and when other sexual opportunities are not available, figure 26-6.

You may feel uncomfortable when you notice such an activity going on, but it is not your right to interfere. You must:

- treat the situation calmly
- draw the curtains to provide privacy or move the resident to a more private area, figure 26-7
- not criticize or make fun of the resident

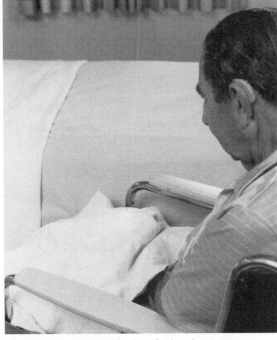

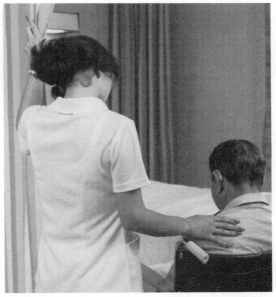

FIGURE 26-7. If you notice a resident stimulating himself provide privacy.

FIGURE 26-6. Self-stimulation is one way some elderly find to reduce built up sexual tension.

If this is a constant activity you might try occupying the resident in some other way. If your attitude is negative, this can make a difficult situation impossible or uncontrollable.

You may wish to review Lesson 14, which deals with the emotional and psychological needs of the resident and the importance of human sexual expression.

OTHER FORMS OF SEXUAL EXPRESSION

Sexual expression takes many forms.

Remember, sexual expression may take many forms other than sexual intercourse. Genital and non-genital caressing, touching one another, tender communications, masturbation (self-stimulation), and mental imaging (**fantasizing**) are examples of ways that people use to satisfy their sexual needs, figure 26–8.

Residents in a facility have little privacy, opportunity, or support that recognizes their need for sexual expression.

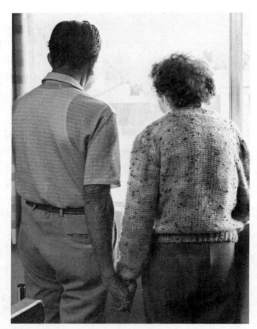

FIGURE 26–28. Sexual expression takes many forms including holding hands.

Limits to Sexual Expression

Unfortunately, many care givers are uncomfortable with the awareness that older people even in their 80s are still interested and capable of a real sexual expression or experience. Some care givers ignore the needs or pretend they don't exist. Others feel that there is something wrong or childish about residents who masturbate or touch one another. You must think honestly about your own sexuality and your attitude in regard to the sexuality of the elderly people in your care.

You must never encourage activities by residents that are not sought by other residents. However, if it is the policy in your facility to provide privacy for sexual activity, try to be open and supportive.

RELATED SURGICAL PROCEDURES ████████████████████████

None of these procedures interfere with the use of the sexual organs for pleasure.

Penile Implants_____

Impotence is the inability to have an erection. Erection may be difficult for some elderly men due to disease or medication. It is possible today for some men to have surgery in which special tubes are implanted in the penis to make erection possible.

Vasectomy_____

Vasectomy is a surgical procedure in which part of the male reproductive tubes (the vas deferens) is cut so that living sperm is no longer released during ejaculation and therefore pregnancy cannot occur. Following a vasectomy, a man is sterile.

Tubal Ligations_____

Women also may undergo surgical procedures that alter the reproductive organs. In a **tubal ligation**, the fallopian tubes are cut and tied. This prevents pregnancy. A woman becomes sterile following this procedure.

Hysterectomy_____

A **hysterectomy** is a fairly common operation in which the uterus is removed. Without a uterus, of course, the woman cannot bear children.

RELATED CONDITIONS ████████████████████████████

Malignancy_____

Malignancies of the male and female organs are fairly common. Be sure to report any bleeding or discharge from the reproductive tract of either male or female.

In the female, frequent sites include:

- the uterine wall
- ovaries
- cervix

In the male, malignancies are often found in the:

- prostate gland
- testes

Radiation, surgery, and chemotherapy may be used alone or in combination to treat these lesions.

Any condition that affects the reproductive organs threatens the individual's self-concept and sense of sexual identity. In addition to the fear inherent in a malignant diagnosis, the resident must also face the fear that he or she will lose his or her ability to fully function as a sexual human being.

You will need much understanding as you offer emotional support to those who suffer from reproductive malignancies.

Procidentia_____

Throughout life many women experience injury to the pelvic organs and pelvic floor. Repeated pregnancies, injury during childbirth, and aging contribute to a weakening of the supportive pelvic structures, resulting in the condition known as **procidentia**, or *prolapsed uterus*. In this condition:

- The uterus drops down from its normal position causing pressure in the vagina.
- There is a feeling of weight in the pelvic area.
- Urinary incontinence or retention occurs.
- The person is predisposed to urinary infections.

To treat procidentia, the uterus may have to be repositioned or removed. Both treatments require surgical intervention.

Vaginitis_____

Vaginitis is fairly common in older women because of the diminished protection offered by the thinner vaginal wall. Infections tend to be chronic and difficult to control.

Senile vaginitis responds to estrogen therapy, vaginal suppositories and mild *douches* to wash out the canal. Each of these therapies requires a specific physician's order.

▓▓▓ PROCEDURE: Giving Nonsterile Vaginal Douche ▪▪▪▪▪▪▪▪▪▪▪▪▪▪▪▪▪▪▪▪▪

1. Wash hands. Obtain disposable douche and bring to bedside with the following equipment:
   a. irrigating standard
   b. bed protector
   c. disposable gloves
   d. Monel cup with cotton balls
   e. disinfectant solution or powder
   f. toilet tissue
   g. bedpan and cover
   h. bath blanket
   i. plastic bag
2. Identify resident and explain what you plan to do.
3. Pour a small amount of specified disinfecting solution over cotton balls in Monel cup.
4. Hang douche container from standard. Close clamp on tubing.
5. Measure water in douche container. Temperature should be about 105°F. Add powder or solution as ordered.
6. Assemble the remaining equipment conveniently at bedside and screen unit.
7. If patient is wearing perineal pad, remove from front to back and discard in plastic bag.
8. Give bedpan to resident and ask her to void. After resident voids, empty and rinse bedpan, measuring urine if ordered. Return bedpan to bedside.
9. Drape resident with bath blanket. Fanfold top bedclothes to foot of bed.
10. Assist resident into dorsal recumbent position.
11. Place bed protector beneath resident's buttocks.
12. Place bedpan under resident.
13. Wash hands. Put on gloves.
14. Cleanse perineum, using one cotton ball with disinfectant for each stroke. Cleanse from vulva toward anus. Cleanse labia minora first. Expose labia minora with thumb and forefinger and cleanse. Give special attention to folds. Discard cotton balls in plastic bag.
15. Open clamp of tubing to expel air. Remove protector from sterile tip.
16. Allow small amount of solution to flow over inner thigh and then over vulva. Do not touch vulva with nozzle.
17. Allowing solution to continue to flow, insert nozzle slowly and gently about 3 inches into vagina with an upward and backward movement.
18. Rotate nozzle from side to side as solution flows.
19. When all solution has been used, remove nozzle slowly and clamp tubing.
20. Have resident sit up on bedpan to allow all solution to be expelled.
21. Remove douche bag from standard and place on paper towels.
22. Dry perineum with tissue. Discard tissue in bedpan.
23. Remove bedpan, cover, and place on chair.

24. Have resident turn on side. Dry buttocks with tissue.
25. Place clean perineal pad over vulva from front to back.
26. Remove bed protector and bath blanket. Replace top bedclothes.
27. Make resident comfortable and leave unit in order.
28. Observe contents of bedpan. Note character and amount of discharge, if any. Remove gloves and discard properly.

29. Clean and return equipment according to facility policy. Wash hands.
30. Report and record completion of procedure, including:
    a. date and time
    b. procedure: Vaginal irrigation (type, amount and temperature of solution)
    c. resident's reaction
    d. your observations regarding douche returns

Pruritus_____

Itching (**pruritus**) of the vulva (*pruritus vulvae*) and anus (*pruritus ani*) is a common complaint of older women. Continual irritation can cause tissue breakdown and permit bacteria to enter and cause infection. Since there are many factors which can contribute to pruritus, a search must be made for the cause, and then steps must be taken to correct the condition. For example, if soaps are irritating, they should not be used; if incontinence allows acid urine to irritate the tissues, then regular routine perineal care can eliminate the problem.

Be alert to the resident who scratches herself or seems irritated before the condition progresses too far.

Benign Prostatic Hypertrophy_____

Benign prostatic hypertrophy is a common problem for elderly men. It is a non-malignant enlargement of the prostate gland. Remember, the urethra passes through the center of this gland, so it is understandable that as the gland enlarges it closes off the flow of urine.

Residents with this condition may have difficulty starting and stopping the stream of urine. They may not be able to empty their bladder completely, which can lead to bladder infections. Frequency, nocturia, and poor urinary control, such as dribbling, are signs that need to be investigated.

To release the obstruction, a surgical procedure may be performed by entering through the urethra. This is called a **transurethral prostatectomy** (TURP). Although some surgical procedures on the prostate gland can result in **impotence**, this is not a complication of the transurethral approach.

VOCABULARY

amenorrhea	ejaculate	gonads
benign prostatic hypertrophy	ejaculation	hysterectomy
	ejaculatory duct	impotence
bulbourethral glands	endometrium	labia majora
climacteric	engorge	labia minora
climax	epididymis	masturbation
clitoris	erection	menopause
coitus	fantasizing	menstruation
copulation	fetus	orgasm
Cowper's glands	foreskin	ovaries
douche	genitalia	oviduct

ovulation	puberty	tubal ligation
ovum	scrotum	urethra
penis	seminal vesicles	uterine tubes
perineum	sexuality	vagina
prepuce	sperm	vaginitis
procidentia	testes	vas deferens
prostate	testicles	vasectomy
prostatectomy	testosterone	vulva
pruritus	transurethral	womb

SUGGESTED ACTIVITIES

1. Using charts and diagrams, study the parts of the male and female reproductive organs.

2. Write a short statement beginning with "When I think about older people and sex, I ———."

3. Discuss your feelings with your classmates about anything in this particular lesson that you have learned about and want to discuss.

4. Using a manikin, practice giving a nonsterile douche.

REVIEW

Brief Answer/Fill in the Blanks

1. Three functions of both male and female reproductive organs are:

   a. _____

   b. _____

   c. _____

2. Seminal fluid leaves the male body as _____.

3. Elderly female residents will already have passed through the climacteric, which is also known as _____.

4. Coitus has both _____ and _____ benefits.

5. The need for sexual expression does not necessarily _____ with age.

6. Surgery of the reproductive organs often threatens the individual's sense of _____.

7. Procidentia is also known as _____ uterus.

8. The temperature of a nonsterile douche solution should be about _____.

9. The douche nozzle should be inserted about _____ into the vagina.

10. When removing a perineal pad, you should never touch the _____ of the pad with your _____.

CLINICAL SITUATION

Gloria Laxamana, age 87, has been diagnosed as having a malignancy of the uterus and adjacent pelvic structures. A course of radiation has failed to control the process. She has a brownish discharge from the vagina and a nonsterile douche has been ordered for comfort. What equipment would you assemble to carry out this procedure?

Answer: _____

_____

_____

LESSON 27 The Nervous System

OBJECTIVES

After studying this lesson, you should be able to:

- Name the parts and functions of the nervous system and special senses.
- Identify and locate the special sense organs.
- Describe normal changes in the nervous system as they relate to the aging process.
- Recognize major health problems related to the aging nervous system.
- Provide for the safety of the confused resident.
- Define and spell all the vocabulary words and terms.

COMPONENTS OF THE NERVOUS SYSTEM

The nervous system controls activities by sending electrical messages called **nervous impulses** throughout the body. The two parts of the nervous system are the:

The nervous system is the body's communication network.

- **peripheral nervous system (PNS)** — includes the nerves outside the brain and spinal cord
- **central nervous system (CNS)** — includes the brain and spinal cord

Special sense organs receive information from the environment. The information travels along the cranial or spinal nerves to reach the brain and spinal cord, where the sensation is interpreted. The sensory receptors include the:

- eyes
- ears
- taste buds
- special receptors in the nose (**olfactory**) for smell
- multiple nerve endings (receptors) found in the skin, muscles, joints, and tendons

The nerve endings in the skin pick up sensations of pain, pressure, and variations in temperature. Receptors in the muscle, tendons, and joints carry information about the degree of muscle contraction and position of body parts. Other receptors in the walls of body organs carry information related to hunger, thirst, and **visceral** (organ) pain.

Neurons_____

Neurons are special strange-looking cells that carry messages, figure 27–1. The neurons and other supporting cells make up the nervous tissue of the brain, spinal cord, and peripheral nerves.

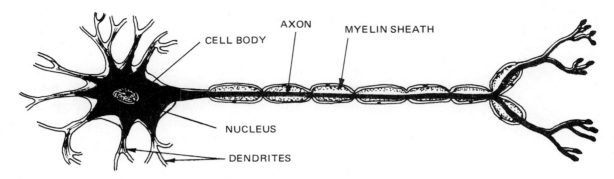

FIGURE 27–1. The neuron is the conducting cell of the nervous system.

Neurons are composed of:

- a central area, called the body
- one or more **dendrites** — processes that receive messages and carry them toward the cell body
- an **axon** — the process that carries messages away from the cell body

Axons and dendrites are called cell processes or **nerve fibers**. A message or nerve impulse begins in the dendrites and is carried along the cell body and then to the axon. It takes more than one neuron to carry the message from where it begins to where it can be carried out or interpreted. The neurons do not actually touch each other. The little space between the axon of one neuron and the dendrites of the next is called the **synapse**.

Neurotransmitters_____

Neurotransmitters are chemicals that make it possible to pass messages (nerve impulses) from one cell to another, figure 27–2. If the chemicals are not produced in adequate amounts, the message pathway becomes confused or blocked.

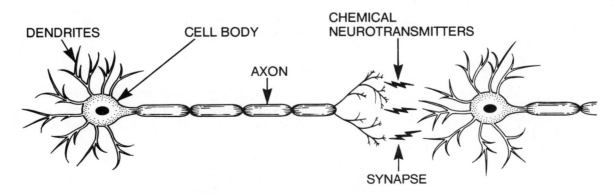

FIGURE 27–2. Chemicals (neurotransmitters) are needed to pass the nerve message across the synapse from one neuron to the next.

Nerves_____

Nerves are bundles of nerve fibers (axons and or dendrites) that connect the body with the central nervous system. Nerves are named according to the type of message they carry and the direction in which they carry the message. The two general types are:

- **sensory nerves**
- **motor nerves**

Sensory Nerves. Sensory nerves carry messages about pain, temperature change, changes in body position, taste, touch, sound and sight. They carry messages toward the brain and spinal cord. When sensory nerves are damaged, the ability to receive messages and interpret sensations is lost.

Motor Nerves. Motor nerves carry messages from the brain and spinal cord to muscles and glands to bring about body responses. When motor nerves are damaged, the person loses the ability to voluntarily control body functions. This condition is called **paralysis**. Paralysis may be complete with no movement possible or partial, so that there is a weaker response.

Peripheral Nerves. Throughout the body, mixed bundles of nerves carrying both sensory and motor fibers form the peripheral nerves. Just as a telephone cable with many insulated lines can carry messages going in different directions at the same time, the peripheral nerves carry both incoming and outgoing information in the same bundle. There are 31 pairs of spinal nerves that carry messages into and out of the spinal cord; 12 pairs of cranial nerves carry messages into and out of the brain.

The peripheral nervous system (PNS) is made up of the spinal nerves and cranial nerves.

CENTRAL NERVOUS SYSTEM ■■■■■■■■■■■■■■■■■■■■■■■■■■■■■■■

The central nervous system (CNS) is made up of the spinal cord and brain.

The central nervous system (CNS) is made up of the brain and spinal cord, figure 27–3. These tissues are very delicate and are protected by the bones of the skull and vertebral column. A triple-layered membrane, the **meninges**, also protects the brain and spinal cord.

The Spinal Cord_____

The spinal cord is about 18 inches long, and extends from the brain downward to just above the small of the back. The 31 pairs of spinal nerves enter and leave the spinal cord, carrying messages to and from the body.

The spinal cord:

- carries messages to and from the brain and relays them to the body through the spinal nerves, figure 27–4
- handles certain special responses called **reflexes**

A reflex occurs when an incoming message becomes an outgoing command without needing to go to a higher conscious level. For example, if you touch something hot, you immediately pull your hand back. You may then realize what you have done, but pulling back your hand first was a reflex response handled by the spinal cord.

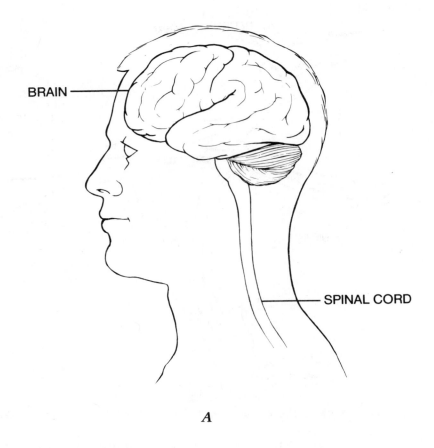

A

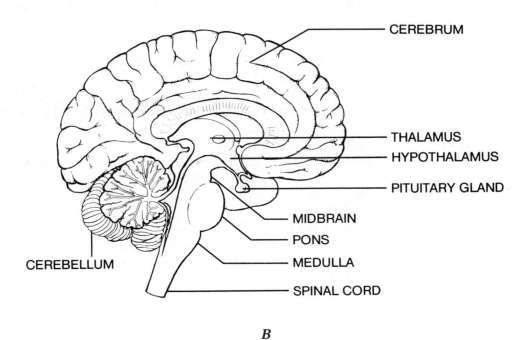

B

FIGURE 27–3. *The central nervous system includes the brain and spinal cord.*

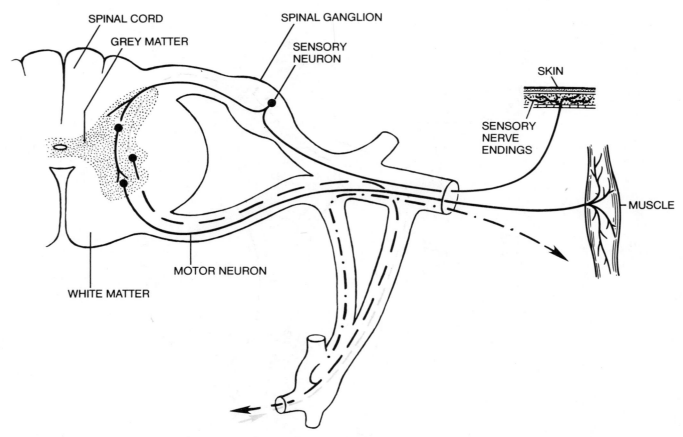

FIGURE 27–4. Sensory receptors carry the message into the spinal cord and a motor response follows.

The Brain

The brain has several parts, each with a special function.

The brain is the most complex organ in the entire body, figure 27–5. The neurons of the brain carry out complex functions such as:

- reasoning
- thinking
- forming and recalling memories
- making judgments
- controlling body functions
- interpreting all the sensations that are brought in by the nerves from outside

The brain can be divided into several parts for study.

Cerebrum. The cerebrum is the largest part of the brain. It is divided into two halves, or *hemispheres*. The outer part of the cerebrum is called the cortex. It is made up of many folds, or deep grooves, called *sulci*. Because the cerebrum is filled with cell bodies, the cortex appears gray (hence the term "gray matter").

The surface of the cerebrum forms lobes that have the same names as the bones under which they are found. They are the:

- frontal lobes
- parietal lobes
- temporal lobes
- occipital lobes

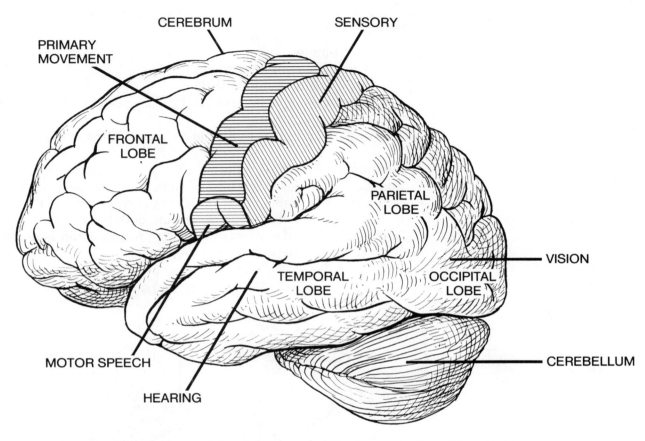

FIGURE 27-5. Different parts of the brain are specialized to control specific activities.

The interior of the cerebrum is composed of the long axons of the neurons. Deep inside the brain are vast interconnections. Different parts of the cerebrum are known to carry out one specific activity. For example:

- Motor control of one side of the body is managed by cells in the opposite side of the frontal lobe.
- Sensations originating on one side of the body are interpreted on the opposite side of the parietal lobe.
- Vision is interpreted in the occipital lobe.
- Hearing is in the temporal lobe.

Cerebellum. The **cerebellum** is called the little brain. It lies beneath the occipital lobes of the cerebrum. This part of the brain coordinates muscular activities and maintains balance.

The Brain Stem. The **brain stem** is that portion of the brain which is connected to the spinal cord. It is composed of the

- medulla oblongata
- pons varolii
- mesencephalon

Special groups of nerve cells called nervous centers control the vital (living) functions of the body. The vital functions that are controlled include:

- respiration
- heart rate and rhythm
- size of the blood vessels
- functioning of internal body organs such as the digestive tract

Most of the 12 pairs of cranial nerves are attached to the brain stem.

Cerebrospinal Fluid. This fluid (CSF) is a clear, colorless fluid derived from the blood (plasma). It fills a system of cavities (**ventricles**), figure 27–6, within the brain and circulates in the central canal of the spinal cord. It acts as a watery cushion around both brain and spinal cord. Cerebrospinal fluid is constantly being produced and is reabsorbed at the same rate back into the bloodstream.

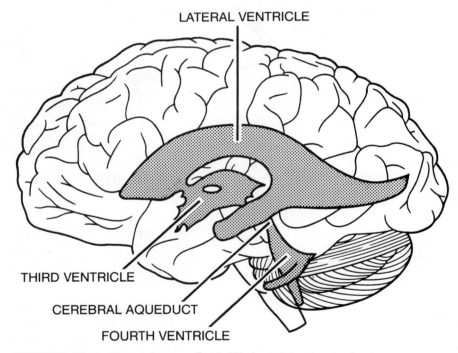

LATERAL VENTRICLE

THIRD VENTRICLE

CEREBRAL AQUEDUCT

FOURTH VENTRICLE

FIGURE 27–6. Ventricles are fluid-filled cavities in the brain.

AUTONOMIC NERVOUS SYSTEM

The autonomic branches control visceral functions.

The autonomic nervous system is part of the PNS and made up of the special nerve pathways that begin in the brain and control heart rate, the secretions of glandular cells, and the contraction of the smooth muscular walls of organs. Two different sets of autonomic fibers reach most body organs.

- **sympathetic fibers** — carry messages that prepare the body for emergency action when under stress
- **parasympathetic fibers** — carry messages that return functions back to normal after the emergency is over

THE SENSE ORGANS

The sense organs carry messages about the external world to the brain. The receptors of sensations are delicate dendrites and are sometimes protected by elaborate structures such as the eye and ear.

The Eye

Sense organs carry messages about
- touch
- temperature
- pain
- vision
- hearing
- taste
- smell
- equilibrium

The eye is protected by the bony eye cavity called the **orbit**. Muscles move the eyes in a coordinated way. The eyelids and eye are covered by a mucous membrane called the **conjunctiva**. Mucus and tears keep the normal eye moist, figure 27–7. Excess tears drain into the nose and sometimes from the eyes to the outside.

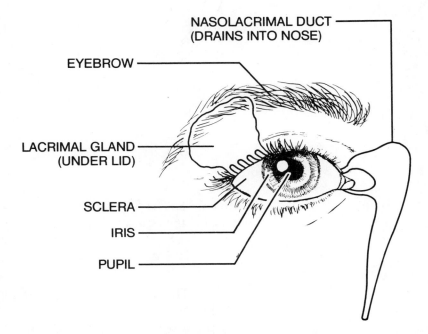

NASOLACRIMAL DUCT (DRAINS INTO NOSE)

EYEBROW

LACRIMAL GLAND (UNDER LID)

SCLERA

IRIS

PUPIL

FIGURE 27–7. Tears (lacrimal secretions) wash across the eye keeping the eye moist.

The eye itself is a nearly spherical, ball-shaped, fluid-filled organ made up of three layers (figure 27–8). These are the:
- **sclera** — the outer white protective cover. The front of the sclera forms the transparent **cornea**.
- **choroid** — the middle layer, which also contains the ciliary body and **iris**. It has many blood vessels and provides nourishment for the eye tissues.
- **retina** — the innermost layer. This is the nervous layer, composed of special receptor neurons that are sensitive to light.

The colored portion of the eye is called the **iris**. It is found behind the cornea. The center, which appears black, is really an opening called the **pupil**, which can open wider or become smaller. It controls the amount of light entering the eye.

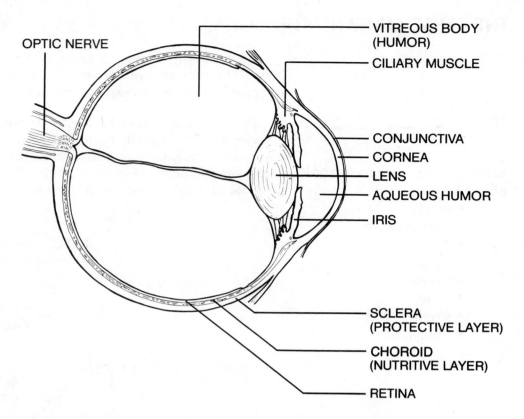

FIGURE 27–8. *The fluid within the eye bends the light rays to focus on the inner lining called the retina.*

The **lens** is located just behind the iris. It is normally clear and bends the light rays that pass through it and directs them toward the photoreceptors of the retina.

Seeing. Light rays are reflected from the object being seen. They pass through the cornea and pupil and are bent to focus on the retina. Once the photoreceptors of the retina are stimulated, the image they receive is transmitted over the **optic nerve** to the brain for vision interpretation. (The optic nerve is one of the cranial nerves.)

The Ear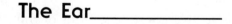

The ear is also a complex receptor sense organ, figure 27–9. It not only enables us to hear, but it also controls **equilibrium**, which allows us to maintain our sense of balance. The ear is made up of the:

- outer ear
- middle ear
- inner ear

The Outer Ear. The part of the ear that you can see is called the **pinna**. Leading inward from the outer ear is the external auditory canal, which carries sound waves toward the eardrum (**tympanic membrane**), which separates the external and middle ear. The sound waves make the eardrum vibrate.

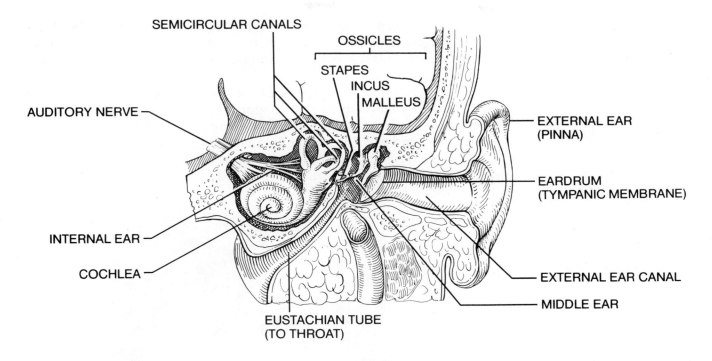

FIGURE 27-9. *The ear.*

The Middle Ear. Three tiny little bones, the **ossicles**, stretch across the middle ear. The first bone is attached to the eardrum and it begins to vibrate as the eardrum moves. The second is attached to the first and the third to the second. Each little bone vibrates in turn at the same rate as the eardrum moves. The third bone attaches to a membraneous opening of the inner ear. Vibrations against this membrane set up fluid vibrations in the inner ear.

The Inner Ear. The inner ear is made up of the:

- **semicircular canals**
- **vestibule**
- **cochlea**

The three semicircular canals pick up information about starting and stopping movements. The vestibule picks up information about the position of the head. Deep within the snail-shaped cochlea are the special hearing receptors that are stimulated by the fluid vibrations, somewhat like a tiny piano keyboard. When these specific receptors are stimulated, the message is picked up and transmitted to the **auditory nerve** and then to the brain for interpretation of sounds which you are hearing.

AGING CHANGES IN THE NERVOUS SYSTEM

Because there are billions of neurons in the nervous system, even though some are lost everyday throughout life, there are still enough to maintain body activities. Some changes, however, do occur with aging:

- Receptors become less sensitive, so that stronger stimuli are needed to get them to respond, figure 27–10. For example, more light is needed to see and louder sound volumes are needed to hear.
- Sensitivity to pain and heat is diminished, so an injury may be ignored; therefore, more protection is needed.
- Reflexes are slowed, so the sense of balance is not as secure and movements are less well coordinated.
- Cerebral activity may not be as swift, but this does not mean that intelligence is diminished.

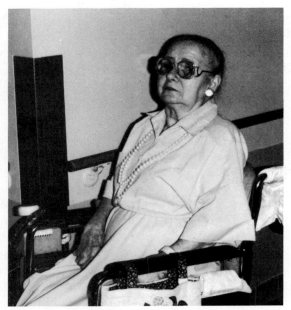

FIGURE 27–10. The lady has sensory losses but still has a keen mind.

These senescent changes are partly due to interference with the normal flow of nourishing blood to the cells and, in some instances, to the diminished production of neurotransmitter chemicals.

NERVOUS SYSTEM DISABILITIES

Many of your residents will suffer from disabilities related to the nervous system. If you review the role of the nervous system in controlling body activities, interpreting sensations, and carrying out mental activities, you can understand how complicated some of these disabilities can be.

The location, cause, and extent of the damage to the nervous tissue determines the type of disability experienced by each resident:

- One resident may suffer from memory loss but be able to walk without assistance.

- Another resident may have competent cerebral functioning, with memory intact, but be unable to move the arm or leg on one side.
- Still another resident may be communicative on one day and confused and disoriented on another.

You will get to know the residents in your care very well. Be alert to changes in their normal behaviors and report and record your observations.

BEHAVIORAL RESPONSE TO STRESS ▪▪▪▪▪▪▪▪▪▪▪▪▪▪▪▪▪▪▪▪▪▪▪▪▪

People handle stress in ways that they have found successful in the past.

Elderly people react to stress in much the same ways as people of other ages, but their tolerance levels to stress are lower. Most older persons will continue the same behavioral patterns they developed and used in their younger years. If childish behavior was a successful basic response to stress in the past, it will be a response that the resident will most likely use throughout his or her lifetime.

How people are treated also helps to determine the way they will behave. For example, if the staff takes for granted that certain residents are incapable of caring for themselves, those residents will behave in dependent ways.

Stress is difficult to manage when a person is young and healthy, but it is much harder to handle when youth is gone and vitality is low. Yet, the majority of older people do manage to stay emotionally and mentally stable most of the time. Very few (1 percent) become **psychotic** (mentally unsound). Keep in mind that the depressed or angry resident may have ample justification for such an emotional response.

BEHAVIORAL DISORDERS ▪▪▪▪▪▪▪▪▪▪▪▪▪▪▪▪▪▪▪▪▪▪▪▪▪▪▪▪▪

Confusion_____

The confused resident needs protection.

Confused or irrational behavior can stem from many situations in the life of the resident as well as from physical changes. Some situations that can lead to confusion are:

- a move to unfamiliar surroundings
- dim light
- diminished oxygen levels because of a respiratory infection
- dehydration
- constipation or inability to empty a full bladder

Confusion may be mild and temporary, making the resident sometimes unaware of who or where he or she is. A mildly confused person may speak without making sense, repeatedly ask the same questions, or may seem withdrawn and less responsive (figure 27-11). He or she may fail to recognize you or may become irritable and negatively resistive to care.

The confusion and disorientation may be more extreme and prolonged. The more disoriented resident may become combative, striking out at others, pulling out tubes, and trying to get out of bed or geri-chair. Such residents need to be protected from themselves and also must be kept from injuring others. Remember, raising your

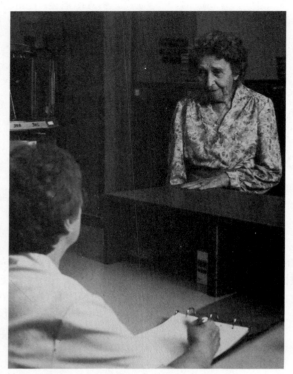

FIGURE 27-11. The confused resident may ask the same questions repeatedly.

voice when speaking to a disoriented, agitated resident may only agitate him or her more.

When in a state of confusion, a resident may misinterpret information because of disorders in his or her sensory perception. The confused resident may suffer from:

- illusions
- delusions
- hallucinations

Illusions. Illusions are false interpretations of sensory input. For example, a resident thinks that he hears people in the corridor who are coming to hurt him; when you explain that he is hearing voices from a radio in another room the resident accepts this explanation and becomes calmer.

Delusions. Like illusions, delusions are mininterpretations of sensory input. However, in this case the false interpretation is maintained despite all evidence to the contrary. The resident who is suffering from delusions cannot accept the real explanation and is unpersuaded by the facts. For example, if the resident described in the preceding paragraph were suffering from delusions (instead of illusions), he would not accept your explanation about the voices he was hearing, and he would continue to be agitated and fearful.

Hallucinations. Hallucinations originate in the resident's mind and have no relationship to reality. For example, a resident sits and talks to her daughter, even though her daugher is several miles away. The resident sees and hears her daughter just as if she were present.

Dementia_____

Dementia is a gradual loss of mental functioning.

Dementia is a progressive loss of mental functioning. The resident becomes more and more confused and is unable to reason accurately. Recent memory is not clear but long-term memory may be quite detailed. For example, you ask a resident if he enjoyed breakfast and he is unable to give you an answer because he can't remember; but when you ask him about some event in his childhood, he gives you a great deal of detailed information.

Residents with dementia become self-centered, tend to be repetitious, and may become agitated because they cannot retain the information that you provide. You may explain to a resident with dementia that it is too early for lunch, only to be asked about lunch five minutes later.

The causes of dementia are not fully known, but many cases are related to arteriosclerotic changes in the vessels supplying the brain, to minor strokes, and to Alzheimer's disease and Parkinson's syndrome. Some cases are due to a combination of conditions.

Mental Breakdown (Psychosis)_____

Excessive pressures can strain the emotional stability of people at any age, but the older one becomes, the less coping ability there is to handle the pressures. Chronic illnesses, organic changes, inability to care for one's basic needs, and the loss of loved ones and familiar surroundings can be overwhelming to a resident.

Emotional responses of anger and frustration, withdrawal, and agitation often precede a complete mental breakdown. Behavioral changes can also give clues that the usual coping mechanisms are failing (figure 27–12). These changes may include incontinence, hoarding of food, or **insomnia** (inability to sleep at night).

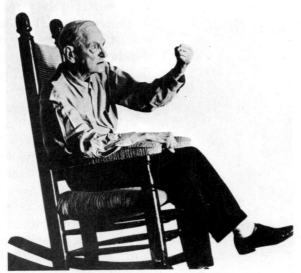

FIGURE 27–12. Be alert to signs of mental breakdown.

The actual breakdown can progress in different ways, but it is common for the individual to:

- become very depressed, crying over minor incidents
- be restless at night
- lose appetite
- be less interested in facility activities
- become hostile toward themselves or others
- speak of suicide and take suicidal steps

A resident who talks about suicide requires professional psychiatric care, which can include medications to overcome the depression.

Your responsibility is to:

- be supportive and observant
- report any suicidal statements, no matter how minor
- communicate with residents in a positive way, accepting the feelings expressed as real and important
- stress the positive aspects of the resident's life
- follow a nursing care plan designed to help the resident reduce and redirect his or her frustrations

Paranoia

The paranoid resident believes everyone is out to get him.

Paranoia is a condition characterized by a heightened, false sense of self-importance and by persistent delusions of being persecuted. A resident with paranoia will believe that everyone is against him or her. He or she may express the idea that the staff is "plotting" against him or her. These feelings tend to intensify, and gradually, as more and more contact with reality is lost, the resident becomes frankly psychotic, and hostility and aggression are pronounced.

Psychiatric care is needed to treat residents with paranoia. Also, care is needed by all confused residents, to protect such residents from self-injury and to protect others from being injured by them.

Care of the Confused Resident

Whatever the cause of confusion, the resident requires special care to protect him or her. You must create and maintain a consistent, quiet environment. You are the resident's link with reality. A bulletin board can help in a small way to keep residents reality-oriented (figure 27-13). Tension between staff members (even the happy stress associated with a holiday celebration) can be upsetting. Changes in routine can cause the resident to become agitated and even more disoriented.

When the resident is confused and forgetful, you must monitor all the resident's daily living activities yourself. Limited attention span and low frustration levels may lead to incomplete dressing, half-eaten meals, and inadequate toilet hygiene. Patience is needed, since the forgetful resident may need repeated reminders. Attention spans and frustration levels are short, so activities need to be carefully supervised. Posting of a daily event board in the facility may help the resident with a short attention span and memory lapses, (figure 27-14). You can best help the resident by:

- reducing stress and keeping to well-set, simple routines
- maintaining orientation by helping the resident keep in touch with reality.
- being calm and gentle in your approach
- monitoring and supporting the resident's daily activities

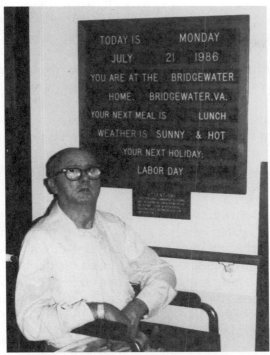

FIGURE 27-13. A bulletin board can help residents with reality orientation.

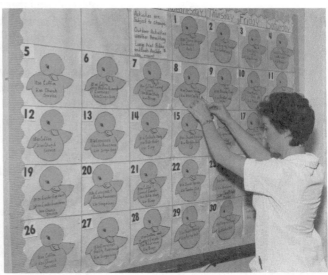

FIGURE 27-14. A daily event board helps forgetful residents keep track of things.

Take every opportunity to orient the resident to reality.

Maintaining Orientation of the Resident. The first indication of **disorientation** may be increasing agitation. Be alert to this change in behavior and intervene. The following steps taken now can limit the disorientation:

- Maintain your routine and call the resident by name.
- Point out familiar belongings.
- Make frequent references to the time of day, date, or season.
- Keep the room well-lighted but minimize noise, especially loud, sudden sounds.
- Give a back rub or soothing bath. This may help the resident to relax.
- Do not add to the confusion by agreeing with the resident when he or she makes inaccurate assumptions.
- Spend as much time with the confused resident as possible, since human contact helps maintain a positive contact with reality.
- Make sure that any sensory aids, such as glasses and hearing aids, are in working order and in place. Confusion is only made worse when sensory information is inaccurate.
- Talk to the resident in a calm manner. Introduce one simple subject, suggestion, or direction at a time. The resident is unable to make any decisions, so do not ask him or her to do so.
- Keep orientation aids such as calendars, clocks, and posters in plain view and point them out as often as you can.

A consistent, positive approach by all staff members can limit the disorientation, helping the confused resident to come back into more accurate reality orientation.

Protection. The confused resident needs to be protected from injury and, in some cases, must be prevented from injuring others. Confusion can lead to misinterpreted interactions, and the resident may become angry and combative. It may be necessary to separate the confused resident from others. Because isolation will compound the confusion, try to place the resident in an area where he or she can be frequently visited and observed and where unit activity can be observed by the resident.

Restraints. Do not restrain a resident unless there is a specific written physician's order and supervision by an RN, and until all other measures to deal with the situation have failed. Restraints or postural supports often increase the agitation of a confused resident, who may interpret their use as a punishment and may struggle against the restraints, thus becoming more and more agitated in the process. Restraints must be checked periodically and removed as soon as the resident's condition permits, figure 27–15.

When restraints are used
- observe carefully
- remove as soon as possible
- do not isolate
- check for circulation
- meet basic needs

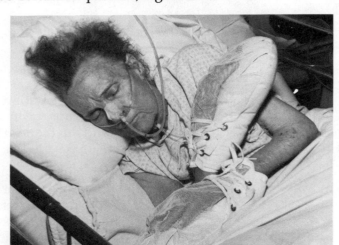

FIGURE 27–15. This resident has hand restraints so she will not pull out her nasogastric tube.

When people are restrained, either because of confusion or simply because they need the support to maintain proper alignment, they are unable to provide for their most basic needs. You must make sure that they receive adequate water and nourishment and are able to meet their elimination needs.

Postural restraints are often used to support residents as they sit in a geri-chair or wheelchair, figure 27–16. Even though a resident is mentally alert, you must be careful in your approach as you apply the support. Remember that body positions need to be checked and changed frequently, since a resident may slip and body pressure will be exerted against the unyielding strap. When in a geri-chair (figure 27–17), the resident may have difficulty reaching water; again, you must be responsible for assuring that basic needs will be met.

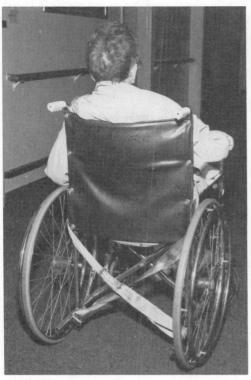

FIGURE 27–16. Note how the postural restraint is secured on the back of the wheelchair.

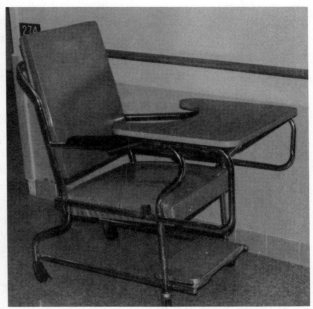

FIGURE 27–17. The geri chair both supports the resident and provides a convenient place for activities.

PROCEDURE: Application of Postural Supports or Restraints

1. Check to be sure the physician has written an order for the resident.
2. Display a positive, gentle attitude.
3. Identify resident and explain what you plan to do and why.
4. Restrain resident only in bed or chairs with wheels.
5. Tie the restraint under the chair out of reach of the patient or to the bed frame.
6. Check resident for proper positioning.
7. Pad areas under restraint to prevent friction.
8. Do *not* use a slip knot to secure ties.
9. Make sure that water and call bell are within reach.
10. Check resident frequently.
11. Remove restraints periodically.
12. Exercise restrained areas regularly.
13. Report and chart:
    a. type of restraint
    b. time of restraint
    c. specific nursing care given
    d. resident's reaction

OTHER CONDITIONS OF THE NERVOUS SYSTEM

Arteriosclerotic Brain Disease

The nervous tissue must be supplied by a constant stream of blood carrying oxygen to remain healthy and functional. **Arteriosclerosis** narrows the blood vessels which in turn causes the brain cells to suffer from lack of oxygen (hypoxia). The resident suffering from this condition may:

- have functional, clear moments between periods of confusion.
- be restless and irritable during confused periods.
- experience lightheadedness and diminished reflexes. This makes the resident prone to falls and injury.
- be aggressive at times. This may lead to unpleasant interactions with staff members or other residents.

Ministrokes

Ministrokes are called **transient ischemic attacks (TIA)** because there is a temporary period of diminished blood flow to the cerebrum. The more often the TIAs occur, the more damage is done to the nerve cells. This situation may lead to dementia, or loss of mental functioning.

Alzheimer's Disease

Residents with neurologic conditions need consistent emotional and physical support.

Alzheimer's disease is a disorder that is slowly progressive, beginning with memory changes that prevent the person from recognizing familiar objects. Within 3 to 10 years of onset, persons suffering with Alzheimer's become unable to reason, control bodily functions, or care for themselves.

Those affected with Alzheimer's disease are usually depressed in the early stages of the disease and as long as they remain aware of their circumstances. Judgment and reasoning ability are progressively lost until all mental abilities cease.

The cause of Alzheimer's disease is not known, but, because of its frequency and devastating effects, much research into the problem is being carried on. Characteristic of the disease process are actual organic changes: the loss of neurons, death of brain cells, and lower levels of neurotransmitters and the enzymes that promote the formation of specific transmitters.

Parkinson's Syndrome

Parkinson's syndrome (**paralysis agitans**) is common in elderly residents. It is believed to be due to insufficient neurotransmitters in the brain stem and cerebellum. The symptoms are progressive over many years, and some residents will show minor changes while others will have much more pronounced symptoms. The signs and symptoms of Parkinson's syndrome include:

- tremors of hands
- muscular rigidity
- difficulty and slowness in carrying out voluntary muscular activities (**akinesia**)
- loss of autonomic nervous control
- mood swings and gradual behavioral changes

Tremors of the hands commonly affect the fingers and thumb in such a way that an affected resident will appear to be rolling a small object such as a pill between them. These tremors occur frequently, usually beginning in the fingers, then involving the entire hand and arm, and finally affecting an entire side of the body. Starting on one side, the tremors eventually involve both sides of the body.

The muscular rigidity and tremors are more evident when the resident is inactive but seem to disappear when the resident sleeps or is engaged in activities such as walking or other exercises that require large muscle involvement. The rigidity makes the resident with Parkinson's syndrome more prone to falls and injury. Eventually, the hand affected with tremors is drawn down and joints form fixed positions.

Persons with advanced Parkinson's typically have a shuffling manner of walking and have difficulty starting the process; and, once started, have difficulty stopping smoothly. Speech may also be affected, causing words to be slurred and poorly spoken. Facial muscles lose their expressiveness, and a resident appears to have no emotional response.

Because of loss of autonomic nervous control, persons with Parkinson's may drool, become incontinent or constipated, or may retain urine. You may notice that the resident with Parkinson's experiences mood swings, appearing up and positive one moment and then depressed. The depression tends to be progressive, and personality and behavioral changes may occur, which cause psychotic breakdowns.

Today, drug therapy — and, for some younger persons surgery — is the treatment of choice for Parkinson's syndrome, but a major area of therapy is designed to limit the muscular rigidity and to meet the basic physical and emotional needs of the resident with this disease. A calm environment is essential, since the symptoms are more intense when the resident is under stress.

You will need to assist and supervise the activities of daily living. For example, directing food into the mouth and then keeping it there to be chewed and swallowed is very difficult for many residents with Parkinson's. Residents with this disorder will need much emotional support and encouragement to carry out general exercise programs and specific exercises to improve mobility. When confused, residents with Parkinson's syndrome will need to be protected and cared for, following the principles outlined.

Seizures

Seizures, or **convulsions**, create an emergency situation. They may be associated with specific conditions such as a cerebrovascular accident, injury to the skull and brain, or the presence of tumors in the brain. Any condition that injures the delicate brain tissue or creates excessive pressure within the bony cranium can cause changes in motor or sensory control referred to as a seizure.

Not all seizures occur in exactly the same way. The major types are:

- **petite mal seizure**
- **jacksonian seizure**
- **grand mal seizure**

Petite Mal Seizure. In this type of seizure, there may be only a momentary loss of consciousness, and such seizures often occur unnoticed until they increase in frequency. The resident having a petite mal seizure may seem to be "day dreaming."

Jacksonian Seizure. This is usually the result of injury to cells in a localized area of the brain. There is one-sided loss of muscular control that can involve both the arm and leg on the affected side or a more limited area.

Grand Mal Seizure. This is the most dramatic seizure. In this form, the resident may experience some form of sensory awareness before loss of consciousness occurs and involuntary movements begin. This sensory awareness, which may be a specific smell or taste or bright light, is called an **aura**. It is part of the convulsive pattern.

A person having a grand mal seizure loses consciousness and becomes rigid; he or she may froth at the mouth, stop breathing temporarily, and become cyanotic. Arms and legs move uncontrollably. Gradually the individual stops moving and regains consciousness. He or she may be confused following a seizure, with no memory of the event.

Nursing Assistant Responsibilities When a Seizure Occurs

If you should witness seizures of any kind:

- Stay with the resident.
- Note the time and type of seizure.
- Do not try to restrain the resident but move any objects away that might cause injury.
- Loosen any constricting clothing, especially around the neck.
- If possible, place a pillow under the resident's head and turn the face to one side so that the saliva will drain out.
- Summon help.

After the seizure, the resident should be allowed to rest. Make sure that side rails are up and secure before leaving to report and record your observations.

EYE DISORDERS

Cataracts

Cataracts cause a loss of vision because the lens of the eye becomes opaque and light rays cannot pass through it to reach the retina. Cataracts tend to develop slowly and can be corrected with surgery on an out-patient basis in an acute care facility, figure 27–18.

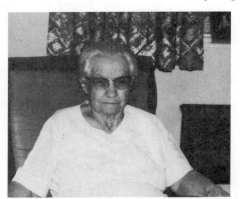

FIGURE 27–18. This resident has lost much of her vision due to cataracts but surgery will soon restore much of it.

Residents returning to your facility following cataract surgery will need to be protected while they ambulate, since the vision will not be balanced for some time. Corrective glasses, or lens implants done at the time of surgery, can solve this problem.

Glaucoma

Glaucoma is the result of improper balance of the aqueous humor, a fluid found in the anterior eye cavity. Poor drainage of this fluid causes pressure within the eye to build up. The pressure against the lens causes damage to the retina. Side vision is lost, and eventually, if uncorrected, the total visual field is destroyed. Treated early, the condition can be controlled with medication.

Since this condition can go undetected for a long period of time, you must be aware of any vision disturbances or irregularity in the eye itself. Be sure to report:

- redness
- tearing
- itching
- complaints of vision changes

Acute glaucoma can develop rapidly. Its onset is signalled by nausea and intense pain. If this occurs, keep the resident quiet and report to the nurse right away.

Blindness

Cataracts, glaucoma, eye infections, and other eye conditions, such as an ocular tumor, can cause blindness. People who are legally blind may still have some vision left and the degree of visual limitation must be taken into account when giving care. It is also important to consider the resident's attitude to his or her disability. Adjustment to blindness is both a physical and an emotional process.

Allow the blind or nearly blind person the opportunity to do as much as possible for himself or herself. Many blind people are very capable and independent.

Permit the blind resident to remain as independent as possible.

You should:

- Orient the blind person to anything new which you introduce into the environment (figure 27–19).

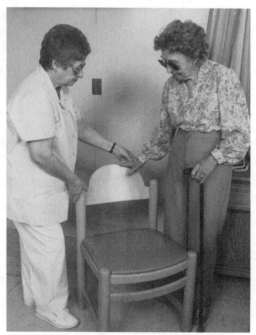

FIGURE 27-19. *The blind resident needs to be oriented to the location of the furniture.*

- Try to place furniture in the most simple arrangement possible.
- Provide support until the resident is thoroughly familiar with the physical arrangement of the living space.
- Return all personal belongings to their proper place.
- When serving food, describe the food and its placement on the plate as if the plate were the face of a clock.

Most blind residents do very well with minimal help and support once they fully orient themselves to their surroundings.

VOCABULARY

akinesia
Alzheimer's disease
arteriosclerosis
auditory nerve
aura
axon
brain stem
cataract
central nervous system (CNS)
cerebellum
cerebrospinal fluid
cerebrum
choroid
cochlea
conjunctiva
convulsions
cornea
cortex
delusion
dementia
dendrites
disorientation

epilepsy
equilibrium
glaucoma
grand mal seizure
hallucination
illusion
insomnia
iris
jacksonian seizure
lens
meninges
ministrokes
motor
nerve
nerve fiber
nerve impulse
neuron
neurotransmitter
olfactory
optic nerve
orbit
ossicles
paralysis agitans

paranoia
parasympathetic fibers
Parkinson's syndrome
peripheral nervous system (PNS)
petite mal seizure
pinna
psychotic
pupil
reflex
retina
sclera
seizure
semicircular canal
sympathetic fibers
synapse
transient ischemic attach (TIA)
tympanic membrane
ventricles
vestibule
visceral

SUGGESTED ACTIVITIES

1. Using models, charts or diagrams, learn the parts of the nervous system.

2. Role play with classmates an assistant caring for a confused resident and an assistant caring for someone who is blind or deaf.

3. Under supervision, give care to a resident with Parkinson's syndrome, to a depressed resident, or to a resident who is confused.

REVIEW

A. Brief Answer/Fill in the Blanks

1. The _____ and the _____ make up the central nervous system.

2. Special sensory receptors that carry information for vision are found in the _____.

3. List three changes that normally take place in the aging nervous system:

   a. _____

   b. _____

   c. _____

4. List three situations that can cause a resident to become temporarily confused:

   a. _____

   b. _____

   c. _____

5. Illusions and delusions are both false interpretations of sensory input, but illusions differ from delusions because a person with illusions will _____ the explanation for them.

6. Residents suffering from dementia experience progressive loss of _____ functioning.

7. List three steps you might take to help a resident become reality oriented:

   a. _____

   b. _____

   c. _____

8. Residents may be restrained to prevent injury to _____ or to _____ only under the orders of a _____.

9. Seizures are also called _____ and are associated with injury to the _____.

10. Name three things you can do to assist a resident who is convulsing.

   a. _____

   b. _____

   c. _____

B. **Matching.** Match the words on the left with the correct term on the right.

   1. _____ mental breakdown

   2. _____ postural support

   3. _____ delusions of persecution

   4. _____ temporary cerebral ischemia

   5. _____ lens of eye becomes opaque

   6. _____ fixed ideas with no relationship to reality

   7. _____ excessive fluid pressure in eye

   8. _____ nervous layer of eye

   9. _____ inability to control motor movements

   10. _____ slowness in carrying out complicated muscular activities

   a. paralysis
   b. TIA
   c. cataract
   d. glaucoma
   e. psychosis
   f. paranoia
   g. hallucination
   h. restraint
   i. retina
   j. akinesia

CLINICAL SITUATION

Katie Murphy has been a resident in your facility for almost two years. She spent many productive years teaching nutrition at Wilton College.

About ten years ago, she began to realize that she couldn't remember details as accurately as she once had. Gradually, her mental and emotional condition deteriorated. She retired and her husband, an engineer, employed a housekeeper to remain at home with her.

This arrangement was maintained for four years, until Mr. Murphy had a heart attack and died. Family members felt admission to a long term care facility was the only answer.

Mrs. Murphy suffers from Alzheimer's disease. What can you do to make this resident more comfortable?

Answer: _____

_____

_____

_____

A. **True or False.** Answer the following questions true (T) or false (F).

1. _____ Urine is stored in the gallbladder.

2. _____ Normal urine is a pale yellow.

3. _____ Micturition is another term for voiding.

4. _____ As one ages the ability to concentrate urine decreases.

5. _____ The gases exchanged in respirations are oxygen and hydrogen.

6. _____ A resident has been spitting up blood. You would best report and chart this as hemoptysis.

7. _____ Hypoglycemic drugs increase the blood sugar level.

8. _____ All people in their 80's have lost interest in sex.

9. _____ The sexual response of elderly persons is just as strong and quick as in early years.

10. _____ A resident can be easily talked out of hallucinations.

11. _____ Lack of routine adds to a resident's confusion.

12. _____ You may apply restraints whenever a resident is, in your opinion, unreasonable.

B. **Multiple Choice.** Select the one best answer and circle the letter (a–e) preceding the correct statement.

1. After collecting a female mid-stream urine specimen, you
   a. clean the vulva from back to front
   b. use a circular motion to clean the vulva
   c. clean the vulva from front to back
   d. use one gauze sponge only
   e. clean only the meatus

2. In the same procedure listed above, you should
   a. allow some urine to flow before collecting the sample
   b. collect the last drops of urine
   c. collect the first drops of urine
   d. position yourself on the left side of the resident
   e. position yourself on the right side of the resident

3. The best position for the male to urinate is
   a. flat on his back
   b. sitting with feet flat on floor
   c. standing
   d. positioned on his knees
   e. lying on his side

4. You can best assist the resident undergoing bladder retraining by
   a. making the evaluation on your own
   b. keeping track of incontinence periods
   c. inserting a catheter
   d. emptying the drainage bag
   e. applying external drainage pressure

5. Urinary incontinence may be related to
   a. emotional stress
   b. inability to reach the facilities
   c. fecal impaction
   d. brain damage
   e. all of the above

6. Senescent changes in the larynx cause
   a. muscles to tighten
   b. the voice to become higher pitched
   c. the blood pressure to rise
   d. urine output to decrease
   e. the resident to become confused

7. Esophageal speech is performed by
   a. replacing the trachea with the esophagus
   b. using a tracheostomy
   c. swallowing and regurgitating air
   d. directing air into the esophagus with a small tube
   e. none of the above

8. You would expect esophageal speech to
   a. sound like ordinary speech
   b. take more time than ordinary speech
   c. be more rapid than ordinary speech
   d. raise the resident's voice level
   e. all of the above

9. A resident with a tracheostomy requires
   a. special mouth care
   b. protection against aspiration
   c. suctioning for nasal congestion
   d. all of the above
   e. none of the above

10. The resident suffering from emphysema has difficulty
    a. with expiration
    b. with inspiration
    c. coughing
    d. sneezing
    e. swallowing

11. The best position for a resident in respiratory distress is
    a. prone
    b. dorsal recumbent
    c. orthopneic
    d. Sims'
    e. Trendelenberg

12. Your resident is an insulin-dependent diabetic. You should report
    a. mental confusion
    b. dizziness
    c. sweating
    d. drowsiness
    e. all of the above

13. A diet for a diabetic resident would *not* include
    a. coffee
    b. fresh fruit
    c. raw carrots
    d. scrambled eggs
    e. candy

14. Your resident is being treated with insulin. Your responsibilities include
    a. giving the insulin
    b. checking the injection site
    c. seeing that all pills are taken
    d. giving the resident sweet treats
    e. none of the above

15. Your resident has diabetes mellitus. Because you understand the possible complications of this condition, you will
    a. wash the resident's feet twice a week
    b. cut her toenails
    c. massage her feet regularly
    d. make sure shoes are tied tightly
    e. allow moisture to collect between the toes

16. One of the residents in your care is masturbating in the day room. You should
    a. ignore the matter
    b. tactfully move the resident to another, more private area
    c. slap his hand
    d. make fun of him so he will stop
    e. call attention of others in the room to the situation

17. A resident is making sexual advances to another, confused resident. You had best
    a. intervene calmly
    b. gently separate the residents
    c. involve the aggressive resident in some other activity
    d. calm the confused resident
    e. all of the above

18. Which best describes the person with Alzheimer's disease?
    a. Walks rapidly and surely.
    b. Has tremors of the hands and muscular rigidity.
    c. Speaks clearly but is confused.
    d. Has good memory patterns.
    e. None of the above.

19. The resident suffering from Parkinson's syndrome requires special attention since they may
   a. slur words, making it difficult to communicate
   b. fall more easily because of muscular rigidity
   c. have difficulty starting and stopping movements
   d. experience mood swings
   e. all of the above

C. **Matching.** Match the words on the right with the correct statement on the left.

		Choices
1. _____ functional unit of the kidney		a. catheter
2. _____ tube placed into urinary bladder to drain urine		b. trachea
		c. stoma
3. _____ inability to predict and control voiding		d. retention
		e. polyphagia
4. _____ inability to expel urine		f. carbon dioxide narcosis
5. _____ membrane covering the lung		g. procidentia
		h. nephron
6. _____ the windpipe		i. retina
		j. pleura
7. _____ an artificial opening in the body		k. hyperglycemia
		l. incontinence
8. _____ results from increased levels of carbon dioxide in the blood		m. illusion
		n. TURP
9. _____ excess level of blood sugar		o. glycosuria
		p. dementia
10. _____ excessive hunger		
11. _____ sugar in the urine		
12. _____ removal of the prostate gland		
13. _____ falsely interpreted sensory input		
14. _____ nervous layer of the eye		
15. _____ prolapsed uterus		

D. **Word Search.** Find the word in the diagram that is a synonym for the terms below. Circle it.

1. unit equal to 1 milliliter
2. rapid respiratory rate
3. word meaning for breathing
4. male organ of copulation
5. external female reproductive organs
6. sense of smell
7. urination at night

8. male reproductive cell
9. sensation that sometimes precedes a seizure
10. sugar in the urine
11. results from renal shutdown
12. excess urine
13. coughing up blood
14. word meaning reproductive organs
15. frequent voiding
16. loss of mental faculties

A	O	P	C	E	U	B	Q	X	D	E	M	E	N	T	I	A	Y
T	C	R	E	S	P	I	R	A	T	I	O	N	A	D	P	U	Z
Q	N	O	M	E	F	B	C	G	F	P	Z	V	X	W	N	R	P
A	D	M	B	C	R	G	D	N	T	B	A	N	U	R	I	A	E
V	U	I	O	P	E	N	I	S	A	E	D	O	I	O	D	M	N
Y	T	Z	A	D	Q	G	H	B	Q	B	N	C	T	P	U	I	Q
A	G	F	H	I	U	D	H	E	M	O	P	T	Y	S	I	S	T
B	E	Q	U	S	E	T	N	F	B	A	Q	U	C	W	G	P	E
Q	N	D	C	E	N	T	I	M	E	T	E	R	X	S	Y	E	A
A	I	B	O	P	C	D	R	N	I	B	Q	I	W	Z	Y	R	T
X	T	A	C	H	Y	P	N	E	A	C	O	A	T	P	C	M	R
C	A	D	O	R	B	W	B	N	Q	S	A	B	D	C	O	Z	W
P	L	R	V	Z	T	C	Q	N	L	J	H	C	T	R	S	A	K
B	I	C	O	D	X	V	U	L	V	A	P	W	E	A	U	D	O
Y	A	X	Q	C	B	A	P	O	L	F	A	C	T	O	R	Y	I
V	Y	A	D	Q	X	E	I	R	N	B	X	W	E	D	I	R	T
A	D	O	S	G	T	M	B	P	O	L	Y	U	R	I	A	Z	E

E. Label the Diagram.

1. Identify the organs of the respiratory system:

   a. _____

   b. _____

   c. _____

   d. _____

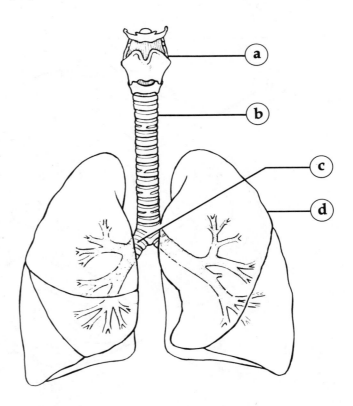

2. Identify organs of the urinary system:

a. _____

b. _____

c. _____

d. _____

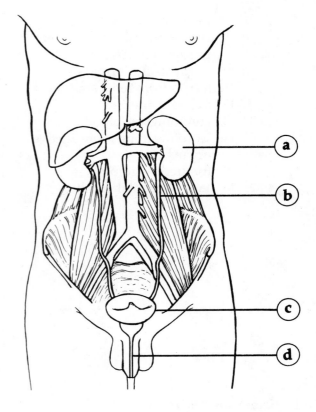

3. Identify the lobes of the brain:

a. _____

b. _____

c. _____

d. _____

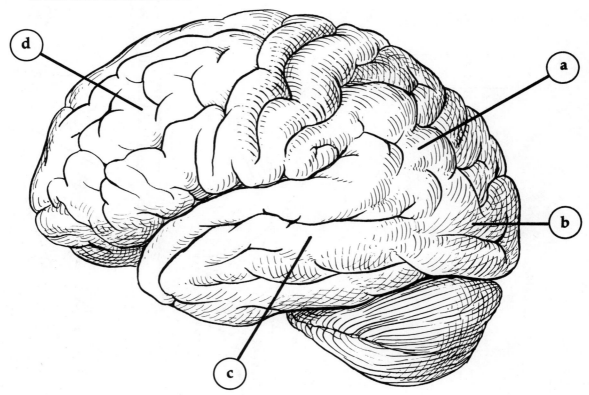

F. **Brief Answer/Fill in the Blanks**

1. Properly compute the following amount of liquid in this diet in milliliters (ml).

	Amount in ounces (oz)	**ml**
7:30 a.m. -	4 oz of orange juice	_____
	8 oz of coffee	_____
9:30 a.m. -	2 oz of water	_____
11:45 a.m. -	6 oz of tea	_____
	1 serving of jello (4 oz)	_____
	4 oz of soup	_____
2:30 p.m. -	4 oz of cranberry juice	_____
	Total ml =	_____

2. Describe the precautions you should take when caring for a resident who is receiving oxygen from a tank.

   a. _____

   b. _____

   c. _____

   d. _____

   e. _____

3. Describe the signs and symptoms you might notice in a resident who has diabetes mellitus of the non–insulin-dependent type.

   a. _____

   b. _____

   c. _____

   d. _____

   e. _____

   f. _____

4. Describe the direction and depth of inserting a douche nozzle.

   a. _____

   b. _____

   c. _____

5. Describe five actions you should take when coming upon a resident experiencing a seizure.

   a. _____

   b. _____

   c. _____

   d. _____

   e. _____

SECTION VI EMPLOYMENT

LESSON 28 Seeking Employment

OBJECTIVES

After studying this lesson, you should be able to:

- List sources of nurse assistant employment.
- Develop a résumé.
- Prepare for an interview.
- Define and spell all the vocabulary words and terms.

CONGRATULATIONS ARE IN ORDER

You have done it! You have passed the written tests and have proven your capability in the clinical area. Now you have your certificate (figure 28–1) and are ready to make your contribution to the care of residents in a long term care facility.

The next thing to do is to find out just where that right position might be located and prepare yourself to apply for it. There are several things that you can do to make the search easier and more productive.

STEP 1 — SELF-APPRAISAL

The first step is to take an honest look at your own assets and limits, figure 28–2. You can do this by making a list.

On one side of a piece of paper, list all the things you have to offer an employer. For example, you are well-trained in nursing assistant skills. Be as specific as you can be about personal as well as educational attributes. Your personal appearance — are you clean and neat at all times? Are you a punctual person? Do you have a caring attitude? These and more are important characteristics in a successful nursing assistant.

Identify your assets.

On the other side of the paper, list any restrictions to your employment. For example, are there hours when you cannot work — for example, when you must be home to care for children? Do you have to work within a specific area because you need to rely on public transportation? Do you have any responsibility that might interfere

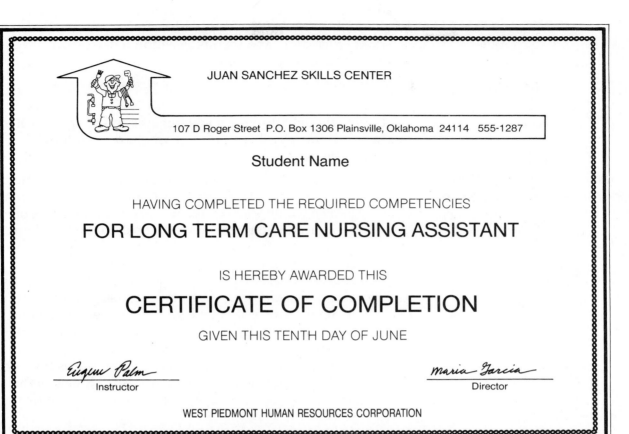

JUAN SANCHEZ SKILLS CENTER

107 D Roger Street P.O. Box 1306 Plainsville, Oklahoma 24114   555-1287

Student Name

HAVING COMPLETED THE REQUIRED COMPETENCIES

FOR LONG TERM CARE NURSING ASSISTANT

IS HEREBY AWARDED THIS

CERTIFICATE OF COMPLETION

GIVEN THIS TENTH DAY OF JUNE

_____
Instructor

_____
Director

WEST PIEDMONT HUMAN RESOURCES CORPORATION

FIGURE 28–1. Certificate of completion.

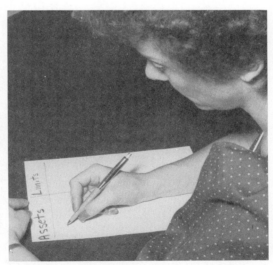

FIGURE 28–2. Be honest as you list your strengths and weaknesses.

with the performance of a job? If so, try to think of ways to handle those responsibilities so that they will not interfere with your employability. For example, if you have an elderly parent of your own living with you and must be there to prepare meals, is there a neighbor or other family member who could come in and prepare these meals on the days or hours that you work?

Put the list away and then review it in a day or two. There may be items you will want to add.

STEP II — POSSIBILITY SEARCH

Having thought through your strengths and limitations, it is time to search for job possibilities — but where do you look?

Suggestions:

Investigate many sources for employment possibilities.

1. *Start with the newspapers.* The classified advertisements are your best bet here, figure 28–3. Circle those that list positions located within your desired work area and that have openings for the shift you need to work. Look in the telephone book for facilities in your area. List names, numbers, and addresses. Follow up and contact them.

2. *Another possibility is to investigate the facility in which you had your clinical experience.* Many times nursing administrators will invite nursing assistants who have trained in their facility to join the staff upon completion of training. There are advantages to this policy. For one thing, since you have already spent time in the facility there is less time needed to orient you as a new employee. Also, the staff has had time to evaluate you while observing you during your training period.

3. *Networking is a valuable technique that can open doors and reveal opportunities.* Let friends and colleagues know of your desire for employment. Networking means forming a network of people with similar needs and interests to provide opportunity to learn about working conditions, job openings, and special ways of carrying out your responsibilities. Many jobs have been located on the recommendation of friends.

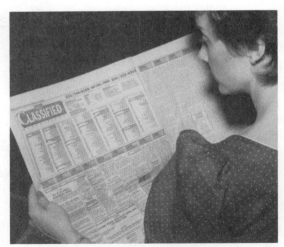

FIGURE 28–3. The classified ads are a good place to start your job search.

STEP III — THE RÉSUMÉ ■■■■■■■■■■■■■■■■■■■■■■■■■■■■■■■

The résumé should make an employer want to meet you.

Develop a summary, called a **résumé**, of your prior work experiences, figure 28–4. This need not be a very formal paper, but it is helpful to a prospective employer to have the résumé before and after your interview is held.

When an employer interviews many applicants, it is sometimes difficult to remember all the information given during a particular conversation. A note on your résumé by the interviewer can make all the difference between being hired and not being hired.

The résumé should include:

1. Your name, address, and telephone number.
2. Your educational background. List your most recent education first, giving dates and a brief summary of the content.
3. Your work history, especially if it gives evidence of successful experience in the same or related areas as the position for which you are applying. Include your work history over the past five years.
4. Other experiences you have had can be valuable. Jobs that show initiative, reliability, or trustworthiness are a plus and should be included. If you have not had paid employment, indicate how you spent your time. Taking care of children or finishing school are worthwhile endeavors and ought to be included.
5. List three **references** (people who know you and can vouch for your character and abilities) that can provide information about you. *Note:* You must get permission from your references before using their names.
6. Include some personal information, such as hobbies and other interests. It is not necessary to include your ethnic origin or religion, or even your age and marital status. *Note:* This is not required. Some people feel that to include such personal information as height, weight, sex, marital status, or religious affiliation is an invasion of privacy. Some of this information may be discussed during the interview, but it is not necessary to include it on your résumé.

Prepare several copies of your résumé. Always keep the original so that you can make more copies if necessary, and a copy for yourself. A typed résumé always makes a better impression. Carry a copy of your résumé whenever you seek employment. It is a ready reference as you fill out forms.

STEP IV — REFERENCES ■■■■■■■■■■■■■■■■■■■■■■■■■■■■■■■

Always get permission to use the names of references.

References are people who know you and who are willing to comment either in writing or verbally over the telephone about you and your abilities. Although the references need to know you well enough to make an honest evaluation, they should not be part of your family. Always get permission to use their names before listing references in your résumé. This is a matter of courtesy and ethics.

PRACTICAL NURSING PROGRAM
Application for Employment

1. Full Name: Miss
   Mrs.
   Mr.
   _____
   Last   First   Middle   Maiden
   _____
   Street and Number or Rural Route
   _____
   City, State and ZIP Code
   _____
   County   Telephone or nearest - Specify
   Social Security Number _____

2. Birth Date_____ Age_____ Birthplace_____

3. Physical Data: Height_____ Weight_____

4. Family and Marital Status: Single__ Married__ Widowed__ Separated__ Divorced__
   Husband or Wife's Name_____
   Are you self-supporting?_____ Number of children and ages_____
   Other dependents (specify)_____

5. Person to notify in case of emergency:
   Name_____   Name of parents_____
   Address_____   Address_____
   _____   _____
   Telephone_____   Telephone_____
   Relationship_____

6. Education: List in this order - High School, College. You must give complete addresses. Also please note if you did not graduate from high school whether or not you have a GED certificate.

School	Address	City	State	Year

7. Work or Vocational Experience: Give most recent first.

Name of Institution or Company	Complete Address	Type of Work	Dates

8. Have you ever been arrested for anything other than minor traffic violations? Yes___ No___
   If yes, explain.

9. Are you now or have you been addicted to the use of alcohol or habit-forming drugs?
   Yes___ No___ If yes, explain.

10. References: Name three people who know your qualifications or who know your character.
               They must not be related to you.

    Name_____
    Address_____

    Name_____
    Address_____

    Name_____
    Address_____

11. What are your reasons for wishing to work at this facility? Please answer this question in a paragraph form on the back of this application.

FIGURE 28–4. Sample résumé.

You may want to refresh the memory of your references about dates of employment or experiences that you have listed in your résumé. Be sure to include accurate titles, names, addresses and telephone numbers when listing these references.

STEP V — TAKING THE STEP

You have made your assessment of your strengths, limitations, and needs; you have searched the market for opportunities and prepared your résumé. Now it is time to take the plunge and apply for a job:

1. Select three facilities that you are most interested in.
2. Call and ask for the Director of Nursing or Personnel Department.
3. When someone answers, tell them you wish to know if there are any openings for a nursing assistant, and if so, what application procedure is to be followed.

The person in charge of hiring may ask you some questions about your preparation and experience, so be prepared to answer in a positive manner. He or she may set up an appointment for an **interview** during your telephone conversation. So before you call, it is helpful if you know when you will be available and have transportation available to keep such an appointment.

Before hanging up, be sure to get the name of the person to whom you are speaking and to thank this person by name.

STEP VI — THE INTERVIEW (Putting Your Best Foot Forward)

Put your best foot forward during the interview.

Prepare for the interview before it takes place by:

1. planning what you will wear.
2. not overdressing, but being neat and clean — for example, polishing your shoes.
3. checking your clothes for loose or lost buttons or stains.
4. being sure to use deodorant.
5. making sure your hair is neat.
6. if you have a beard or a mustache, making sure that it is trimmed.

Remember, you must sell yourself. Be careful of your body language.

Next, make a list of information you want the interviewer to learn about you and that you want to share with him or her (figure 28–5). You will of course share your background and answer questions the interview will ask.

You, in turn, will want to learn the following:

1. starting salary
2. schedule of raises
3. fringe benefits
   a. holiday pay and/or overtime
   b. health benefits

4. hours of work
5. responsibilities (ask for a job description)
6. uniform regulations
7. opportunities for growth (inservice education and orientation process)

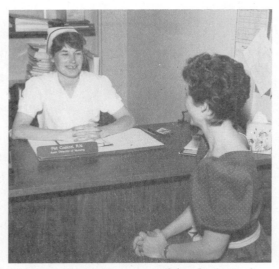

FIGURE 28–5. *Be prepared for the interview. Know what you want to learn and what you want to share.*

Be on time for your interview. Promptness indicates interest. Stand until you are invited to sit down — then do so. At the end of the interview, whether you are hired or not, thank the interviewer(s). Leave a copy of your résumé, if you have not already done so, so that if an opening occurs in the near future your file is there and you will be remembered.

After the interview, go home and congratulate yourself if you were hired. If you were not, don't be discouraged. Think through the interview and plan to make any changes in your answers that you might deem advisable or necessary for the next interview. Send a short thank-you note to the person who interviewed you, thanking them for giving you the opportunity of being interviewed for the job.

Job hunting isn't easy. It is emotionally trying and can be physically exhausting, but keep trying and you will find the perfect position for you. Good luck!

KEEPING THE JOB

Getting the job was only the beginning; now you must keep it. You can secure your position if you:

1. Arrive on time.
2. Perform your work as taught and be flexible to change.
3. Follow the rules of ethical and legal conduct.
4. Maintain an open positive attitude; be ready to learn and grow. Remember — learning is a lifelong challenge.

GROWING ▪▪▪▪▪▪▪▪▪▪▪▪▪▪▪▪▪▪▪▪▪▪▪▪▪▪▪▪▪▪▪▪▪▪▪▪

Learning is a life-long challenge.

You will continue to grow if you take advantage of each new experience and of the opportunities you find.

1. Seek out knowledgeable staff members and watch and learn by their example.
2. Don't be afraid to ask questions at the appropriate times.
3. Use the nursing and medical literature that is available to learn more about the conditions of the residents.
4. Participate in the Care Conferences with an open mind so that each can become a learning experience for you.

Investigate the possibilities of advancing your education. You might consider:

- a general education course offered at the high school or college in your area.
- courses in communication, listening, English and psychology. These can be very helpful in your field.
- inservice education programs at your facility or at nearby hospitals. Many of these programs are free.
- courses that are offered for continuing education credit for nurses which are sometimes available, without credit, and at a reduced price, for non-licensed persons.
- mini-courses offered by hospitals on subjects of general public interest, such as hypertension, weight control, and diabetes.
- selecting books at the library that pertain to aging and the aging process.
- programs that can prepare you for professional advancement into the ranks of LPN or RN.

RESIGNING ▪▪▪▪▪▪▪▪▪▪▪▪▪▪▪▪▪▪▪▪▪▪▪▪▪▪▪▪▪▪▪▪▪▪▪

When you resign from a job, leave as good an impression as when you began the job.

The time may come when you find it necessary to leave your place of current employment. To do this properly, you should give notice as early as possible and submit a letter of resignation at the time. Appropriate notice is usually equal to the time of a pay period.

Your letter of resignation should include:

1. the date.
2. a salutation to the Director of Nursing.
3. a brief explanation of your reasons for leaving. *Note:* Even if you feel upset by something that happened, make your reasons positive in nature.
4. the date your resignation is to be effective.
5. a thank-you for the opportunity to have worked and grown with the experience of working at that facility.
6. your signature.

VOCABULARY

interview   references

networking   résumé

SUGGESTED ACTIVITIES

1. Gather newspapers and nursing magazines and cut out or circle ads for nursing assistant positions.
2. Call several nursing homes in the area and find out their beginning wage and employment requirements.
3. Role play an interview for employment.
4. Practice writing a résumé.

REVIEW

Brief Answer/Fill in the Blanks

1. The first step in preparing to find a job is to carry out a _____.
2. List three positive attitudes that might improve job prospects:

   a. _____

   b. _____

   c. _____

3. List two factors that might limit your selection of work sites:

   a. _____

   b. _____

4. You might start to look for a job by examining the_____.
5. Two advantages of obtaining employment in the same facility in which you trained are:

   a. _____

   b. _____

6. Sharing information with others who have common interests or needs is called _____.
7. A summary of your experiences and personal information is called a _____.
8. You should include people who know you and your abilities as references, but they should not be members of your _____.
9. To help you make the most of an interview, you should make a list of _____ before the interview takes place.
10. Three things you should learn during the interview are:

    a. _____

    b. _____

    c. _____

CLINICAL SITUATION

You have just completed a course that has prepared you to function as a nurse assistant in a long term care facility. List ways you will approach the problem of getting a job.

Answer: _____

_____

_____

PROCEDURE COMPETENCY EVALUATIONS

LESSON 3

PERFORMANCE CHECKLIST			S = Satisfactory U = Unsatisfactory
Charting	S	U	Comments
Checks to insure that it is the right chart.			
Fills out new chart headings completely; uses the correct color ink.			
Prints or writes clearly, using correct spelling; dates and gives time of each entry.			
Leaves no blank lines or spaces between entries.			
Corrects errors by drawing a line through the errors; prints the word "error" above incorrect entry and adds her or his' initials.			
Uses phrases; does not name resident or use that term; makes entries brief but complete and accurate.			
Signs each entry properly and uses proper job classification.			

PROCEDURE COMPETENCY EVALUATIONS

LESSON 7

PERFORMANCE CHECKLIST			S = Satisfactory U = Unsatisfactory
Assisting the Conscious Choking Person (Heimlich Maneuver)	S	U	Comments
Stands behind and to one side of the victim.			
Waits if person starts to cough.			
Clenches fist, keeping thumb straight.			
Places fist, thumb side in, against abdomen between naval and tip of sternum.			
Grasps clenched fist with opposite hand.			
Pushes forcefully with thumb side of the fist against midline of abdomen, inward and upward 6 to 10 times.			
If victim becomes unconscious, places victim flat on floor on back; kneeling and straddling victim, places one hand flat on stomach between waist and sternum; places other hand at right angles to the first; pushes in and up in quick movements.			
Care of the Resident Who Is Bleeding (Hemorrhage)			
Identifies location of bleeding area.			
Applies continuous, direct pressure over bleeding area with a pad or hand.			
If seepage occurs, increases the padding and pressure.			
If there are no broken bones and no pain, raises wounded area above the level of heart.			
Supports the elevated area.			
Uses binding of some kind to hold padded pressure if there is bleeding from more than one area.			
Applies pressure over the appropriate vessel to stem hemorrhage.			

PERFORMANCE CHECKLIST			S = Satisfactory U = Unsatisfactory
Care of the Resident Who Is Bleeding (Hemorrhage) (cont.)	S	U	Comments
Keeps resident comfortably warm and quiet until help arrives.			
Signals for help but stays with resident.			
Handwashing			
Assembles the following equipment: a. soap b. paper towels c. wastebasket			
Turns the faucet on with a paper towel held between the hand and the faucet; drops towel in wastebasket.			
Wets hands with the fingertips pointed downward.			
Picks up soap, rinses and lathers hands well; rinses soap and replaces in soap dish or applies liquid soap and lathers well.			
Rubs hands together in a circular motion and by interlacing fingers; cleans fingernails; rinses and repeats.			
Rinses hands, fingertips down, and dries them thoroughly.			
Turns off faucet with another paper towel; drops the paper towel into wastebasket.			
Opening a Sterile Package			
1. **Article wrapped in paper:**			
Washes hands.			
Checks seal to be sure it is intact.			
With two hands, grasps each side of separated end and gently pulls apart.			
Does not open until nurse or doctor is ready to use article.			
If the article is to be taken by nurse or doctor, opens only enough to expose the end sufficiently to be withdrawn without contamination.			
2. **Article double-wrapped in cloth:**			
Washes hands.			
Checks tape seal to be sure color change indicating sterility has taken place.			
Places package fold side up on flat surface.			
Removes tape.			

PERFORMANCE CHECKLIST

S = Satisfactory
U = Unsatisfactory

Opening a Sterile Package (cont.)	S	U	Comments
Unfolds flap farthest away by grasping outer surface only between thumb and forefinger.			
Opens left flap with left hand using same technique.			
Opens right flap with right hand, using same technique.			
Opens final flap (nearest you); touches only the outside of flap; is careful not to stand too close; does not allow uniform to touch flap as it is lifted free; is sure flaps are pulled open completely to prevent them from folding back up over the sterile field.			
Isolation Techniques			
1. Outside the Door:			
Places a ''Barrier,'' ''Isolation,'' or ''Precaution'' sign on door.			
Places bedside table or cart beside door and supplies with: a. isolation gowns, masks, gloves (if ordered) b. waxed paper bag and/or plastic bags c. large laundry bags specially marked as ''Isolation''.			
2. Inside the Room:			
Lines wastebasket with plastic bag.			
Supplies laundry hamper with waterproof laundry bag in it.			
Checks supply of paper towels and liquid soap in foot-operated dispenser.			
3. Donning Clean Mask, Gown, and Gloves:			
Washes hands.			
Adjusts mask over nose and mouth and ties securely.			
Puts on gown, slipping arms into sleeves.			
Slips fingers under inside of neckband and grasps ties in the back; secures in bow-knot.			
Reaches behind and overlaps edges of gown to cover uniform completely; secures waist ties in a bow-knot.			
Puts on non-sterile disposable gloves.			

PERFORMANCE CHECKLIST			S = Satisfactory U = Unsatisfactory
Isolation Techniques (cont.)	S	U	Comments
4. Removing Contaminated Gown, Gloves, and Mask:			
Removes gloves, turning inside out and disposes in receptable.			
Undoes waist ties and loosens gown at waist.			
Turns faucets on with clean paper towel; discards towel in wastebasket.			
Washes hands carefully; dries with paper towels.			
Turns off faucets with dry paper towel.			
Undoes mask; holding by ties only, deposits in proper container.			
Undoes neck ties; loosens gown at shoulders.			
Slips fingers of right hand inside left cuff without touching out-side of the gown; pulls gown down and over left hand.			
Pulls gown down over right hand with gown-covered left hand.			
Folds gown with contaminated side inward; rolls and deposits in laundry bag or waste container, if disposable.			
Rewashes hands, using proper technique.			
Removes watch from paper towel; touches only clean side of paper towel and deposits it in wastebasket.			
Opens door with clean paper towel; props door open with foot and drops paper in wastebasket.			
5.Transferring Food and Disposable Equipment **Outside the Isolation Unit:**			
a. **Inside ("Contaminated") Person**			
Disposes of left-over liquids and food in toilet without splashing.			
Wraps hard foods in plastic (double).			
Opens door with paper towel with propped foot.			
Puts disposables in waste container in room.			
Seals dressings in plastic before transferring to outside ("clean") person.			
b. **Outside ("Clean") Person**			
Holds cuffed plastic bag over hands to receive tray.			
Secures top of plastic bag tightly.			

PERFORMANCE CHECKLIST

S = Satisfactory
U = Unsatisfactory

Isolation Techniques (cont.)	S	U	Comments
Receives dressings by holding cuffed plastic bag.			
Secures top of plastic bag tightly.			
6. Transferring Nondisposable Equipment Outside the Isolation Unit:			
Washes and soaks some equipment in a disinfectant solution in room before sending for sterilization.			
Double-bags items in paper and labels ''Isolation''; sends to the central service for sterilization of equipment that must be reused.			
7. Collecting a Specimen in the Isolation Unit:			
Brings clean specimen container and covers into unit and places on clean paper towel.			
Places specimen into container without touching container.			
After caring for receptacle in which specimen was collected, washes hands thoroughly.			
Covers and labels specimen; double-bags specimen, as with equipment.			
Attaches requisition with clip and takes to laboratory.			
8. Care of Laundry in the Isolation Unit (Double-Bagging):			
Brings clean linen to unit as needed.			
Closes top of bag in laundry hamper when it is one half to two thirds full; clean person cuffs and holds specially marked laundry bag outside room and receives closed laundry bag.			
Securely ties covers of outside bag and deposits linen in accord with facility policy.			
9. Transporting the Resident in Isolation:			
Notifies the department or charge nurse that resident from isolation is on the way.			
Covers wheelchair or stretcher with clean sheets and wheels into room.			
Identifies resident and explains what is planned and how resident can help.			
Puts on gown and assists resident into wheelchair or onto stretcher.			
Masks resident if deemed necessary.			

PERFORMANCE CHECKLIST

Isolation Techniques (cont.)	S	U	Comments
			S = Satisfactory
			U = Unsatisfactory
Wraps resident in a sheet and instructs him or her not to touch the wheelchair or stretcher.			
Removes gown after leaving unit, following proper techniques.			
10. **Donning Sterile Disposable Gloves:**			
Washes hands and dries thoroughly.			
Picks up two unsterile plastic gloves.			
Lays gloves on table so thumbs are pointed in opposite directions; turns one glove inside out if necessary.			
Makes cuff on each glove.			
Grasps left glove by cuff with right thumb and fingers.			
Brings left thumb toward palm of hand.			
Slips fingers into glove, easing glove over hand and fingers as glove is pulled on with opposite hand.			
Picks up right glove with left hand by slipping fingers of gloved hand under cuff.			
Curves fingers of right hand, bending thumb slightly forward, and inserts into glove.			
Spreads fingers slightly to slide into proper areas, using cuff on glove.			
Adjusts cuff on gloves by interlacing fingers.			
11. **Removing Contaminated Disposable Gloves:**			
Slips glove-covered fingers of right hand under cuff of opposite hand, touching glove only.			
Pulls glove down to fingers, exposing thumb.			
Slips uncovered thumb into opposite cuff.			
Allows glove-covered fingers of left hand to touch only the outer portion of soiled glove.			
Pulls glove down over right hand almost to fingertips and slips glove onto other hand.			
With right hand touching only inside of left glove or hand, continues pulling left glove over right hand until only clean (inside) surface is outermost.			
Disposes of gloves according to facility policy.			
Washes hands thoroughly.			

PROCEDURE COMPETENCY EVALUATIONS

LESSON 8

PERFORMANCE CHECKLIST	S	U	S = Satisfactory U = Unsatisfactory
Making Unoccupied Bed	S	U	Comments
Washes hands and assembles linen.			
Locks bed wheels at side of bed.			
Arranges linen on chair in order in which it is to be used.			
Positions mattress to head of bed by grasping handles on sides of mattress.			
Places mattress cover on mattress and adjusts it smoothly at corners.			
Works entirely from one side of the bed until that side is completed.			
Places and unfolds bottom sheet, smooth side (hem side) up with wide hem at the top, and center fold at center of bed and tucks in lower fitted sheet on one side.			
Tucks 12 to 18 inches of sheet smoothly over top of mattress.			
Makes mitered or square corner.			
Tucks in sheet on one side, keeping it straight; works from head to foot of bed.			
Unfolds top sheet and places wrong side up, hem even with upper edge of mattress, and center fold in center of bed.			
Spreads blanket over top sheet and foot of mattress, keeping blanket centered.			
Tucks top sheet and blanket under mattress at foot of bed as far as center only and makes mitered or square corner.			
Places spread with top hem even with head of mattress.			
Unfolds spread to foot of bed.			
Tucks spread under mattress at foot of bed and makes mitered or squared corners.			

PERFORMANCE CHECKLIST

S = Satisfactory
U = Unsatisfactory

Making Unoccupied Bed (cont.)	S	U	Comments
Goes to other side of bed and fanfolds top covers to the center of bed.			
Tucks bottom sheet under head of mattress and makes mitered or square corners.			
Tucks in top sheet and blanket pleats.			
Folds top sheet back over blanket, making 8-inch cuff.			
Tucks in spread at foot of bed and makes mitered or square corners.			
Brings top of spread to head of mattress.			
Inserts pillow in case properly.			
Places pillow at head of bed with open end away from door.			
Lowers bed to lowest horizontal position.			
Replaces equipment properly; washes hands.			
Reports completion of task.			

Making Occupied Bed

	S	U	Comments
Washes hands and assembles clean linen and a laundry hamper.			
Identifies the resident and explains what is to be done.			
Places bedside chair at foot of bed.			
Arranges linen on chair in order in which it is to be used.			
Screens unit for privacy.			
Raises bed to working height and locks wheels; lowers side rail.			
Loosens bedclothes on all sides by lifting edge of mattress with one hand and drawing bedclothes out with other hand.			
Does not shake linen.			
Adjusts mattress to head of bed.			
Removes top covers except for top sheet and places over back of chair.			
Places clean sheet over top sheet properly.			
Slides the soiled top sheet out, from top to bottom. Discards in hamper.			
Asks resident to roll toward her or him and assists if necessary; moves one pillow with resident and removes other pillow; pulls up side rail.			

PERFORMANCE CHECKLIST

S = Satisfactory
U = Unsatisfactory

Making Occupied Bed (cont.)	S	U	Comments
Goes to other side of bed; lowers side rail; fanfolds cotton drawsheet, if used, and bottom sheet close to resident.			
Straightens out mattress pad; places clean bottom sheet on bed so that narrow hem comes to edge of mattress at foot of bed and lengthwise center fold of sheet is at center of bed.			
Tucks top of sheet under head of mattress.			
Makes mitered or squared corner.			
Tucks side of sheet under mattress, working toward foot of bed.			
Positions fresh turning sheet and tucks under mattress.			
Asks resident to roll toward him or her and assists as needed, moving pillow with resident.			
Raises side rail; goes to the other side of the bed and removes the soiled linen by rolling the edges inward and places in hamper; is careful not to let soiled linen touch uniform.			
Completes making bed as for unoccupied bed.			
Asks resident to turn on back and assists as necessary; places clean case on pillow not being used; replaces pillow; changes other pillowcase.			
Adjusts bed position for resident's comfort.			
Checks to be sure side rails are up and secure; lowers bed to lowest position.			
Places signal cord within resident's reach.			
Replaces bedside table and chair; removes hamper.			
Washes hands.			
Reports completion of task.			

Terminal Cleaning of Resident Unit			
Assembles the following equipment: a. basin of warm water b. soap c. brush d. cleaning cloths e. disinfectant solution f. laundry hamper g. newspaper for waste h. scouring powder i. stretcher j. radiator brush			

PERFORMANCE CHECKLIST

S = Satisfactory
U = Unsatisfactory

Terminal Cleaning of Resident Unit (cont.)	S	U	Comments
Removes any special equipment; makes sure it is clean and returns it to proper area.			
Removes all disposable material from bedside table and wraps it in newspaper to be burned.			
Removes all basic equipment from bedside stand; washes with hot water and detergent; sterilizes equipment according to facility policy.			
Strips bed and discards linen in laundry hamper; places pillows on chair.			
Takes rubber drawsheet, if used, to utility room and washes with soap, water, and disinfectant solution; allows to dry thoroughly.			
Moves stretcher to side of bed; with help, lifts mattress from bed to stretcher.			
Dry-dusts coils of bedsprings, using long-handled radiator brush.			
Using cleaning cloth and disinfectant solution, proceeds as follows: a. Washes plastic cover on mattress with damp cloth and damp-dusts pillow surface. b. Washes framework of bed, including bedsprings; removes parts for thorough cleaning. c. Washes bedside table inside and out; leaves drawers open to air. d. Washes bedside chair after placing pillows on mattress. e. Washes lamp and call bell cord.			
Damp-dusts all surfaces of mattress and pillows.			
Places clean equipment in stand and stocks bedside table according to facility policy.			
Airs bed as long as possible to be sure all moisture has evaporated.			
Replaces mattress.			
Makes closed bed; puts bed in lowest horizontal position.			
Places bedside table on right side of bed at head; places chair at foot on same side; places overbed table across from chair; checks other equipment; leaves unit orderly.			
Washes hands; returns cleaning supplies.			
Reports completion of task.			

PROCEDURE COMPETENCY EVALUATIONS

LESSON 9

PERFORMANCE CHECKLIST			S = Satisfactory U = Unsatisfactory
Hearing Aids	**S**	**U**	**Comments**
1. **Caring for Resident with Hearing Aid:**			
Faces resident and speaks slowly and distinctly.			
Forms words carefully; keeps sentences short.			
Rephrases words as needed.			
Makes sure any light source is behind resident.			
Uses facial expressions or gestures to help express meaning.			
Encourages lip reading.			
Diminishes outside noise or distractions.			
2. **Care of Hearing Aid:**			
Keeps hearing aid in safe, dry place when not in use.			
Keeps ear mold clean by disconnecting mold from hearing aid when not in use.			
Inserts needle or pipe cleaner gently in opening of mold and rotates to remove wax.			
Washes mold gently in warm, soapy water.			
Rinses and allows to air-dry thoroughly before reconnecting to hearing aid.			
3. **Applying Behind-the-Ear Hearing Aid:**			
Washes hands and explains what is going to be done.			
Assists resident to comfortable position with head turned to opposite side.			
Picks up hearing aid and checks to be sure it is off, that volume is at lowest level, and that there are no chips or breaks in equipment; checks tubing for bends or kinks.			
Places aid over resident's ear, allowing ear mold to hang free.			

PERFORMANCE CHECKLIST

S = Satisfactory
U = Unsatisfactory

Hearing Aids (cont.)	S	U	Comments
3. **Applying Behind-the-Ear Hearing Aid** (cont.)			
Adjusts hearing aid behind resident's ear; grasps ear mold and gently inserts tapered end into ear canal.			
Gently twists ear mold into curve of ear, pushing upward and inward on bottom of ear mold while pulling gently on earlobe with the other hand.			
Turns on control switch so sound is at comfortable level.			
Washes hands and records procedure.			
4. **Removing Behind-the-Ear Hearing Aid:**			
Washes hands and explains to resident what is to be done.			
Turns off hearing aid; gently loosens outer portion of ear mold by gently pulling on upper part of ear; lifts ear mold upward and outward.			
Stores in safe area.			
Washes hands and records procedure.			
Care Of Eyeglasses			
Washes hands and assembles the following equipment: a. resident's eyeglasses b. cleaning solution c. clear water d. soft cleaning tissue			
Explains what is to be done.			
Handles glasses by frames only.			
Cleans glasses with cleaning solution or clear water.			
Dries with tissues.			
Returns eyeglasses to resident or places in case on bedside table.			

PROCEDURE COMPETENCY EVALUATIONS

LESSON 13

PERFORMANCE CHECKLIST			S = Satisfactory U = Unsatisfactory
Feeding the Resident	S	U	Comments
Identifies resident; assists resident to wash hands and face.			
Offers bedpan or assists resident to bathroom; washes hands.			
If permitted, raises head of the bed or adjusts position of resident through use of pillows.			
If permitted, assists resident to sit in a chair.			
Clears overbed table.			
Removes unpleasant articles from sight.			
Obtains correct tray. Checks identification.			
Identifies foods and their placement on the tray to resident if necessary.			
Assists by cutting meat, pouring liquids, or buttering bread.			
Allows resident to do as much for himself or herself as possible.			
Is pleasant and unhurried.			
Assisting Resident Who Can Feed Himself or Herself			
Identifies resident and explains what is to be done.			
Offers bedpan or urinal or assists resident to the bathroom.			
Washes hands and encourages resident to do the same.			
If permitted, elevates head of bed or assists out of bed.			
Clears and positions overbed table in front of resident.			
Removes unpleasant equipment from sight.			
Checks dietary name tag against resident's identification.			
Places tray on overbed table and arranges food in a convenient manner.			

PERFORMANCE CHECKLIST			S = Satisfactory U = Unsatisfactory
Assisting Resident Who Can Feed Himself or Herself (cont.)	**S**	**U**	**Comments**
Assists in food preparation as needed.			
Encourages the resident to do as much for himself or herself as possible.			
Removes tray as soon as resident is finished.			
Notes what resident has and has not eaten. Records fluids on intake record if necessary.			
Pushes overbed table out of the way and assists resident to return to bed or places in a comfortable position before leaving room.			
Leaves call bell and water within reach; leaves room tidy.			
Washes hands.			
Feeding the Helpless Resident			
Washes hands and checks diet order.			
Checks name card against resident's identification.			
Removes unnecessary articles from overbed table.			
Adjusts resident to a comfortable position.			
Places napkin under resident's chin.			
Butters bread and cuts meat. Does not pour hot beverage until resident is ready for it.			
Holding spoon at right angle, feeds solid foods from point of spoon.			
Alternates liquids and solids.			
Describes or shows resident what kind of food is being served.			
Tests hot foods by dropping small amount on inside of wrist before feeding it to resident.			
Allows resident to hold bread or assist to the extent that is possible.			
Uses napkin to wipe resident's mouth as often as necessary.			
Removes tray as soon as resident is finished.			
Makes sure to note what resident did or did not eat; records fluids on intake record if necessary.			
Washes hands.			

PERFORMANCE CHECKLIST

S = Satisfactory
U = Unsatisfactory

Serving Supplementary Nourishments	S	U	Comments
Washes hands.			
Checks nourishment list of each resident for any limitations or special dietary instructions.			
Allows resident to choose from available nourishments whenever possible.			
Assists those who are unable to take nourishment alone.			
Removes used glasses and dishes after the resident has finished.			
Records fluids on I&O sheet if required.			
Changing Water			
Checks to be sure that resident is drinking proper amount of fluids. If ''forced fluids'' are mandated, encourages resident to intake more fluids.			
Washes hands.			
Checks whether resident is allowed ice or tap water.			
Washes, refills, and returns pitcher to resident's bedside table.			
Leaves clean glass beside pitcher.			
Places bendable straw beside glass.			
Makes sure water is close at hand.			

PROCEDURE COMPETENCY EVALUATIONS

LESSON 16

PERFORMANCE CHECKLIST			S=Satisfactory U=Unsatisfactory
Post Mortem Care	S	U	Comments
Washes hands and assembles the following equipment: a. shroud or clean sheet b. basin with warm water c. washcloth d. towels e. identification cards (3) f. cotton g. bandages as needed h. pads as needed			
Closes door or screens off unit.			
Removes all equipment and used articles.			
Works quickly and quietly; maintains an attitude of respect.			
Places body on back, with head and shoulders elevated; closes eyes by grasping eyelashes; replaces dentures, if necessary; secures jaw if needed.			
Bathes as necessary; removes any soiled dressings and replaces with clean ones.			
Places cotton pads between the ankles and knees. Ties lightly.			
Pads anal area in case of drainage.			
Puts shroud on body.			
Collects, wraps, and labels all belongs.			
Fills out identification cards and fastens as follows: a. one on body b. one on the resident's clothing and valuables (securely wrapped) c. one on morgue compartment (see below)			
Closes doors and empties corridor of residents and visitors. With assistance, places body on gurney; covers with sheet and takes to the morgue; places identification card on morgue compartment.			

PROCEDURE COMPETENCY EVALUATIONS

LESSON 17

PERFORMANCE CHECKLIST	S	U	S = Satisfactory U = Unsatisfactory
Admitting a Resident	**S**	**U**	**Comments**
Washes hands and assembles the following equipment: a. pad and pencil b. resident's record c. stethoscope d. blood pressure cuff e. equipment for taking temperature f. watch with second hand g. equipment for urine specimen			
Prepares unit for resident by making sure that all necessary equipment and furniture are in proper places; checks for adequate lighting and provides ventilation.			
Identifies new resident by asking his or her name and checking identification.			
Introduces self and takes resident and family to unit; behaves in a courteous manner. Asks family to go to the lounge or lobby while carrying out this procedure.			
Screens the unit. Asks new resident to be seated or, if ordered, after helping resident to undress, assists him or her into bed from stretcher or wheelchair, and adjusts side rails. Otherwise, resident is encouraged to stay up and in their own clothes.			
Unscreens unit. Introduces resident to others in the room.			
Explains signal system and standard regulations.			
Insofar as it is permitted, explains what will happen in the next hour.			
Has family return to unit; screens unit.			
Cares for clothing and personal articles according to facility policy.			
Lists valuables or jewelry that have not been left at the office. Asks resident to sign list, if possible.			

PERFORMANCE CHECKLIST

Admitting a Resident (cont.)	S	U	Comments
S = Satisfactory			
U = Unsatisfactory			
Has family members also sign list; take valuables home or place them in the safe.			
Checks and records resident's weight and height.			
Measures and records resident's temperature, pulse, respiration, and blood pressure.			
Cleans and replaces equipment, according to facility policy.			
Leaves fresh water, if permitted.			
Leaves call bell close at hand.			
Records information, according to facility policy, on resident's chart.			
Measuring Oral Temperature (Glass Thermometer)			
Washes hands and assembles the following equipment on a tray: a. pad and pencil b. watch with second hand c. container with tissues d. container for soiled tissues e. container with clean thermometers f. container for used thermometers			
Identifies resident and explains what is to be done.			
Has resident rest in comfortable position in bed or chair.			
Removes thermometer from container by holding stem end; wipes with tissue and checks to be sure that thermometer is intact.			
Reads mercury column. If necessary, shakes down to below 96°F.			
Inserts bulb end of thermometer under resident's tongue, toward side of mouth. Tells resident to hold thermometer gently with lips closed for 3 minutes.			
After 3 minutes, removes thermometer, holding by stem; wipes with tissue from stem toward bulb end; discards tissue in proper container.			
Reads thermometer and records on pad.			
Places thermometer in container for used thermometers; if thermometer is to be reused for this resident, washes it with soap and cold water and dries it; returns thermometer to individual disinfectant-filled holder.			

PERFORMANCE CHECKLIST

S = Satisfactory
U = Unsatisfactory

Measuring Oral Temperature (Glass Thermometer) (cont.)	S	U	Comments
Cleans and replaces equipment according to facility policy.			
Records temperture on resident's chart; reports any unusual variation in reading immediately to supervising nurse.			

Measuring Rectal Temperature (Glass Thermometer)	S	U	Comments
Washes hands and assembles equipment as for oral temperature, except uses rectal thermometer with rounded bulb and assembles lubricant.			
Identifies resident and explains what is to be done.			
Screens unit.			
Lowers back rest of bed; asks resident to turn on side, assisting if necessary.			
Places small amount of lubricant on tissue.			
Removes thermometer from container by holding stem end; reads mercury column; shakes down if necessary so that it registers below 96°F; checks condition of thermometer.			
Applies lubricant on tissue to bulb.			
Folds top bedclothes back to expose anal area.			
Separates buttocks with one hand. Inserts the thermometer gently 1½ inches into rectum.			
Holds in place for 2 minutes. Replaces bedclothes as soon as thermometer is inserted.			
After 2 minutes, removes thermometer; reads temperature and records on pad.			
Places thermometer in container for used thermometers. If thermometer is to be reused for this resident, washes it with soap and cold water and dries it; returns thermometer to individual disinfectant-filled holder.			
Cleans and replaces equipment according to facility policy.			
Records temperature on resident's chart, with the letter "R" beside the reading; reports any unusual variation in reading immediately to supervising nurse.			

PERFORMANCE CHECKLIST

S = Satisfactory
U = Unsatisfactory

Measuring Axillary or Groin Temperature (Glass Thermometer)	S	U	Comments
Washes hands and assembles equipment as for oral temperature.			
Identifies resident and explains what is to be done.			
Wipes axillary or groin area dry and places thermometer. Holds in place 10 minutes.			
Removes thermometer and reads at once.			
Cleans or disposes of thermometer per facility policy.			
Washes hands.			
Records temperature, with the letters "AX" for axillary temperature and "GR" for groin temperature; reports any unusual variation in reading immediately to supervising nurse.			
Measuring Oral Temperature Using Electronic Thermometer			
Washes hands and assembles the following equipment: a. electronic thermometer b. protective sheath			
Identifies resident and explains what is to be done.			
Covers probe with protective sheath.			
Inserts covered probe under resident's tongue toward side of mouth; holds probe in position.			
When buzzer signals that temperature has been determined, takes reading and records on pad.			
Discards sheath in wastebasket by pushing release. Does not touch sheath.			
Returns probe to proper position and entire unit to charging stand. Washes hands.			
Records temperature on the resident's chart and notes time when it was taken.			
Reports any unusual variations in reading immediately to supervising nurse.			
Measuring Rectal Temperature Using Electronic Thermometer			
Washes hands and assembles the following equipment: a. electronic thermometer b. disposable sheaths c. lubricant			

PERFORMANCE CHECKLIST			S = Satisfactory U = Unsatisfactory
Measuring Rectal Temperature Using Electronic Thermometer (cont.)	S	U	Comments
Identifies resident and explains what is to be done.			
Screens unit.			
Lowers back rest of bed; asks resident to turn on side, assisting if necessary.			
Puts sheath over tip of the thermometer; places a small amount of lubricant on the tip of sheath.			
Folds top bedclothes back to expose anal area.			
Separates buttocks with one hand; inserts sheath-covered probe about ½ inch into rectum and holds in place; replaces bedclothes as soon as thermometer is inserted.			
Reads temperature when registered on digital display and notes on pad.			
Removes probe and discards sheath.			
Assists resident to comfortable position.			
Returns probe to proper position and entire unit to charging stand.			
Washes hands and returns equipment to proper location.			
Records temperature reading on graph, placing an ''R'' after the reading.			
Measuring Axillary Temperature Using Electronic Thermometer			
Washes hands and assembles equipment as for procedure using oral thermometer but substitutes oral electronic thermometer with an oral probe (blue) and disposable sheaths.			
Identifies the resident and explains what is to be done.			
Wipes axillary area dry and places covered probe in place; keeps resident's arm close to body; holds probe in place until temperature is registered on digital display; notes on pad.			
Removes probe and disposes of sheath. Returns probe to proper position and entire unit to charging stand.			
Washes hands and returns equipment to proper location.			
Records axillary temperature, placing the letters ''AX'' after the reading on the graphic chart.			

PERFORMANCE CHECKLIST		S = Satisfactory U = Unsatisfactory	
Measuring Apical Pulse	S	U	**Comments**
Washes hands and takes stethoscope to bedside.			
Identifies resident and explains what is to be done.			
Cleans and places stethoscope earpieces in ears.			
Places stethoscope diaphragm or bell over apex of heart.			
Listens carefully for the heartbeat.			
Counts beats for 1 minute.			
Checks radial pulse for 1 minute.			
Compares results. Charts apical pulse over the radial pulse.			
Cleans earpieces. Returns stethoscope. Washes hands.			
Reports apical/radial differential to nurse.			
Measuring Radial Pulse			
Washes hands.			
Identifies resident and explains what is to be done.			
Assists resident to a comfortable position, with arm resting across chest and palm of hand down.			
Locates pulse on thumb side of wrist with tips of first three fingers.			
Exerts slight pressure when pulse is felt.			
Using second hand of watch, counts pulse rate for 1 minute.			
Records rate and character of pulse.			
Counting Respirations			
After measuring radial pulse, leaves fingers in place on wrist.			
Begins counting the number of times that chest rises and falls during 1 minute.			
Notes depth and regularity of respirations.			
Records time, rate, depth, and regularity of respirations.			
Measuring Blood Pressure			
Washes hands and collects the following equipment: a. sphygmomanometer b. stethoscope			
Identifies resident and explains what is to be done; positions resident comfortably.			

PERFORMANCE CHECKLIST

S = Satisfactory
U = Unsatisfactory

Measuring Blood Pressure (cont.)	S	U	Comments
Instructs the resident to rest arm, palm upward, on bed or table. Uses same arm for all readings.			
Rolls resident's sleeve up about 5 inches above elbow; makes sure it is not tight on arm.			
Applies cuff around upper arm just above elbow.			
Wraps armband smoothly around arm. Tucks ends under fold; hooks or simply presses if Velcro is used to secure.			
Checks that cuff is secure but not too tight.			
Cleans stethoscope earpieces with antiseptic solution and places in ears.			
Locates brachial artery with fingers; places stethoscope head directly over artery.			
Closes valve attached to hand pump (air bulb) and inflates cuff until indicator registers 20 mm above point where pulse ceases to be heard.			
Opens valve of pump and lets air escape slowly until the first sound is heard; notes reading at first regular sound on manometer as systolic pressure.			
Continues to release air pressure slowly until there is an abrupt change in the sound from very loud to soft; notes reading at second sound as diastolic pressure.			
Removes cuff, expels air.			
Cleans earpieces of stethoscope with antiseptic solution and returns to proper place; replaces equipment.			
Records time and blood pressure reading.			
Weighing and Measuring Resident Using Upright Scale			
Identifies resident and explains what is to be done. Escorts resident to scale.			
Places paper towel on platform of scale.			
Checks to be sure that weights are at extreme left and that balance bar hangs free.			
Helps resident remove shoes and step onto scale platform. Stands close for support.			
Moves large weight to the closest estimated weight.			

PERFORMANCE CHECKLIST

S = Satisfactory
U = Unsatisfactory

Weighing and Measuring Resident Using Upright Scale (cont.)	S	U	Comments
Moves the small weight to right until balance bar hangs free halfway between upper and lower bar guides.			
Adds two figures and notes total weight in pounds or kilograms, according to facility policy, on pad.			
Raises height bar until it rests level on top of resident's head.			
Makes reading at movable point of ruler; on pad, notes height in inches, feet and inches, or centimeters, according to facility policy.			
Helps resident step off scales and put on shoes.			
Enters height and weight in the appropriate place on the resident's record.			
Weighing Resident Using Mechanical Lift			
Washes hands and assembles equipment.			
Checks slings and straps for frayed areas or poorly closing clasps.			
Identifies the resident and explains what is to be done; takes scale and lift to resident's bedside and screens unit.			
Locks bed and rolls resident toward self.			
Positions slings beneath resident's body behind shoulders and buttocks.			
Rolls resident back onto the sling and positions properly.			
Attaches suspension straps to sling; checks fasteners for security.			
Positions lift frame over bed with base legs in maximum open position; locks frame.			
Elevates head of bed and brings resident to a semi-sitting position.			
Attaches suspension straps to frame; positions resident's arm inside straps.			
Secures restraint straps if needed.			
While talking to resident, slowly lifts the resident free of bed.			
Guides lift away from bed so that no part of resident touches bed.			
Adjusts weights to balance scale; notes weight on pad.			
Lowers resident to bed by releasing knob.			

PERFORMANCE CHECKLIST	S	U	S = Satisfactory U = Unsatisfactory
Weighing Resident Using Mechanical Lift (cont.)	**S**	**U**	**Comments**
Detaches hooks and rolls resident towards self; folds sling under resident, rolls resident away from self, and removes sling.			
Repositions resident comfortably with call bell close at hand and side rails up.			
Returns equipment to proper location.			
Washes hands.			
Records weight on resident's chart in pounds or kilograms, according to facility policy.			
Measuring Height of Resident Who Must Remain in Bed			
Positions resident flat in bed with legs extended.			
Marks sheet at the top of resident's head and at heels.			
Uses a tape measure to determine the distance between the two marks; this is the resident's height.			
Records resident's height in inches, feet and inches or centimeters, according to facility policy.			
Transfer of the Resident			
Identifies resident and explains what is to be done.			
Checks to be sure that resident is clean and well groomed.			
Gathers all personal belongings.			
Compares the articles with those listed in original inventory.			
Secures valuables in a sealed envelope, listing articles on outside and has person receiving them sign for them; gives them to family member, if possible. Checks with charge nurse for special instructions.			
Escorts resident to doorway of facility.			
Signs chart off including: a. time of transfer b. date of transfer c. method of transport d. destination of transfer e. resident's reactions f. signature			

PROCEDURE COMPETENCY EVALUATIONS

LESSON 18

PERFORMANCE CHECKLIST			S = Satisfactory U = Unsatisfactory
Applying an Aquamatic K-Pad	S	U	Comments
Washes hands and assembles the following equipment: a. K-Pad and control unit b. covering for pad c. distilled water			
Identifies resident and explains what is to be done.			
Places control unit on bedside stand.			
Removes cover of water container and fills unit with distilled water to fill line.			
Screws cover in place and loosens it one-quarter turn.			
Covers pad and places it on resident.			
Coils tubing on bed keeping it at bed level.			
Turns on unit. Sets temperature at 95° to 100°F and removes key.			
Leaves pad in place for prescribed time, checking resident frequently.			
Removes pad, replacing it according to policy. Assists resident to comfortable position.			
Washes hands.			
Records procedure on resident's chart.			
Applying a Heat Lamp			
Washes hands and assembles the following equipment: a. bath blanket b. heat lamp c. tape measure			
Identifies resident and explains what is to be done.			
Screens unit.			

PERFORMANCE CHECKLIST

S = Satisfactory
U = Unsatisfactory

Applying a Heat Lamp (cont.)	S	U	Comments
Positions resident and drapes with bath blanket so that only the area to be treated is exposed.			
Positions the lamp at least 18 inches from the resident; checks distance with tape measure.			
Turns lamp on, noting time.			
Checks resident every 5 minutes, observing skin carefully for signs of redness or burning.			
Discontinues procedure after prescribed time.			
Assists resident to comfortable position.			
Adjusts bedding and removes bath blanket.			
If procedure is to be repeated, folds and leaves bath blanket in bedside table.			
Leaves unit tidy.			
Cleans and returns equipment according to facility policy.			
Washes hands.			
Reports and records procedure properly.			

Assisting with Hot Arm Soak

	S	U	Comments
Washes hands and assembles the following equipment on a tray: a. bath thermometer b. pitcher c. arm soak basin			
Collects and brings to bedside: a. a large plastic sheet b. bath blanket c. bath towel			
Brings tray to bedside; identifies resident and explains what is to be done.			
Screens unit and places equipment on overbed table.			
Covers resident with bath blanket; fanfolds top bedclothes to foot of bed.			
Exposes arm to be soaked.			
Elevates head of bed to sitting position, if permitted.			
Helps resident to move to far side of bed, opposite arm to be soaked.			

PERFORMANCE CHECKLIST

Assisting with Hot Arm Soak (cont.)	S	U	S = Satisfactory U = Unsatisfactory Comments
Checks to be sure side rail is up and secure.			
Covers bed with plastic sheeting and towel.			
Fills arm soak basin half full with water at prescribed temperature; checks temperature with bath thermometer.			
Takes arm soak basin from overbed table and positions on bed protector.			
Assists resident to place arm gradually in basin.			
Checks temperature every 5 minutes.			
Uses pitcher to get additional water and adds to arm soak basin to maintain proper temperature; removes body part before adding hot solution.			
Discontinues procedure at end of prescribed time by lifting resident's arm out of basin; slips basin forward and allows arm to rest on bath towel; places basin on overbed table and gently pats arm dry with towel.			
Removes plastic sheeting and towel; adjusts bedding and removes bath blanket. If treatment is to be repeated puts blanket in bedside table.			
Lowers head of bed and makes resident comfortable.			
Leaves unit tidy and call bell within reach.			
Takes equipment to utility room; cleans and stores according to facility policy.			
Washes hands.			
Records and reports procedure properly.			
Assisting with Hot Foot Soak			
Washes hands and assembles the following equipment on a tray: a. bath thermometer b. solution, as ordered in container c. extra pitcher of hot water			
Places tray on overbed table.			
Brings following equipment to bedside: a. large rubber or plastic sheet b. 2 bath blankets c. 2 bath towels d. tub or basin of appropriate size e. filled hot water bottle			
Screens unit; identifies resident and explains what is to be done.			

PERFORMANCE CHECKLIST

S = Satisfactory
U = Unsatisfactory

Assisting with Hot Foot Soak (cont.)	S	U	Comments
Has resident flex knees; loosens top bedclothes at foot of bed and folds them back to just below resident's knees.			
Makes a bed protector by placing rubber sheet across foot of bed; places bath blanket folded in half with top half fanfolded toward foot of bed, over rubber sheet; places towel on blanket and hot water bottle at lower edge of towel.			
Raising resident's feet, draws rubber sheet, blanket and bath towel up under legs and feet; brings upper half of bath blanket over feet.			
Fills tub half full of water and places it lengthwise at the foot of bed; checks temperature with bath thermometer.			
Raising resident's feet with one hand, draws tub under them and gradually immerses feet; places towel between edge of tub and legs.			
Draws bath blanket up over knees and folds it over from each side. Brings top covers over foot of bed to retain heat.			
Replenishes water as necessary to maintain desired temperature.			
Discontinues treatment within 15 or 20 minutes.			
Removes resident's feet from tub and moves them to towel with hot water bottle under it. Covers feet.			
Removes tub to table or chair.			
Dries and powders feet.			
Removes bath blanket, rubber sheet, and towel; draws down top covers and tucks in at foot.			
Cleans and replaces equipment according to facility policy.			
Washes hands.			
Records and reports properly.			

Applying a Moist Compress

	S	U	Comments
Washes hands and assembles the following equipment on a tray: a. Asepto syringe b. basin with prescribed solution at temperature ordered c. bath thermometer d. bed protector e. binder or towel f. compresses g. pins or bandage h. hot water bag filled with water at ordered temperature			

PERFORMANCE CHECKLIST

S = Satisfactory
U = Unsatisfactory

Applying a Moist Compress (cont.)	S	U	Comments
Identifies resident and explains what is to be done.			
Brings equipment to bedside and screens unit.			
Exposes only the area to be treated.			
Protects bed and resident's clothing with bed protector (e.g. Chux).			
Moistens compresses; removes excess liquid; applies to treatment area.			
Secures compresses with bandage or binder, making sure compresses are in contact with skin.			
Helps resident to maintain a comfortable position throughout treatment.			
Keeps compresses moist or hot water bag hot or cold as prescribed.			
Checks skin several times each day.			
Removes dressings when ordered and discards.			
Cleans and replaces equipment according to facility policy.			
Washes hands.			
Records completion of procedure on resident's chart.			
Applying a Hot Water Bag			
Washes hands and assembles the following equipment in the utility room: a. hot water bag b. cover c. thermometer d. paper towels e. container for hot water			
Fills container with water and tests for correct temperature.			
Fills hot water bag one third to half full to avoid unnecessary weight.			
Expels air by placing hot water bag horizontally on flat surface; holds neck of bag upright until water reaches neck; closes top when all air has been expelled.			
Wipes bag dry with paper towels and turns upside down to check for leakage.			
Places cover on hot water bag so that resident's skin does not come in contact with rubber or plastic.			

PERFORMANCE CHECKLIST

S = Satisfactory
U = Unsatisfactory

Applying a Hot Water Bag (cont.)	S	U	Comments
Takes equipment to bedside on tray.			
Identifies resident and explains what is to be done.			
Applies hot water bag to affected area, as ordered.			
Checks resident's condition at 15 to 20 minute intervals.			
Removes bag at end of prescribed time; removes cover and places in laundry hamper.			
Cleans and replaces equipment according to facility policy.			
Repeats procedure as necessary. Checks condition of skin with each reapplication.			
Washes hands.			
Records procedure on resident's chart; reports any unusual observations immediately to supervising nurse.			

Assisting with Sitz Bath (Portable Unit)

	S	U	Comments
Washes hands, assembles following equipment and takes to bathroom: a. bath thermometer b. bath towel, face cloth c. bath blanket d. clean gown e. safety pin f. portable sitz unit			
Adjusts temperature of bathroom to between 78° to 80°F; cleans tub.			
Identifies resident and explains what is to be done. Escorts resident to bathroom.			
Fills tub half full.			
Adjusts water temperature to 105°F; checks temperature with bath thermometer.			
Assists resident to remove robe and slippers and assists to sit; resident may keep slippers on.			
Covers resident's shoulders with the bath blanket.			
Places cool compresses on resident's forehead.			
Stays with resident during procedure.			
Allows some water to run out of tub; replaces it to maintain constant temperature.			

PERFORMANCE CHECKLIST

S = Satisfactory
U = Unsatisfactory

Assisting with Sitz Bath (cont.)	S	U	Comments
After 10 to 20 minutes, assists resident to stand.			
Helps resident to towel-dry and put on clean gown.			
Assists resident to return to bed.			
Cleans unit and replaces it according to facility policy.			
Washes hands; records procedure on resident's chart.			

Applying a Disposable Cold Pack

	S	U	Comments
Washes hands and assembles the following equipment: a. disposable cold pack b. cloth covering (towel, hot water bag cover) c. tape or rolls of gauze			
Identifies resident and explains what is to be done.			
Screens unit.			
Exposes area to be treated; notes condition of area.			
Places cold pack in cloth covering.			
Strikes or squeezes cold pack to activate chemicals.			
Places covered cold pack on proper area; secures with tape or gauze.			
Notes time of application.			
Leaves resident in comfortable position with signal cord within easy reach.			
Returns to bedside every 10 minutes and checks area being treated for discoloration or numbness; reports to supervisor if these signs and symptoms occur.			
Removes pack in 30 minutes; notes condition of area being treated.			
Applies new pack if treatment is to be continued.			
Removes cover from pack; discards used pack according to facility policy; puts cover in laundry hamper.			
Leaves resident comfortable and unit tidy.			
Washes hands; records and reports procedure.			

PERFORMANCE CHECKLIST

S = Satisfactory
U = Unsatisfactory

Applying an Ice Bag	S	U	Comments
Washes hands and assembles the following equipment in the utility room: a. ice bag or collar b. ice scoop or large spoon c. cover (usually muslin) d. ice cubes or crushed ice e. paper towels			
If ice cubes are used, rinses them in water to remove sharp edges.			
Fills ice bag half full, using ice scoop or large spoon; avoids making ice bags too heavy.			
Expels air by resting ice bag on table in horizontal position with top in place but not screwed on; squeezes bag until air has been removed.			
Fastens top securely; tests for leakage.			
Wipes ice bag dry with paper towels; places muslin cover on bag so that rubber or plastic will not touch resident's skin.			
Takes equipment to bedside on tray.			
Identifies resident and explains what is to be done.			
Applies ice bag to affected part with metal top away from resident.			
Refills bag before all ice is melted.			
Checks skin area with each application; if skin is discolored or white or if resident reports that skin is numb, reports observations to nurse immediately.			
Removes ice bag after prescribed period of time; washes bag with soap and water; drains and screws top on loosely after use; leaves air in bag to prevent sticking.			
Washes hands. Records procedure on resident's chart.			

Giving a Cooling Bath	S	U	Comments
Washes hands and assembles the following equipment: a. 2 bath towels b. 2 bath blankets c. 1 washcloth d. basin of tap water (ice cubes if ordered) e. covered ice bag, filled f. 5 covered, filled hot water bottles g. alcohol (70%) if ordered			

PERFORMANCE CHECKLIST

S = Satisfactory
U = Unsatisfactory

Giving a Cooling Bath (cont.)	S	U	Comments
Identifies resident and explains what is to be done.			
Screens unit for privacy and to prevent drafts.			
Takes the resident's temperature and records on chart.			
Fanfolds top bedding to foot of bed; positions one bath blanket under resident.			
Covers resident with the other bath blanket; removes gown.			
Adds alcohol, if ordered, to basin of water, which is about 70°F.			
Applies ice bag to head; applies one hot water bottle each to feet, groin, and axillary areas.			
Places washcloth in basin, removes washcloth and squeezes out excess water; sponges body with washcloth, exposing only one area at a time.			
Covers sponged area; allows to air-dry.			
Sponges with strokes in direction of heart for approximately 20 minutes.			
Bathes entire body, except for eyes and genitals.			
Removes ice bag and hot water bottles; replaces gown and top bedding; removes bath blankets and discards in hamper.			
Cleans equipment according to facility policy.			
Takes vital signs 10 minutes after sponge bath; records procedure and vital signs on resident's chart.			

PROCEDURE COMPETENCY EVALUATIONS

LESSON 19

PERFORMANCE CHECKLIST		S=Satisfactory U=Unsatisfactory	
Range of Motion (ROM) Exercises	**S**	**U**	**Comments**
ROM for the Neck			
Supports the head and turns gently from side to side.			
Supports the head; bends head toward right shoulder and then left.			
Supports the head; brings chin toward chest. Returns head to straight position.			
Places pillow under shoulders and supports head in a backward tilt.			
ROM for Upper Extremities: Shoulder and Elbow			
Supports the elbow and wrist and brings the entire arm out at right angles to the body.			
Supports the elbow and wrist and brings the entire arm back against the body.			
With shoulder in abduction, flexes the elbow and raises the entire arm over the resident's head.			
Supports upper arm and wrist and bends elbow toward shoulder.			
Supports upper arm and wrist and straightens elbow.			
Positions arm flat on bed with palm of hand up.			
With arm flat on bed, rotates forearm until palm of hand is down.			
ROM for Upper Extremities: Wrist and Fingers			
Supporting arm and hand, flexes wrist.			
Supporting wrist, arm and hand, straightens wrist.			

PERFORMANCE CHECKLIST			S = Satisfactory U = Unsatisfactory
Range of Motion (ROM) Exercises (cont.)	**S**	**U**	**Comments**
ROM for Upper Extremities: Wrist and Fingers (cont.)			
Supporting hand, points hand in suppination toward thumb side.			
Supporting hand, points hand in suppination toward little finger side.			
Covers resident's fingers and makes a fist.			
Covers resident's fist and gently straightens them out.			
Supports the hand and touches the thumb to each fingertip.			
Supports the hand and moves each finger in turn, including the thumb, away from the middle finger.			
Supports the hand and moves each finger in turn, including the thumb, toward the middle finger.			
ROM for Lower Extremities: Hip and Knee			
Supports knee and ankle and moves entire leg away from body center.			
Supporting knee and ankle, moves entire leg back to body center.			
Supporting knee and ankle, flexes knee and hip.			
Supporting knee and ankle, straightens hip and knee.			
Supporting ankle and thigh, flexes knee and rotates leg medially.			
Supporting ankle and thigh, flexes knee and rotates leg laterally.			
Supporting ankle and thigh, bends knee and leg is raised from the bed.			
Supporting ankle and thigh, straightens knee out as leg is lowered to bed.			
ROM for Lower Extremities: Ankle, Foot and Toes			
Supporting ankle and toes, brings toes toward knee.			
Supporting ankle and toes, brings toes toward foot of bed.			
Grasping foot, gently turns it outward.			
Grasping foot, gently turns it inward.			
Supporting foot, moves each toe away from the second toe.			
Supporting foot, moves each toe back toward second toe.			

PERFORMANCE CHECKLIST	S	U	S=Satisfactory U=Unsatisfactory
Range of Motion (ROM) Exercises (cont.)	**S**	**U**	**Comments**
ROM for Lower Extremities: Ankle, Foot and Toes (cont.)			
Placing fingers over toes, bends them gently.			
Placing fingers over toes, straightens them gently.			
Assisting Resident to Get Out of Bed and Ambulate			
Washes hands.			
Checks orders for ambulatory aid.			
Secures correct aid and checks for defects; reports defects and replaces if necessary.			
Identifies resident and explains what will be done and how the resident can help.			
Has resident's slippers and robe or clothing ready.			
Places chair at right angles beside the bed, facing the head; screens unit.			
Lowers side rails.			
Drapes resident with bath blanket and fanfolds top bedclothes to foot of bed.			
Gradually elevates head of bed.			
Helps resident to dress or put on robe.			
Allows resident to sit on edge of bed for a few minutes; notes color, pulse, and response.			
Puts on shoes or slippers.			
Tells resident to swing legs over side of bed; if resident becomes dizzy, returns resident to bed, secures side rail and reports to nurse immediately.			
Lowers bed to lowest position, if previous step is well tolerated by resident.			
Helps resident to stand for a few minutes; if resident becomes or feels weak or tired, seats resident in chair or returns resident to bed.			
Supports chair by placing one foot behind chair to keep it from moving; allows resident to rest and then stand.			
Transfers arm behind the resident's waist and turns so both face in the same direction.			

PERFORMANCE CHECKLIST

S = Satisfactory
U = Unsatisfactory

Assisting Resident to Get Out of Bed and Ambulate (cont.)	S	U	Comments
Assists resident to transfer weight to aid, if used.			
Follows, walking behind and to one side, until resident is stable.			
Observes frequently.			
Reports and records completion of task.			
Log Rolling the Resident			
Washes hands.			
Asks another assistant to help.			
Identifies resident and explains what is to be done.			
Screens unit.			
Elevates bed to waist-high horizontal position and locks wheels. Checks that side rails are secure.			
Lowers side rail on opposite side to which resident will be turned. Both assistants should be on the same side of bed.			
Moves the resident as a unit toward self; places pillow lengthwise between resident's legs; folds resident's arms over chest.			
Raises side rail and checks for security.			
Goes to opposite side of bed and lowers side rail.			
Turns resident to his or her side by using turning sheet that has been previously placed under the resident; reaching over resident, grasps and rolls turning sheet toward resident.			
One assistant should be positioned beside resident to keep shoulders and hips straight; second assistant should be positioned to keep thighs and lower legs straight. If turning sheet is not in position, first assistant positions hands on far shoulder and hips; second assistant positions hands on far thigh and lower leg.			
At specified signal, resident is drawn toward both assistants in a single movement, keeping spine, head, and legs in straight position.			
Places additional pillows behind resident to maintain position.			
Checks resident for comfort, alignment, and support; leaves signal cord within reach and unit tidy.			
Raises side rail and lowers bed.			
Washes hands and reports completion of task to nurse.			

PERFORMANCE CHECKLIST

S = Satisfactory
U = Unsatisfactory

Assisting Resident into Chair or Wheelchair	S	U	Comments
Washes hands.			
Identifies resident and explains what is to be done and how resident can help. Has resident's slippers and robe nearby.			
Screens unit for privacy.			
Covers chair or wheelchair with cotton blanket.			
Places chair or wheelchair near head of bed facing foot of bed; locks wheelchair and raises foot rests.			
Locks bed and elevates head. Lowers bed to lowest horizontal position.			
Drapes resident with bath blanket and fanfolds bedclothes to foot of bed.			
Assists resident to a sitting position by placing arm (the one closest to the head of the bed) around resident's shoulders; places other arm under resident's knees and pivots (rotates) resident toward side of bed slowly and smoothly; remains facing the resident to prevent a fall.			
Assists resident to put on robe and slippers.			
Still facing resident, checks to be sure he or she is ready to stand.			
Has resident place feet on floor or on footstool with both hands on assistant's shoulders; places hands under resident's arms; raises resident slightly and helps resident to slide off edge of bed gradually to a standing position.			
Keeping hands in same position, helps resident to turn slowly until resident's back is toward chair.			
Has another person hold chair or moves to side of resident, placing one foot behind front leg of chair; lowers resident gradually to a sitting position in chair, bending at hips and knees; while doing this, keeps back straight.			
Arranges robe or blanket smoothly; if resident is in a wheelchair, places both feet on the foot rests and locks the wheelchair securely. Covers resident with bath blanket.			
Stays with the resident until sure that there are no adverse side effects; reports anything unusual to supervising nurse.			
Leaves signal cord and drinking water within reach; makes sure that bed and unit are tidy.			
Washes hands and reports completion of task to supervisor.			

PERFORMANCE CHECKLIST

Moving Helpless Resident to Head of Bed	S	U	Comments
Washes hands.			
Asks co-worker to assist from opposite side of bed.			
Identifies resident and explains what is to be done.			
Locks wheels of bed; raises bed to high horizontal position and lowers side rails.			
Removes pillow and places on chair or at the head of the bed on its edge, for safety.			
Lifts top bedclothes and exposes draw sheet; loosens both sides of draw sheet.			
Rolls edges close to both sides of resident's body.			
Faces the head of bed, grasping the roll with the hand closest to resident.			
Positions resident's feet twelve inches apart with the foot that is farthest from bed edge forward.			
Places free hand and arm under resident's neck and shoulders, cradling head from both sides.			
Bends from hips slightly.			
Together, on a count of three, raises—with co-worker—resident's hips and back with the draw sheet, while supporting head and shoulders; moves resident smoothly toward head of bed.			
Replaces pillow under resident's head.			
Tightens and tucks in draw sheet.			
Checks resident for proper body alignment.			
Adjusts bedding.			
Raises side rails and lowers bed; leaves unit tidy.			
Washes hands and reports completion of task to nurse; records, if necessary.			

S = Satisfactory
U = Unsatisfactory

Care of the Falling Resident

	S	U	Comments
Keeps own back straight and base of support broad as resident falls.			
Eases resident to the floor, protecting head.			
Stays with resident.			
Calls for help.			

PERFORMANCE CHECKLIST

S = Satisfactory
U = Unsatisfactory

Care of the Falling Resident (cont.)	S	U	Comments
Does not move resident until he or she has been examined.			
Assists in returning resident to bed.			
Washes hands.			
Reports and records incident on resident's chart.			
Assisting Resident Who Is Out of Bed to Ambulate			
Checks that orders permit ambulation.			
Washes hands.			
Secures proper ambulation aids; checks aids for support.			
Identifies resident and explains what is to be done and how resident can help.			
Assists resident slowly to standing position.			
Keeps one hand under the resident's bent arm for support.			
Adjusts aids.			
If gait belt is used, checks for security; grasps gait belt with hand firmly.			
Walks behind and to one side of resident during ambulation.			
Encourages resident to use hand rails.			
Watches for signs of fatigue; if resident becomes fatigued, assists resident to sit down.			
Talks to resident during procedure and is on guard for anything in the way that might contribute to fall.			
Washes hands.			
Records and reports completion of task.			
Lifting Resident Using Lift Sheet			
Washes hands.			
Asks co-worker to assist.			
Identifies resident and explains what is to be done and how resident can help.			
Stands on one side of the bed; has assisting person stand on opposite side of bed.			
Elevates bed to working height; locks bed wheels; drops side rails.			

PERFORMANCE CHECKLIST

S = Satisfactory
U = Unsatisfactory

Lifting Resident Using Lift Sheet (cont.)	S	U	Comments
Rolls lift sheet close to resident's body.			
Grasps rolled sheet with hand closest to resident.			
Facing head of bed, flexes knees, keeping feet separated and back straight; places other hand under resident's head and neck.			
Instructs assisting person to assume similar position.			
On count of three, together with assisting person, lifts sheet and resident, moving toward head of bed.			
Positions resident comfortably, leaving lift sheet in place.			
Lowers bed and secures side rails.			
Leaves call bell within reach.			
Washes hands and reports completion of task.			
Lifting Resident Without Lift Sheet			
Washes hands.			
Asks co-worker to help.			
Identifies resident and explains what is to be done and how resident can help.			
Stands on one side of bed; assisting person stands on opposite side of bed.			
Elevates bed to working height; locks bed wheels; drops side rails.			
Stands close to bed.			
Facing head of bed, knees flexed, keeping feet separated and back straight; slips one hand and arm under resident's head and shoulders; places other hand and arm under resident's buttocks.			
Instructs assisting person to assume similar position.			
On the count of three, together with co-worker, lifts resident, moving to the head of the bed.			
Positions resident comfortably.			
Lowers bed and secures side rails.			
Leaves call bell within reach.			
Washes hands and reports completion of task.			

PERFORMANCE CHECKLIST			S = Satisfactory U = Unsatisfactory
Care of Resident in a Cast	S	U	Comments
Provides overbed trapeze, if available.			
Handles the cast material by supporting the area with the palms of the hands.			
Maintains good alignment with pillows under the cast.			
Keeps the cast uncovered.			
Checks area around cast for circulation by noting warmth, color, and pulse; reports coldness, color change, or numbness immediately.			
Observes for drainage and odors.			
Turns resident frequently to permit air to circulate.			
Pads rough edges of cast to prevent irritation.			
Reports and records observations.			
Turning Resident Toward You			
Washes hands.			
Identifies resident and explains what is to be done.			
Locks bed wheels and elevates bed to working height.			
Crosses resident's far leg over other leg.			
Places hand nearest head of bed on resident's far shoulder; places other hand on resident's hip on the far side; braces self against side of bed.			
Rolls resident toward self slowly, gently, and smoothly; helps resident bring upper leg toward self and bend comfortably.			
Raises side rail; checks to be sure it is secure.			
Goes to opposite side of bed.			
Places one hand under the resident's shoulders and the other under the resident's hips; pulls resident toward center of bed.			
Makes sure that resident's body is properly aligned and safely supported and positioned.			
If resident is unstable to move self, positions resident's legs and supports with pillows; if resident has an indwelling catheter, makes sure that tubing is not between the legs.			
Places pillow behind resident's back. Secures it by pushing near side under the resident to form a roll.			
Washes hands and reports completion of task to superivsor.			

PERFORMANCE CHECKLIST

S=Satisfactory
U=Unsatisfactory

Turning Resident Away from You	S	U	Comments
Washes hands.			
Identifies resident and explains what is to be done.			
Locks bed wheels and raises side rail on opposite side of bed; raises bed to working horizontal height.			
Has resident bend knees, if able; crosses resident's arms on chest.			
Places arm nearest head of bed under resident's head and shoulders and other hand and forearm under small of his or her back. Practices good body mechanics bending body at hips and knees and keeping back straight; pulls resident toward self.			
Places forearms under resident's hips and pulls hips toward self.			
Moves resident's ankles and knees toward self by placing one hand under the resident's shoulder and one under the knees.			
Crosses resident's nearer leg over other leg at ankles.			
Rolls resident away from self, slowly and carefully, by placing one hand under the resident's shoulder and one hand under hips.			
Places hands under resident's head and shoulders and draws them back toward center of the bed.			
Moves resident's hips to center of bed.			
Places pillow for support behind resident's back.			
Makes sure that resident's body is in good alignment; supports upper legs with pillow.			
Replaces side rail on near side of bed and returns bed to lowest position.			
Washes hands and reports completion of procedure to supervisor.			

Assisting Resident into Bed from Chair or Wheelchair

	S	U	Comments
Washes hands. Identifies resident and explains what is to be done.			
Screens unit.			
Checks to see that bed is in lowest horizontal position and that wheels are locked; raises head of bed, fanfolds top bedclothes to foot, and raises opposite side rail.			

PERFORMANCE CHECKLIST

S = Satisfactory
U = Unsatisfactory

Assisting Resident into Bed from Chair or Wheelchair (cont.)	S	U	Comments
Positions chair or wheelchair at foot of bed; locks wheels of wheelchair and lifts foot rests.			
Has resident place feet flat on floor.			
Removes bath blanket, folds, and returns to bedside stand.			
Stands in front of resident; practices good body mechanics, keeping back straight and base of support broad.			
Places hands on either side of resident's chest; has resident place his or her hands on assistant's shoulders. Assists resident to stand.			
Pivots resident toward bed slowly and smoothly; assists resident to sit on edge of bed.			
Assists resident to remove robe and slippers.			
Places one arm around resident's shoulders and one arm under resident's legs and swings resident's legs onto the bed.			
Lowers head of bed and assists resident to move into center of bed.			
Draws top bedclothes over resident; remakes bed if necessary.			
Makes resident comfortable; places signal cord within reach.			
Washes hands.			
Reports completion of assignment.			
Care of Resident in Traction			
While giving care, examines the traction lines to find the primary traction lines; locates support lines.			
Does not disturb weights or permit them to swing.			
Checks under belts for areas of pressure or irritation.			
Makes sure that straps, belts, or halters are smooth, straight and properly secured.			
Assisting Resident Who Ambulates with Cane or Walker			
Washes hands.			
Secures appliance (cane or walker); checks appliance for worn areas or loose parts.			
Identifies resident and explains what is to be done.			

PERFORMANCE CHECKLIST			S = Satisfactory U = Unsatisfactory
Assisting Resident Who Ambulates with Cane or Walker (cont.)	S	U	Comments
Lowers bed to lowest horizontal position; lowers side rail.			
Raises head of bed and assists resident to a sitting position.			
Assists resident to swing legs over edge of bed to allow feet to rest on floor; assists resident to put on robe and slippers.			
If necessary, applies gait belt around resident's waist.			
Places walker or cane within easy reach; assists resident to standing position.			
Has resident grasp walker or cane to maintain balance.			
Walks beside resident, grasping transfer belt for additional support.			
After ambulation, returns resident to bed by reversing the procedure.			
Leaves resident in comfortable position; raises side rail and checks that it is secure.			
Washes hands.			
Records completion of task on chart, including: a. date and time b. procedure: Assisting to ambulate with cane (or walker) c. resident's reaction			
Transferring Resident Using a Mechanical Lift			
Washes hands and assembles equipment.			
Checks slings and straps for frayed areas or poorly closing clasps.			
Takes lift to resident's bedside and screens unit.			
Identifies resident and explains what is to be done.			
Places wheelchair or chair at right angles to foot of bed, facing head.			
Locks bed wheels and rolls resident toward self.			
Positions slings beneath resident's body behind shoulders and buttocks; makes sure that sling is smooth.			
Rolls resident back onto sling and positions properly.			
Attaches suspension straps to sling; checks fasteners for security.			
Positions lift frame over bed with base legs in maximum open position; locks frame.			

PERFORMANCE CHECKLIST

S = Satisfactory
U = Unsatisfactory

Transferring Resident Using a Mechanical Lift (cont.)	S	U	Comments
Elevates head of bed and brings resident to semi-sitting position.			
Attaches suspension straps to frame; positions resident's arms inside straps; secures restraint straps if needed.			
Talking to resident, slowly lifts him or her free of bed; guides lift away from bed.			
Positions resident close to chair or wheelchair (with wheels locked); slowly lowers resident into chair or wheelchair.			
Unhooks suspension straps and removes lift.			
Makes resident comfortable and secure before leaving.			
Washes hands.			
Records procedure on resident's chart.			
Transferring Dependent Resident			
Washes hands; identifies patient and explains what is going to be done.			
Locks wheels of bed; raises bed to horizontal position equal to height of stretcher. Fanfolds bedding to foot of bed.			
Enlists help from two co-workers; positions one assisting person next to opposite side of bed and one at foot of stretcher; positions self on opposite side of stretcher.			
Positions stretcher against bed; locks wheels and lowers side rails of stretcher.			
Loosens stretcher restraints and bath blanket covering resident; rolls turning sheet close to resident's body.			
Instructs assisting person on opposite side of bed to use both hands to grasp turning sheet, and to lift and draw resident onto bed.			
Instructs assisting person at foot of bed to lift resident's feet and legs.			
Standing opposite stretcher, places one arm for support under head and shoulders of resident and with the other hand grasps turning sheet to guide resident.			
All assistants must coordinate their activities and move together as a signal is given.			
Moves stretcher out of way.			
Using turning sheet, positions resident in bed.			

PERFORMANCE CHECKLIST			S = Satisfactory U = Unsatisfactory
Transferring Dependent Resident (cont.)	S	U	Comments
Pulls top bedclothes up over resident and slips bath blanket from underneath.			
Raises side rails; returns bed to lowest horizontal position.			
Washes hands.			
Reports the return of resident to nurse.			
Assisting Resident to Move to Head of Bed			
Washes hands.			
Identifies resident, explains what is to be done, and how to aid assistant at the count of three.			
Locks wheels of bed; raises bed to high horizontal position and lowers side rail on side nearest self.			
Removes pillow and places on chair or at the head of bed on its edge for safety.			
Faces head of bed, positioning the foot that is farthest from the bed approximately 12 inches in front of other foot.			
Places arm nearest head of the bed under resident's head and shoulders; locks other arm with resident's arm.			
Instructs resident to bend knees and press in with heels; as resident does this, begins count, lifts shoulders and moves resident smoothly toward head of bed reaching it on a count of three.			
May use alternate method as follows: Places pillow at head of bed on its edge; has resident grasp head of bed; slips hands under resident's back and buttocks; as resident presses in with heels; assists resident to raise his or her hips and move to head of bed.			
Replaces pillow under resident's head and makes resident comfortable.			
Lowers bed and raises side rail; leaves unit tidy.			
Washes hands and reports completion of task to nurse.			

PROCEDURE COMPETENCY EVALUATIONS

LESSON 20

PERFORMANCE CHECKLIST			S = Satisfactory U = Unsatisfactory
Dressing and Undressing Resident	S	U	Comments
Washes hands.			
Identifies resident and explains what is to be done.			
Helps resident to select appropriate clothing; encourages resident to help in the selection; arranges clothing in order of application.			
Screens unit for privacy.			
Raises bed to comfortable working height; elevates head of bed to sitting position.			
Covers resident with bath blanket; fanfolds top bedclothes to the foot of the bed; assists resident to comfortable sitting position.			
Removes night clothing, keeping resident covered with bath blanket.			
Gathers undershirt or other garment and slips over resident's head; or helps hook bra.			
Grasps resident's hand and guides it through armhole by reaching into armhole from outside; repeats procedure with opposite hand.			
Assists resident to sit forward, adjusting shirt or dress so it is smooth and covers upper body.			
Helps resident to put on shirt or button-front dress by inserting hand through sleeve of shirt or dress and grasping the hand of the resident, drawing the sleeve over your hand and resident's hand.			
Adjusts sleeves at shoulder.			
Assists the resident to sit forward and arranges clothing across back. Buttons or secures front of shirt or dress.			
Slips underwear over feet and draws as high up on the legs as possible; assists resident to raise buttocks to draw underwear up to waist.			

PERFORMANCE CHECKLIST

S = Satisfactory
U = Unsatisfactory

Dressing and Undressing Resident (cont.)	S	U	Comments
For a male resident, repeats process with trousers; helps to fasten or zip trousers.			
Puts on socks or assists female resident to put on panty hose, using same technique as for underwear.			
Puts on and secures shoes.			
Assists resident to a comfortable position out of bed; leaves call bell within reach.			
When undressing the resident, reverses the procedure.			
Leaves unit tidy.			
Washes hands.			
Reports completion of task and any observations to nurse.			

Assisting with Special Oral Hygiene

	S	U	Comments
Washes hands and assembles the following equipment: a. mouthwash or solution in cup; or mixture of glycerine in lemon juice b. emesis basin c. bath towel d. plastic bag e. applicators f. tissues g. tongue depressor h. lubricant for lips			
Identifies resident and explains what is to be done; screens unit.			
Covers pillow with towel and turns resident's head to side; places emesis basin under resident's chin.			
Opens mouth gently with tongue depressor; dips applicators into mouthwash solution or glycerine mixture.			
Using moistened applicators, wipes gums, teeth, tongue, and inside of mouth; discards used applicators in plastic bag.			
Lubricates lips with cold cream or petroleum jelly.			
Cleans and replaces equipment according to facility policy.			
Washes hands.			
Reports and records completion of task.			

Assisting Resident to Brush Teeth

	S	U	Comments
Washes hands and assembles the following equipment: a. emesis basin b. toothbrush and toothpaste c. glass of cool water d. mouthwash (if permitted) e. hand towel f. bed protector g. dental floss			

PERFORMANCE CHECKLIST

S = Satisfactory
U = Unsatisfactory

Assisting Resident to Brush Teeth (cont.)	S	U	Comments
Identifies resident and explains what is to be done and how resident can help; screens unit.			
Elevates head of bed; helps resident into comfortable sitting position.			
Lowers side rails; positions overbed table across resident's lap; covers table with plastic protector.			
Places emesis basin and glass of water on overbed table; places towel across resident's chest.			
Is prepared to help as resident brushes and flosses teeth.			
When resident has completed oral care, pushes overbed table to the foot of the bed; removes towel, folds and places on table.			
Lowers head of bed; helps resident to assume a comfortable position; adjusts bedding; raises side rails; leaves unit tidy.			
Cleans and stores equipment according to facility policy; discards soiled linen in proper receptacle.			
Washes hands.			
Reports completion of task and observations to nurse.			

Caring for Dentures

	S	U	Comments
Washes hands and assembles the following equipment: a. tissues e. gauze squared b. emesis basin f. denture cup c. toothbrush or denture brush g. mouthwash d. toothpaste or powder			
Identifies resident and explains what is to be done.			
Screens unit.			
Allows resident to clean dentures if able to do so; if resident cannot do it, gives tissue to resident and asks that the dentures be removed; assists if necessary.			
Places dentures in denture cup padded with gauze squares; takes to bathroom or utility room.			
Puts toothpaste or tooth powder on toothbrush; places dentures in palm of hand and holds them under gentle stream of warm water; brushes until all surfaces are clean.			
Rinses dentures thoroughly under cold running water; rinses denture cup.			

PERFORMANCE CHECKLIST

S = Satisfactory
U = Unsatisfactory

Caring for Dentures (cont.)	S	U	Comments
Places fresh gauze in denture cup; places dentures in cup and takes to bedside.			
Assists resident to rinse mouth with mouthwash.			
Uses tissue or gauze to hand clean dentures to resident; inserts if necessary.			
Cleans and replaces equipment according to facility policy.			
Washes hands.			

Giving Foot and Toenail Care

	S	U	Comments
Washes hands and assembles the following equipment: a. wash basin e. disposable bed protector b. soap f. bath towel and washcloth c. bath mat g. orangewood stick d. lotion			
Identifies resident and explains what is to be done.			
Assists resident out of bed and into chair, if permitted.			
Places bath mat on floor in front of resident.			
Fills basin with warm water (105°F); puts basin on bath mat.			
Removes slippers and instructs resident to place feet in water; covers with bath towel to help retain the heat.			
Soaks feet approximately 20 minutes; adds warm water as necessary; lifts feet from water while warm water is being added.			
At end of soak period, washes feet with soap. Uses washcloth to scrub roughened areas; rinses and dries feet; notes any abnormalities, such as corns or callouses, and reports to supervisor.			
Removes basin, covering feet with towel.			
Uses orangewood stick to gently clean toenails. Dry feet.			
Pours lotion into palms of hands; holds hands together to warm lotion and applies to resident's feet.			
Assists resident into slippers and returns resident to bed, unless ambulatory; makes resident comfortable.			
Gathers equipment, cleans, and stores, according to facility policy; leaves unit tidy.			
Washes hands.			
Reports completion of task and observations to nurse.			

PERFORMANCE CHECKLIST

S = Satisfactory
U = Unsatisfactory

Giving Hand and Fingernail Care	S	U	Comments
Washes hands and assembles the following equipment: a. basin b. soap c. bath towel and washcloth d. lotion e. plastic protector f. nail clippers g. nail file h. orangewood stick			
Identifies resident and explains what is to be done.			
Screens unit.			
Elevates head of bed, if permitted, and adjusts overbed table in front of resident; if resident is allowed out of bed, assists to transfer to a chair and positions overbed table waist-high across resident's lap.			
Places plastic protector over bedside table.			
Fills basin with warm water at approximately 105°F and places on overbed table.			
Instructs resident to put hands in basin and soak for approximately 20 minutes; places towel over basin to help retain heat; adds warm water if necessary; remembers to remove the resident's hands before adding warm water.			
Washes hands; pushes cuticles back gently with washcloth.			
Lifts hands out of basin and dries with towel.			
Uses nail clippers to cut fingernails straight across; shapes and smooths fingernails with nail file.			
Pours small amount of lotion in palm of hands and gently smoothes on resident's hands.			
Empties basin of water; gathers equipment, cleans, and stores, according to facility policy.			
Returns overbed table to foot of bed; if resident has been sitting up for procedure, assists resident into bed.			
Lowers head of bed and makes resident comfortable; leaves call bell within easy reach; makes sure that bed is in lowest position and side rails are up and secure.			
Leaves unit tidy.			
Washes hands.			
Reports completion of task and any observations to the nurse.			

PERFORMANCE CHECKLIST

S = Satisfactory
U = Unsatisfactory

Giving Female Perineal Care	S	U	Comments
Washes hands and assembles the following equipment: a. bath blanket b. bedpan and cover c. graduate pitcher d. cotton balls e. disposable gloves f. bed protector or bath towel g. ordered solution (if other than water) h. plastic bag to dispose of used cotton balls i. perineal pad and belt, if needed			
Identifies resident and explains what is to be done.			
Fills pitcher with warm water (or ordered solution) at approximately 100°F and takes to bedside.			
Screens unit.			
Lowers side rail and positions bed protector (or towel) under resident's buttocks.			
Fanfolds spread to foot of bed; covers resident with bath blanket and fanfolds top sheet to foot of bed.			
Positions resident on bedpan.			
Puts on disposable gloves.			
Has resident flex and separate knees; draws bath blanket upward to expose perineal area only.			
Unfastens perineal pad if in use, touching only outside; notes amount and color of discharge; folds pad with insides together and places in plastic bag.			
Holding pitcher of water approximately 5 inches above pubis, allows water to flow downward over vulva and into bedpan.			
Dries vulva, using cotton balls in proper manner.			
Removes and disposes of disposable gloves.			
Asks resident to raise hips and carefully removes bedpan; covers and places on chair.			
Applies perineal pad, if needed, and secures to belt, using proper techniques.			
Removes bath towel or disposable pad and disposes according to facility policy.			
Draws sheet and spread up over resident and removes bath blanket; folds bath blanket and stores in bedside stand.			

PERFORMANCE CHECKLIST

S = Satisfactory
U = Unsatisfactory

Giving Female Perineal Care (cont.)	S	U	Comments
Makes resident comfortable and leaves unit tidy.			
Cleans equipment and discards disposables, according to facility policy.			
Washes hands.			
Reports completion of task and observations to the nurse.			
Giving Male Perineal Care			
Washes hands and assembles the following equipment: a. bath blanket b. urinal and cover c. soap, washcloth and towel d. disposable gloves and plastic bag e. bed protector or bath towel f. ordered solution (if other than water)			
Identifies resident and explains what is to be done.			
Fills basin with warm water at approximately 100°F and takes to bedside.			
Screens unit.			
Lowers side rail and positions bed protector (or towel) under resident's buttocks.			
Fanfolds spread to foot of bed; covers resident with bath blanket and fanfolds top sheet to foot of bed.			
Offers resident urinal; empties and cleans before proceeding with perineal care.			
Washes hands, puts on disposable gloves.			
Has resident flex and separate knees; draws bath blanket upward to expose genital area only.			
With washcloth, water, and soap, washes pubis, penis, and scrotum; gently draws foreskin back and cleans glans; rinses area well and dries; makes sure prepuce is properly positioned.			
Turns resident on side away from self; washes, rinses and dries area under scrotum and around anus; repositions resident.			
Removes and disposes of disposable gloves; removes bath towel or disposable pad and disposes, according to facility policy.			
Draws sheet and spread up over resident and removes bath blanket; folds bath blanket and stores in bedside stand.			
Makes resident comfortable and leaves unit tidy.			
Cleans equipment and discards disposables according to facility policy.			

PERFORMANCE CHECKLIST

S = Satisfactory
U = Unsatisfactory

Giving Male Perineal Care (cont.)	S	U	Comments
Washes hands.			
Reports completion of task and observations to nurse.			
Giving a Partial Bath			
Washes hands and assembles the following equipment: a. bed linen b. bath blanket c. bath thermometer d. soap and soap dish e. washcloth, bath towel and face towel f. gown or robe g. laundry bag or hamper h. bath basin and water 105°F i. alcohol or lotion; powder j. equipment for oral hygiene k. nail brush and emery board l. brush, comb, and deodorant m. bedpan or urinal and cover n. paper towels or protector			
Identifies resident and explains what is to be done.			
Makes sure that windows and door are closed to prevent chilling of the resident; screens unit.			
Puts towels and linen on chair in order of their use; places laundry bag or hamper conveniently close.			
Offers bedpan or urinal; empties and cleans before proceeding with bath; washes hands.			
Elevates head rest, if permitted, to comfortable position.			
Loosens top bedclothes; removes and folds blanket and spread; places bath blanket over top sheet and removes sheet by sliding it out from under bath blanket.			
Leaves one pillow under resident's head; places other pillow on chair.			
Assists resident to remove gown and places in laundry bag or hamper. Wraps bath blanket around resident.			
Places paper towels or bed protector on overbed table.			
Fills bath basin two thirds full with water at 105°F; places on overbed table.			
Pushes overbed table comfortably close to resident; places towels, washcloth, and soap on overbed table.			
Instructs resident to wash as much as he or she is able; returns to complete the bath as necessary.			
Places call bell within easy reach; asks resident to signal when ready; washes hands and leaves unit.			
Washes hands and returns to unit when resident signals.			

PERFORMANCE CHECKLIST

S = Satisfactory
U = Unsatisfactory

Giving a Partial Bath (cont.)	S	U	Comments
Changes bath water; completes bathing areas the resident couldn't; makes sure that face, hands, axilla, buttocks, back, and genitalia are washed and dried.			
Gives back rub with lotion or alcohol and powder.			
Assists resident to apply deodorant and/or powder and to put on fresh gown.			
Covers pillow with towel and combs or brushes hair; assists with oral hygiene if needed.			
Cleans and replaces equipment according to facility policy.			
Puts clean washcloth and towels in stand or hangs them according to facility policy.			
Changes linen, following occupied bed procedure; replaces and discards soiled linen in laundry bag or hamper.			
Leaves resident comfortably positioned with side rails up and bed in lowest horizontal position; places signal cord and water within reach.			
Replaces furniture; leaves unit in order; turns out ceiling light, if used.			
Washes hands.			
Reports completion of tasks and any observations to nurse.			
Assisting with Tub Bath or Shower			
Washes hands and assembles the following equipment: a. soap f. bath thermometer b. washcloth g. bath powder c. 2 or 3 bath towels h. chair or stool d. bath blanket i. bath mat e. gown, robe, and slippers			
Takes supplies to bathroom and prepares it for the resident. Makes sure tub is clean.			
Fills tub half full of water between 95° and 105°F or adjusts shower flow to a comfortable level; tests bath water with a thermometer and shower temperature with wrist.			
Identifies resident and explains what is to be done.			
Places a towel in bottom of tub or shower to prevent resident from slipping.			
Assists resident with robe and slippers; assists resident to bathroom.			

PERFORMANCE CHECKLIST

S = Satisfactory
U = Unsatisfactory

Assisting with Tub Bath or Shower (cont.)	S	U	Comments
Helps resident to undress; gives male resident a towel to wrap around midriff.			
Assists resident into tub or shower.			
Washes resident's back; provides privacy so that resident may wash genitalia.			
Holds bath blanket around the resident when he or she steps out of tub; male resident may choose to remove wet towel under bath blanket.			
Assists resident to dry, powder, dress, and return to unit.			
Returns supplies to proper areas.			
Cleans bathtub or shower; washes hands.			
Reports completion of task to nurse and records on chart, including: a. date and time b. procedure: tub bath or shower c. resident's reaction			
Bathing Resident in a Century Tub			
Prepares bath before transporting resident by: a. checking to be sure the tub is clean b. filling tub with water at 97°F to approximately 8 inches from top c. checking that room temperature is approximately 70°F d. adding one capful of liquid soap			
Washes hands and assembles the following equipment: a. talcum powder b. deodorant c. 2 bath towels d. 1 bath blanket e. resident's clothing			
Takes Saf-Kary chair to bedside.			
Identifies resident and explains what is to be done.			
Screens unit; assists resident to undress.			
Positions resident in Saf-Kary chair; secures safety straps; covers resident with bath blanket.			
Transports resident to tub room.			
Replaces bath blanket with two towels. Folds blanket for later use.			

PERFORMANCE CHECKLIST

S = Satisfactory
U = Unsatisfactory

Bathing Resident in a Century Tub (cont.)	S	U	Comments
Positions chair with back against left arm; steps on ''up'' pedal of lift to engage seat on Saf-Kary chair; checks to see that both pins are engaged in left arm slots; latches safety latches.			
Raises lift to maximum height; rotates seat on left arm 90 degrees so that resident faces self; faces resident and slowly guides to tub edge so that resident is parallel to and over tub edge.			
Lifts resident's feet and guides over tub edge toward lower well of tub; lowers resident into tub by stepping gently on ''down'' pedal.			
Presses turbine button, activating whirlpool for 5 minutes; bathes face and upper body with a washcloth.			
Steps on ''up'' pedal, raising resident until feet are level with whirlpool outlet; dries upper body.			
Raises lift to maximum height; pulls chair and resident toward self; rotating seat, lifts resident's feet from the tub; dries feet.			
Covers resident with bath blanket.			
Raises safety latch on Saf-Kary chair.			
Applies deodorant and talcum powder; dresses resident.			
Slowly lowers lift and Saf-Kary until chair is flat on floor.			
Returns resident to unit.			
Replaces supplies in resident's unit; returns to tub room and cleans tub.			
Reports and records completion of task.			
Giving a Bed Bath			
Washes hands and assembles the following equipment: a. bed linen b. bath blanket c. laundry bag or hamper d. bath basin and water (about 105°F) e. bath thermometer f. soap and soap dish g. washcloth and face towel h. bath towel i. hospital gown (or resident's bedclothes) j. alcohol or lotion and powder k. equipment for oral hygiene l. nail brush and emery board m. brush and comb n. bedpan or urinal and cover			

PERFORMANCE CHECKLIST

S = Satisfactory
U = Unsatisfactory

Giving a Bed Bath (cont.)	S	U	Comments
Identifies resident and explains what is to be done and how resident can assist.			
Makes sure windows and door are closed to prevent chilling resident.			
Screens unit.			
Puts towel and linen on chair in order of their use; places laundry bag or hamper conveniently.			
Offers bedpan or urinal; empties and cleans before proceeding with bath; washes hands.			
Lowers head of bed and side rails if permitted.			
Loosens top bedclothes; removes and folds blanket and spread; places bath blanket over top sheet and removes sheet by sliding it out from under bath blanket.			
Leaves one pillow under resident's head; places other pillow on chair.			
Removes resident's gown and places gown in laundry bag or hamper.			
If resident has IV line, removes gown as follows: a. Loosens gown from neck. b. Slips gown from arm. c. Makes sure that resident is covered with bath blanket. d. Slips gown away from body toward arm with IV line in place. e. Gathers gown at arm and slips downward over arm and line, being careful not to disturb line. f. Gathers material of gown in one hand so there is no pull or pressure on line; slowly draws gown over tip of fingers. g. With free hand, lifts IV bottle free of standard; slips gown over bottle.			
Fills bath basin two thirds full of water at 105°F.			
Assists resident to move to side of bed nearest self.			
Folds face towel over upper edge of bath blanket.			
Forms a mitten by folding washcloth around hand; wets washcloth and washes eyes, using separate corners of cloth for each eye; does not use soap near eyes.			
Rinses washcloth and applies soap if resident desires; squeezes out excess water; washes and rinses resident's face, ears, and neck; dries with towel.			
Exposes resident's far arm; protects bed with bath towel placed underneath arm; washes, rinses, and dries arm and hand; repeats on other arm.			

PERFORMANCE CHECKLIST

S = Satisfactory
U = Unsatisfactory

Giving a Bed Bath (cont.)	S	U	Comments
Applies deodorant and powder if resident requests them or needs them.			
Cares for hands and nails as necessary; washes each hand carefully and rinses and dries; pushes cuticle back gently with towel while wiping the fingers; cleans under nails and shapes with emery board.			
Puts bath towel over resident's chest; folds blanket to waist; washes, rinses, and dries chest; rinses and dries under breasts of female resident; powders lightly if necessary.			
Folds bath blanket down to pubic area; washes, rinses, and dries abdomen; folds bath blanket up to cover abdomen and chest; slides towel out from under bath blanket.			
Asks resident to flex knees, if possible; folds bath blanket up to expose thigh, leg, and foot.			
Protects bed with bath towel; puts bath basin on towel; places resident's foot in basin; washes and rinses leg and foot, supporting leg properly. Removes basin; dries leg and foot, with special attention to area between toes.			
Moves basin to other side of bed; repeats procedure, bathing and drying other leg and foot.			
Cares for toenails as necessary; files nails straight across; applies lotion to feet. (Note: If resident is diabetic and toenails need trimming, do not file them yourself, but report this to nurse.)			
Changes water, checks temperature with bath thermometer.			
Helps resident to turn on side away from self and to move toward center of bed; places towel lengthwise next to resident's back; washes, rinses, and dries back, neck and buttocks.			
Gives resident back rub.			
Helps resident to turn on back.			
Places towel under buttocks and thighs; places washcloth, soap, basin, and bath towel within convenient reach of resident. Has resident complete bath including washing of genitalia.			
Carries out range-of-motion exercises as ordered.			
Covers pillow with towel and combs and/or brushes hair; assists resident, if necessary, with oral hygiene.			
Assists resident to put on clean gown or clothes.			
Cleans and replaces equipment according to facility policy.			

PERFORMANCE CHECKLIST

S = Satisfactory
U = Unsatisfactory

Giving a Bed Bath (cont.)	S	U	Comments
Changes bed linen following occupied bed procedure. Replaces and discards soiled linen and towels and washcloth in laundry bag or hamper.			
Leaves resident in comfortable position; raises side rails and checks that they are secure.			
Places signal cord and water within reach; replaces furniture; leaves unit tidy; turns out ceiling light, if used.			
Washes hands.			
Reports completion of procedure and any observations to nurse.			
Cleaning and Flossing Resident's Teeth			
Washes hands and assembles the following equipment: a. emesis basin e. mouthwash, if permitted b. toothbrush and tooth paste f. hand towel or powder g. bed protector c. glass of cool water d. dental floss			
Identifies the resident and explains what is to be done.			
Screens unit.			
Elevates head of bed, if permitted; assists resident to a comfortable position.			
Lowers side rails and positions overbed table across resident's lap.			
Places towel or bed protector across resident's chest.			
Places tooth paste or powder on moistened toothbrush; cleans all surfaces of each tooth; has resident rinse mouth using emesis basin.			
Selects a piece of dental floss about 12 inches long; asks resident to open mouth; gently inserts floss between each tooth down to *but* not *into* gumline; asks resident to rinse mouth with water or mouthwash, using emesis basin.			
Wipes resident's face dry with towel on chest.			
Pushes overbed table to foot of bed.			
Positions resident comfortably; makes sure that water and call bell are close at hand.			
Raises and secures side rails.			
Empties emesis basin; gathers equipment; cleans, and stores according to facility policy; discards towel or bed protector in laundry hamper.			

PERFORMANCE CHECKLIST

S = Satisfactory
U = Unsatisfactory

Cleaning and Flossing Resident's Teeth (cont.)	S	U	Comments
Washes hands.			
Reports completion of task and observations to nurse.			
Giving a Bed Shampoo			
Washes hands and assembles the following equipment: a. shampoo tray and shampoo b. washcloth and 3 bath towels c. bath blanket d. basin of water (105°F) e. large, empty basin f. safety pin g. 2 bed protectors h. waterproof covering for pillow i. large basin to collect used water j. hair dryer, if available k. hairbrush and comb l. small pitcher or cup m. large pitcher of water (115°F) to be used if additional water is needed.			
Screens unit.			
Identifies resident and explains what is to be done.			
Places chair beside head of bed; covers seat with bed protector; places large, empty basin on chair.			
Arranges bedside stand within easy reach and puts the following equipment on it: a. basin of water (105°F) b. pitcher of water (115°F) c. washcloth d. 2 bath towels e. shampoo f. small pitcher or cup			
Replaces top bedclothes with bath blanket; replaces pillow case with waterproof covering; covers head of bed with bed protector.			
Asks resident to move to side of bed nearest self.			
Loosens neck ties of gown.			
Places towel under resident's head and shoulders; brushes hair free of tangles, working snarls out carefully.			
Brings towel down around resident's neck and shoulders and pins it securely; positions pillow under shoulders so that head is tilted slightly backward.			
Raises bed to high horizontal position.			

PERFORMANCE CHECKLIST

S = Satisfactory
U = Unsatisfactory

Giving a Bed Shampoo (cont.)	S	U	Comments
Raises resident's head and positions shampoo tray so that drain is over edge of bed directly above empty basin on chair.			
Gives resident washcloth to cover eyes; rechecks temperature of water in basin; using small pitcher or cup, pours small amount of water over hair until thoroughly wet; with one hand, directs flow away from face and ears.			
Applies a small amount shampoo, working up lather; works from scalp to hair ends; massages scalp with tips of fingers; does not use fingernails.			
Rinses thoroughly, pouring from hairline to hair tips and directing flow into drain; uses warm water in pitcher, if needed; checks temperature of water before use.			
Repeats wash and rinse procedure.			
Lifts resident's head; removes tray and bed protector; places tray on basin; adjusts pillow and slips dry bath towel underneath head.			
Wraps hair in towel; dries face, neck, and ears as needed.			
Dries hair with towel or hair dryer.			
Combs and/or brushes hair and removes protective pillow cover; replaces with cloth cover.			
Lowers height of bed to comfortable working position.			
Replaces bedclothes and removes bath blanket; helps resident assume comfortable position; lowers bed to lowest horizontal position; allows resident to rest undisturbed.			
Empties water collected in basin; cleans equipment according to facility policy and returns it to proper area; leaves unit tidy.			
Washes hands.			
Reports and records procedure, including: a. date and time b. procedure: bed shampoo c. resident's reaction			
Giving a Back Rub			
Washes hands and assembles the following equipment: a. basin of water (105°F) b. bath towel c. soap and alcohol or lotion d. body powder			
Identifies resident and tells what is to be done.			

PERFORMANCE CHECKLIST

S = Satisfactory
U = Unsatisfactory

Giving a Back Rub (cont.)	S	U	Comments
Screens unit and raises bed to comfortable work height.			
Places lotion container in basin of water to warm.			
Assists resident to turn facing away from self.			
Exposes and washes back.			
Pours a small amount of lotion into hand; applies to skin and rubs with gentle but firm strokes; gives special attention to all bony prominences.			
Beginning at the base of spine, with long, soothing strokes rubs up the center of back, around shoulders and down sides of back and buttocks.			
Repeats this step 4 times, using long, soothing upward stroke and circular motion on the downward stroke.			
Repeats again, but on downward stroke rubs in a small circular motion with palm of hand; includes area over coccyx.			
Repeats long, soothing strokes to muscles for 3 to 5 minutes.			
Dries area well; if pressure areas are noted, reports these to nurse.			
Straightens draw sheet.			
Changes resident's gown, if needed; positions resident comfortably.			
Replaces equipment according to facility policy.			
Washes hands.			
Reports completion of task and any observations to nurse.			

Daily Care of Hair

	S	U	Comments
Washes hands and assembles the following equipment: a. towel b. comb and brush c. alcohol or petroleum jelly (Vaseline)			
Identifies resident and explains what is to be done.			
Asks resident to move to side of bed nearest self, or assists resident to sit in chair, if permitted.			
Screens unit.			
Covers pillow wih towel.			
Parts or sections hair and combs hair, beginning at scalp.			

PERFORMANCE CHECKLIST

S = Satisfactory
U = Unsatisfactory

Daily Care of Hair (cont.)	S	U	Comments
Brushes hair carefully and thoroughly.			
Has resident turn so hair on back of head can be combed and brushed; if hair is snarled, works section by section, applying alcohol to oily hair or petroleum jelly to dry hair as needed; unsnarls hair, beginning near hair ends and working toward scalp.			
Completes brushing and arranges hair attractively; braids long hair to prevent repeated snarling.			
Cleans and replaces equipment according to facility policy.			
Washes hands.			
Reports completion of task and any observations to nurse.			
Shaving Male Resident			
Washes hands and assembles the following equipment: a. electric shaver or safety razor b. shaving lather or an electric pre-shave lotion c. basin of water (115°F) d. hand towel e. mirror f. after-shave lotion or powder			
Identifies resident and explains what is to be done; lets resident help as much as possible.			
Screens unit.			
Raises head of bed; places equipment on overbed table.			
Places hand towel across resident's chest.			
Moistens face and applies lather if safety razor to be used; otherwise, applies pre-shave electric lotion.			
With safety razor, starts in front of ear; holds skin taut and brings razor down over cheek toward chin; repeats until lather on cheek is removed and area has been shaved; repeats on other cheek. Uses firm, short strokes, rinsing razor frequently.			
Lathers neck area and strokes up toward chin in similar manner.			
Washes face and neck and dries thoroughly.			
Applies after-shave lotion or powder, if resident requests it.			
If skin is nicked, applies pressure directly over area and then applies antiseptic; reports incident to nurse.			
Cleans and replaces equipment according to facility policy.			

PERFORMANCE CHECKLIST			S = Satisfactory U = Unsatisfactory
Shaving Male Resident (cont.)	S	U	Comments
Washes hands.			
Reports completion of task and observations to nurse.			

PROCEDURE COMPETENCY EVALUATIONS

LESSON 21

PERFORMANCE CHECKLIST	S	U	S = Satisfactory U = Unsatisfactory
Application of TED Hose	S	U	Comments
Washes hands.			
Takes elasticized stockings (TED hose) of proper length and size to resident's bedside.			
Identifies resident and explains what is to be done.			
Has resident lie down; exposes one leg at a time.			
Grasps stocking with both hands at top and rolls toward toe end.			
Adjusts over toes, positioning opening at base of toes (unless toes are to be covered).			
Applies stocking to leg by rolling upward toward body.			
Checks to be sure that stocking is applied evenly and smoothly and that there are no wrinkles.			
Repeats procedure on other leg.			
Reports and records completion of task, including: a. date and time b. procedure: Applying TED hose c. any unusual observations			

PROCEDURE COMPETENCY EVALUATIONS

PERFORMANCE CHECKLIST			S = Satisfactory U = Unsatisfactory
Caring for a Stoma	S	U	Comments
Washes hands and assembles the following equipment: a. washcloth and towel b. basin of warm water (105°F) c. bed protector d. bath blanket e. bedpan f. disposable colostomy bag and belt g. disposable gloves h. skin lotion, as directed i. toilet tissue			
Takes equipment to bedside; identifies resident and explains what is to be done.			
Replaces top bedclothes with bath blanket; places bed protector under resident's hips.			
Puts on disposable gloves.			
Removes soiled disposable colostomy bag and places in bedpan; removes belt which holds colostomy bag; saves belt if clean.			
Gently cleans area around stoma with toilet tissue to remove feces and drainage; disposes of soiled tissue in bedpan.			
Washes area around stoma with soap and water; rinses thoroughly and dries.			
Applies skin lotion lightly around stoma, if ordered.			
Positions belt around resident; inspects area for signs of irritation or breakdown.			
Places clean ostomy bag over stoma and secures to belt; removes and disposes of gloves.			
Removes bed protector; checks that bottom sheet is not wet; changes if necessary.			
Replaces bath blanket with top bedclothes; makes resident comfortable.			

PERFORMANCE CHECKLIST	S	U	S=Satisfactory U=Unsatisfactory
Caring for a Stoma (cont.)	**S**	**U**	**Comments**
Gathers soiled linen and equipment and disposes of according to facility policy.			
Cleans bedpan and basin and returns to unit.			
Washes hands.			
Reports and records completion of task and observations.			
Irrigating a Colostomy in Bathroom			
Washes hands.			
Checks orders for colostomy and assembles the following equipment in resident's bathroom: a. irrigating can, tubing, and clamp b. connector and catheter c. disposable gloves d. disposable irrigating apparatus e. dressing for fresh ostomy bag and belt f. pole or other fixture to support irrigating can g. lubricant h. toilet tissue i. washcloth and towel			
Identifies resident and explains what is to be done.			
Assists resident to bathroom.			
Positions resident on toilet and drapes legs with towel.			
Puts on disposable gloves.			
Removes disposable colostomy bag or dressing; cleanses area of stoma with tissue and disposes of tissue in toilet.			
Applies disposable irrigating sleeve by placing face plate directly over stoma; secures with belt; drops end of plastic drainage sheath between resident's legs into toilet.			
Attaches catheter to connector and them to tubing; attaches tubing to irrigating container.			
Fills container with solution, as ordered; allows small amount of fluid to fill tubing and catheter to warm tubing and expel air.			
Squeezes small amount of lubricant onto toilet tissue and applies to tip of catheter; gently inserts catheter 3 to 4 inches into stoma, using rotating motion.			
Slowly releases approximately 500 ml of fluid into ostomy.			
Removes catheter and allows return to flow into toilet; notes character of return.			

PERFORMANCE CHECKLIST

S = Satisfactory
U = Unsatisfactory

Irrigating a Colostomy in Bathroom (cont.)	S	U	Comments
Repeats procedure until returns are clear.			
Detaches irrigating bag from belt; disposes of bag according to facility policy.			
Cleans around stoma area with warm, soapy water; rinses and dries thoroughly; applies small amount of lotion if ordered.			
Applies small dressing or clean ostomy bag and secures with belt.			
Removes gloves; disposes of gloves according to facility policy.			
Assists resident back to bed.			
Cleans equipment and replaces according to facility policy.			
Washes hands.			
Reports and records completion of procedure.			
Irrigating an In-Bed Colostomy			
Washes hands and assembles the following equipment: a. bed protector and bath blanket b. toilet tissue c. lubricant d. basin e. disposable gloves f. emesis basin lined with paper towels g. disposable irrigating apparatus h. IV pole to hang irrigating can i. solution, as ordered j. wash cloth and towel k. irrigating can, tubing, catheter, and connector l. dressing or fresh ostomy bag and belt			
Identifies resident and explains what is to be done.			
Replaces top bedclothes with bath blanket.			
Positions resident close to edge of bed, either sitting or in semi-Fowler's position.			
Places protective bed covering in position on bed.			
Places bedpan on a chair beside bed.			
Attaches tubing, connector, and catheter to irrigating can; clamps tubing.			
Fills irrigating container with solution; allows small amount of fluid to flow through tubing.			

PERFORMANCE CHECKLIST

S = Satisfactory
U = Unsatisfactory

Irrigating an In-Bed Colostomy (cont.)	S	U	Comments
Hangs container from IV standard near bed, approximately 18 inches above stoma.			
Places emesis basin on bed with concave surface facing resident.			
Puts on disposable gloves; removes dressing or disposable ostomy bag and places in emesis basin.			
Cleans stoma area gently with toilet tissue; disposes of tissue in emesis basin.			
Places disposable irrigation bag over stoma, with open end in bedpan.			
Squeezes small amount of lubricant onto toilet tissue and applies to tip of catheter; gently inserts catheter 3 to 4 inches into stoma, using rotating motion.			
Slowly releases approximately 500 ml of fluid into ostomy.			
Removes catheter and allows return to flow into bedpan.			
Repeats procedure until returns are clear.			
Detaches irrigating bag from belt and disposes of according to facility policy.			
Cleans area around stoma with warm, soapy water; rinses and dries thoroughly.			
Applies small amount of lotion, if ordered; applies dressing or clean ostomy bag and secures with belt.			
Removes gloves and disposes of them, according to facility policy.			
Cleans equipment and replaces, according to facility policy.			
Washes hands.			
Reports and records completion of procedure.			
Giving and Receiving Bedpan			
Washes hands and assembles the following equipment: a. bedpan and cover b. toilet tissue c. basin of warm water (105 °F) d. soap e. washcloth and towel			
Identifies resident and explains what is to be done.			
Screens unit for privacy; lowers head of bed, if permitted.			
Places bedpan on chair; puts tissue on bedside table within easy reach of resident; places remainder of articles on bedside table.			

PERFORMANCE CHECKLIST

S = Satisfactory
U = Unsatisfactory

Giving and Receiving Bedpan (cont.)	S	U	Comments
Places bedpan cover at foot of bed between mattress and springs; prepares bedpan properly by heating and drying.			
Folds top bedcloths back. Raises the resident's gown; asks resident to flex knees and rest weight on heels if possible.			
Positions bedpan properly, using proper body mechanics.			
Replaces top bedclothes; raises head of bed to comfortable height.			
Makes sure that signal cord is within easy reach; leaves resident alone unless contraindicated.			
Answers resident's call bell immediately; lowers head of bed; fills basin with warm water.			
Removes bedpan properly, using good body mechanics.			
Assists resident to clean area of bed; discards soiled tissue in bedpan, unless specimen is to be collected; covers bedpan and places on chair; assists resident, if necessary, to cleanse perineal area with warm water and soap.			
Replaces bedclothes; encourages resident to wash hands and freshen up after procedure; changes bed linen or protective pads as necessary.			
Takes bedpan; rinses with cold water and disinfectant, dries and covers.			
Places bedpan in resident's bedside table; cleans and replaces other articles.			
Washes hands, leaves unit in order.			
Reports any unusual observations to the supervisor and charts accordingly.			
Checking for Fecal Impaction			
Washes hands and assembles the following equipment: a. disposable glove b. lubricant c. bed protector d. bath blanket e. toilet tissue f. basin of warm water g. washcloth and towel			
Identifies resident and explains what is to be done.			
Screens unit for privacy.			

PERFORMANCE CHECKLIST

S = Satisfactory
U = Unsatisfactory

Checking for Fecal Impaction (cont.)	S	U	Comments
Raises bed to comfortable working height; lowers side rails on side closest to self.			
Asks resident to raise hips; places bed protector under hips.			
Assists resident to turn to side away from self; instructs resident to bend (flex) knees.			
Covers resident with bath blanket; fanfolds top bedclothes to foot of bed.			
Puts disposable glove on dominant hand; lubricates index finger of that hand.			
Asks resident to take deep breath and bear down; inserts lubricated finger into rectum; checks for impaction; withdraws finger; notes findings.			
Washes resident's buttocks with warm water and soap; assists resident to turn onto back; asks resident to raise hips; withdraws bed protector.			
Folds bed protector and gloves from outside to inside; places on chair.			
Draws up top bedclothes; removes bath blanket; folds bath blanket and places in bedside table.			
Raises side rail; makes resident comfortable; leaves call bell within reach.			
Empties and dries basin; returns to bedside table.			
Puts towel and washcloth in laundry hamper; disposes of protector and glove according to facility policy.			
Washes hands.			
Reports completion of procedure and observations to the nurse.			

Giving Oil-Retention Enema

	S	U	Comments
Washes hands and assembles the following equipment: a. prepackaged oil for retention enema b. bedpan and cover c. bed protector d. toilet tissue e. bath blanket f. towel, soap, and basin with water			
Identifies resident and explains what is to be done.			
Places chair at foot of bed; covers with towel and places bedpan on chair.			

PERFORMANCE CHECKLIST	S	U	S=Satisfactory U=Unsatisfactory
Giving Oil-Retention Enema (cont.)	**S**	**U**	**Comments**
Covers resident with bath blanket and fanfolds top bedclothes to foot of bed.			
Places bed protector under resident's buttocks; helps resident to assume the Sims' position.			
Exposes resident's anus; removes cap from prepackaged oil-retention enema; inserts prelubricated tip into anus as resident takes deep breath.			
Squeezes container until all of solution has entered rectum; removes container and places in package box to be discarded.			
Encourages resident to remain on side; checks resident every 5 minutes until fluid has been retained for 20 minutes.			
Positions resident on bedpan or assists to bathroom			
If resident is on bedpan, raises head of bed to comfortable height; places toilet tissue and signal cord within easy reach of resident.			
If resident is in bathroom, stays nearby.			
Disposes of material according to facility policy.			
Removes bedpan or assists resident to return from bathroom to bed; observes contents of bedpan or toilet; covers pan and disposes of contents or flushes toilet.			
Gives resident soap, water, and towel to wash and dry hands.			
Replaces top bedclothes; removes bath blanket and bed protector and disposes of according to facility policy.			
Washes hands.			
Reports and records completion of task.			
Giving a Soapsuds Enema			
Washes hands and obtains disposable, commercially available, enema, consisting of a plastic container, tubing, clamp, and lubricant. Assembles unit as follows: a. Connects tubing to solution container. b. Adjusts clamp on tubing and snaps shut. c. Fills container with warm water to 1000 ml line. d. Opens packet of liquid soap and puts soap in water. e. Uses tip of tubing to mix the solution gently so no suds form. f. Runs small amount of solution through tube to get rid of air and warm the tube.			

PERFORMANCE CHECKLIST			S=Satisfactory U=Unsatisfactory
Giving a Soapsuds Enema (cont.)	S	U	Comments
If disposable equipment is not available, assembles: a. funnel b. tubing and clamp c. connecting tube d. rectal tube e. graduate pitcher with warm, soapy water.			
Takes following equipment to bedside: a. disposable enema unit or prepared one b. lubricant c. toilet tissue d. bedpan and cover e. towel, soap, and basin with water f. bath blanket g. bed protector e.g., (Chux)			
Identifies resident and explains what is to be done. Screens unit.			
Places chair at foot of bed and covers with towel; places bedpan on towel.			
Covers resident with bath blanket; fanfolds top bedclothes to foot of bed.			
Places bed protector under buttocks; assists resident to turn on left side and flex knees (Sims' position).			
Places container of solution on chair so tubing will reach resident; lubricates tip of rectal tube.			
Adjusts bath blanket to expose anal area; exposes anus by raising upper buttock.			
Never forces tube; gets help if tube cannot be inserted easily.			
Opens clamp and raises container 12 to 15 inches so that fluid flows in slowly; asks resident to take deep breaths to relax abdomen; if resident complains of cramping, clamps tube and waits; then opens tubing to continue fluid flow; when enough solution has been given, clamps tubing.			
Tells resident to hold breath while upper buttock is raised and tube is gently withdrawn.			
Wraps tubing in paper towel; puts in disposable container.			
Places resident on bedpan or assists resident to bathroom; if resident is on bedpan, raises head of bed to comfortable height; places toilet tissue and signal cord within reach of resident; if resident is in bathroom, stays nearby.			

PERFORMANCE CHECKLIST

S = Satisfactory
U = Unsatisfactory

Giving a Soapsuds Enema (cont.)	S	U	Comments
Takes tray to utility room; rinses enema equipment thoroughly in cool water and then washes in warm, soapy water; returns to bedside or discards according to facility policy.			
Removes bedpan or assists resident to return to bed; observes contents of toilet or bedpan; covers bedpan.			
Removes bed protector; gives resident, soap, water and towel to wash hands.			
Replaces top bedclothes and removes bath blanket; folds bath blanket and places in bedside table; airs room; leaves room in order.			
Cleans and replaces all other equipment according to facility policy; washes hands.			
Reports and records completion of procedure and results.			
Inserting a Lubricating Suppository			
Washes hands and assembles the following equipment: a. suppository, as ordered b. lubricant c. toilet tissue d. disposable gloves e. bedpan and cover if needed			
Identifies resident and explains what is to be done.			
Draws curtains for privacy.			
Assists resident to assume the left Sims' position; exposes buttocks only.			
Puts on disposable gloves and unwraps suppository.			
With left hand, separates buttocks, exposing anus; applies small amount of lubricant to anus and inserts suppository.			
Encourages resident to take deep breaths and relax until the need to defecate is experienced.			
Removes and disposes of gloves.			
Adjusts bedding, helping resident assume comfortable position; places call bell within easy reach of resident.			
Checks resident every 5 minutes.			
Provides bedpan when needed or assists resident to toilet.			
Notes, records, and reports results of procedure.			

PERFORMANCE CHECKLIST

S = Satisfactory
U = Unsatisfactory

Collecting a Stool Specimen	S	U	Comments
Washes hands and assembles the following equipment: a. bedpan and cover b. specimen container and cover c. toilet tissue d. tongue blades e. label for container			
Fills out label, including: a. resident's full name and room number b. date and time of collection c. doctor's name d. type of test to be performed e. other information as requested			
Identifies resident and explains what is to be done; screens unit.			
Receives bedpan with specimen; offers wash water to resident; takes covered pan to utility room.			
Uses tongue blades to remove specimen from bedpan and place in specimen container; discards tongue blade.			
Washes hands.			
Covers container and attaches completed label; makes sure that cover is on container tightly.			
Cleans and replaces equipment.			
Takes or sends specimen to laboratory promptly.			
Washes hands.			
Reports and records procedure.			

PROCEDURE COMPETENCY EVALUATIONS

LESSON 23

PERFORMANCE CHECKLIST			S = Satisfactory U = Unsatisfactory
Giving Indwelling Catheter Care	S	U	Comments
Washes hands and collects following equipment: a. disposable gloves e. daily catheter care kit b. bed protector f. antiseptic solution c. bath blanket g. sterile applicators d. plastic bag h. tape			
Identifies resident and explains what is to be done. Screens unit.			
Raises bed to working height and lowers side rail closest to self; assists resident to lie on back, with legs separated and knees bent, if permitted.			
Covers resident with bath blanket and fanfolds top bedclothes to foot of bed; positions bath blanket so that only genitals are exposed.			
Asks resident to raise hips; places bed protector underneath hips.			
Arranges catheter care kit and plastic bag on overbed table.			
Puts on gloves; opens catheter care kit.			
To cleanse genital area of male resident: a. Gently grasps penis and draws foreskin back. b. Dipping fresh applicator in antiseptic solution for each stroke, cleanses from meatus toward shaft for approximately 4 inches. c. Places each applicator in plastic bag after use.			
To cleanse genital area of female resident: a. Separates the labia. b. Using fresh applicator dipped in antiseptic solution for each stroke, cleanses from front to back. c. Places used applicator in plastic bag after use.			
Removes gloves and places in plastic bag.			
Checks that catheter is taped properly; retapes and adjusts for slack, if needed.			

PERFORMANCE CHECKLIST

S = Satisfactory
U = Unsatisfactory

Giving Indwelling Catheter Care (cont.)	S	U	Comments
Checks that tubing is coiled without kinks on bed and hangs straight down into drainage container; checks level of urine in container; empties bag and measures if necessary.			
Replaces bedclothes and removes bath blanket; folds bath blanket and places in bedside table.			
Helps resident to assume comfortable position; checks that call bell is within easy reach.			
Lowers bed and raises and secures side rail; leaves unit tidy.			
Disposes of equipment according to facility policy.			
Washes hands.			
Reports and records completion of task on resident's chart.			
Routine Drainage Check			
Washes hands.			
Identifies resident and explains what is to be done. Screens unit.			
Raises bedding to observe tubing.			
Checks position of catheter and meatus.			
Checks that drainage tube is coiled smoothly on the bed and that there is a direct drop to collection bag.			
If necessary, adjusts collection bag, so that it is below level of resident's hips.			
Checks that end of drainage tube is above urine level in bag.			
Makes sure drainage tube is attached to bed frame.			
Notes color and character and flow of urine; measures urine using proper technique.			
Washes hands.			
Reports and records completion of task and findings.			
Collecting Mid-Stream Urine Specimen			
Washes hands and assembles the following equipment: a. sterile urine specimen container b. gauze squares or cotton, soap and basin of water c. antiseptic solution d. filled out requisition slip and label for container, including: 　1. resident's full name and room number 　2. date and time of collection			

PERFORMANCE CHECKLIST			S=Satisfactory U=Unsatisfactory
Collecting Mid-Stream Urine Specimen (cont.)	S	U	Comments

d. (cont.)
  3. doctor's name
  4. type of test to be performed
  5. other information as requested			

Identifies resident and explains what is to be done. Screens unit.			
Assists resident to bathroom or provides urinal or bedpan.			
Cleanses genital area, or has resident do so using proper technique.			
Instructs resident to void; allows first part of urine stream to escape; then catches urine stream that follows in sterile specimen container; allows last portion of urine stream to escape; measures all urine as output if required.			
Places sterile cap on specimen container immediately to avoid contamination of urine specimen; with cap securely tightened, washes outside of specimen container.			
Allows resident to wash hands.			
Washes hands.			
Labels container as instructed and attaches requisition slip for appropriate test.			
Cleans and replaces equipment according to facility policy.			
Takes or sends specimen to appropriate area immediately.			
Reports completion of task to nurse and properly records procedure on chart.			
Disconnecting a Catheter			
Washes hands.			
Identifies resident and explains what is to be done. Screens unit.			
Clamps catheter; disinfects area around catheter connection.			
Disconnects catheter and drainage tubing; does not put them down or allow them to touch anything.			
Inserts sterile plug in end of catheter; places sterile cap over exposed end of drainage tube.			
Secures drainage tube to bed in such a way that it will not touch floor.			
Washes hands.			
Reverses procedure to reconnect catheter.			
Reports and records completion of task.			

PERFORMANCE CHECKLIST

S = Satisfactory
U = Unsatisfactory

Emptying Urinary Drainage Unit	S	U	Comments
Washes hands.			
Identifies resident and explains what is to be done.			
If drainage bag has opening in bottom, places graduate under it and allows urine to drain.			
If there is no opening, removes tube to empty unit; protects end of drainage tube with sterile cap or sterile gauze sponge.			
Measures urine.			
Removes protective cover from end of tube and reinserts it in bag.			
Washes hands. Reports completion of task.			
Records amount on resident's I&O record and chart.			
Replacing Urinary Condom			
Washes hands and assembles the following equipment: a. basin of warm water f. disposable gloves b. washcloth and towel g. plastic bag c. bed protector h. tincture of benzoin d. bath blanket i. paper towels e. condom with drainage tip			
Identifies resident and explains what is to be done.			
Screens unit and elevates bed to comfortable working height; arranges equipment on overbed table; lowers side rail closest to self.			
Covers resident with bath blanket and fanfolds top bedclothes to foot of bed; places bed protector under resident's hips; adjusts bath blanket to expose genitals only.			
Puts on disposable gloves.			
Removes present condom by rolling it toward tip of penis; places in plastic bag if disposable; if reusable, places on paper towel to be washed and dried.			
Washes and dries penis carefully; observes for signs of irritation.			
Checks to see if condom has "ready-stick" surface; if not, a thin spray of tincture of benzoin may be applied to penis; does not spray on head of penis.			
Applies fresh condom to penis by rolling it toward base of penis; if resident is uncircumcised, checks that foreskin remains in good position.			
Reconnects drainage system.			

PERFORMANCE CHECKLIST

S = Satisfactory
U = Unsatisfactory

Replacing Urinary Condom (cont.)	S	U	Comments
Removes gloves and discards in plastic bag.			
Adjusts bedding and removes bath blanket; folds bath blanket and places in bedside stand.			
Lowers bed and raises side rail; makes resident comfortable; checks that call bell is in easy reach; leaves unit tidy.			
Cleans and replaces equipment and discards disposables according to facility policy.			
Washes hands.			
Reports and records completion of task.			
Measuring and Recording Fluid Output			
Takes urine saved in bedpan or urinal to utility room or resident's bathroom. Has on hand: a. graduate pitcher b. pen for recording c. I&O record			
Pours urine from bedpan or urinal into graduate; measures amount.			
Records amount immediately under output column on I&O record.			
Empties urine into toilet.			
Rinses graduate with cold water; cleans according to facility policy.			
Cleans bedpan or urinal and returns to proper place, according to facility policy.			
Washes hands.			
Copies information on chart from I&O record, according to facility policy.			
Measuring and Recording Fluid Intake			
Washes hands and assembles the following equipment: a. I&O record at bedside b. pen c. graduated pitcher			
Identifies the resident and explains what is to be done.			
Records intake on the I&O record at the bedside.			
Copies information on resident's chart from I&O record, according to facility policy.			

PERFORMANCE CHECKLIST

S = Satisfactory
U = Unsatisfactory

Assisting with Bedside Commode	S	U	Comments
Washes hands and assembles the following equipment: a. portable commode b. basin of warm water c. washcloth and towel d. soap e. toilet tissue			
Identifies resident and explains what is to be done; screens unit.			
Positions commode beside bed, facing head; locks wheels and removes cover; checks that receptacle is in place under seat.			
Lowers side rail nearest to self; lowers bed to lowest horizontal position.			
Assists resident to sitting position; helps resident to swing legs over edge of bed.			
Puts on resident's slippers and robe; assists resident to stand.			
Has resident place hands on shoulders; supports resident under arms; pivots resident to right; lowers resident to commode.			
Leaves call bell and tissue within reach.			
When signaled, returns promptly; draws warm water in basin and brings to bedside along with soap, towel, and washcloth.			
Assists resident to stand.			
Cleanses anus or perineum if resident is unable; allows resident to wash and dry hands.			
Helps resident to return to bed; adjusts bedding and pillows for comfort.			
Puts cover on commode; removes receptacle; covers with bedpan cover.			
Takes receptacle to bathroom; notes contents and measures, if required.			
Empties and cleans receptacle, according to facility policy; replaces receptacle in commode; returns commode to proper place.			
Cleans and replaces remaining equipment, according to facility policy.			
Washes hands.			
Reports and records completion of task.			

PERFORMANCE CHECKLIST

S = Satisfactory
U = Unsatisfactory

Giving and Receiving The Urinal	S	U	Comments
Washes hands and assembles the following equipment: a. urinal and cover b. basin of warm water c. soap, washcloth and towel			
Identifies resident and explains what is to be done.			
Screens unit.			
Lifts top bedcovers and places urinal under covers so that resident may grasp handle.			
Makes sure that signal cord is within easy reach; leaves resident alone if possible.			
Answers resident's signal immediately; takes urinal from resident; covers urinal; fills basin with warm water and lays out soap, washcloth, and towel so that resident can wash and dry hands.			
Takes urinal to bathroom or utility room, observes and notes contents of urinal; measures if required.			
Empties urinal; rinses with cold water and cleans with warm soapy water; rinses, dries, and covers urinal.			
Places urinal inside resident's bedside table; cleans and returns articles to proper place.			
Rearranges bedcovers if necessary; leaves resident comfortable and unit tidy.			
Washes hands.			
Reports any unusual observations to nurse and charts according to facility policy.			
Collecting Routine Urine Specimen			
Washes hands and assembles the following equipment: a. washcloth and towel b. soap and basin of water c. bedpan or urinal and cover d. specimen container and cover e. graduate pitcher f. laboratory requisition slip, properly filled out g. label			
Fills out label, including: a. resident's full name and room number b. date and time of collection c. doctor's name d. type of test to be performed e. other information as requested			

PERFORMANCE CHECKLIST

S = Satisfactory
U = Unsatisfactory

Collecting Routine Urine Specimen (cont.)	S	U	Comments
Identifies resident and explains what is to be done.			
Screens unit; offers bedpan or urinal.			
After resident has voided, takes bedpan or urinal to utility room; offers wash water to resident.			
Pours specimen from bedpan or urinal into graudate; notes amount if resident's intake and output are to be recorded.			
Pours about 120 ml into specimen container. (*Note:* Some facilities require only 10 to 20 ml.)			
Washes hands; is careful not to contaminate outside of container.			
Covers container; attaches label and requisition slip to container.			
Cleans and replaces equipment according to facility policy.			
Takes or sends specimen to laboratory promptly.			
Records completion of task on resident's chart; records fluid output on I&O record, if required.			

PROCEDURE COMPETENCY EVALUATIONS

LESSON 24

PERFORMANCE CHECKLIST			S = Satisfactory U = Unsatisfactory
Collecting Sputum Specimen	S	U	Comments
Washes hands and assembles the following equipment: a. specimen container and cover b. glass of water c. tissues d. emesis basin e. properly filled out requisition slip f. label for container			
Fills out label, including: a. resident's full name and room number b. date and time of collection c. doctor's name d. type of test to be performed e. other information as requested			
Identifies resident and explains what is to be done; screens unit.			
Has resident rinse mouth, using emesis basin.			
Asks resident to cough deeply to bring up sputum and expectorate into specimen container; has resident cover mouth with tissue to prevent spread of infection; collects 1 to 2 tablespoonfuls of sputum, unless otherwise ordered.			
Washes hands; is careful not to contaminate outside of container; covers container tightly and attaches completed label.			
Cleans and replaces equipment according to facility policy.			
Takes or sends specimen to laboratory promptly.			
Records procedure on resident's chart.			
Assisting with Special Oral Hygiene			
Washes hands and assembles the following equipment: a. mouthwash or ordered solution or mixture of glycerine and lemon juice b. emesis basin			

PERFORMANCE CHECKLIST

S = Satisfactory
U = Unsatisfactory

Assisting with Special Oral Hygiene (cont.)	S	U	Comments
Washes hands and assembles the following equipment: (cont.) c. bath towel d. plastic bag e. applicators f. tongue depressor g. cold cream or petroleum jelly to lubricate lips			
Identifies resident and explains what is to be done. Screens unit.			
Covers pillow with bath towel and turns resident's head to one side; places emesis basin under resident's chin.			
Opens resident's mouth gently with tongue depressor.			
Dips applicator into mouthwash, gylcerine mixture or ordered solution; using moistened applicators, wipes gums, teeth, tongue, and inside of mouth.			
Uses new applicator for each stroke; discards used applicators in plastic bag.			
Lubricates lips with cold cream or petroleum jelly; removes emesis basin and towel; rearranges bedclothes as necessary and makes resident comfortable.			
Cleans and replaces equipment and discards disposables, according to facility policy.			
Washes hands.			
Reports and records completion of task.			

PROCEDURE COMPETENCY EVALUATIONS

LESSON 25

PERFORMANCE CHECKLIST			S = Satisfactory U = Unsatisfactory
Urine Testing for Sugar Using Clinitest Tablets	S	U	Comments
Washes hands and assembles following equipment: a. freshly voided urine sample b. Clinitest tablet c. Clinitest color chart d. medicine dropper e. test tube f. water g. watch with second hand			
Reads manufacturer's directions carefully.			
With medicine dropper, places 5 drops of urine in clean, dry test tube; holds medicine dropper upright so urine does not touch sides of tube.			
Rinses medicine dropper in cold water.			
With medicine dropper, adds 10 drops of fresh water to test tube; if miscounts, begins again.			
Removes Clinitest tablet from wrapper; is careful not to touch tablet with fingers; drops tablet into test tube; if bottle of tablets is used, drops tablet into test tube from cover of bottle; covers bottle at once.			
Watches reaction carefully; does not touch tube; 15 seconds after reaction has stopped, shakes test tube gently; compares resulting color with Clinitest color chart and records results.			
Discards urine sample; cleans and replaces equipment, according to facility policy.			
Washes hands.			
Reports and records completion of task.			

PERFORMANCE CHECKLIST			S = Satisfactory U = Unsatisfactory
Urine Testing for Ketone Bodies Using Acetest Tablets	**S**	**U**	**COMMENTS**
Washes hands and assembles the following equipment: a. freshly voided urine sample b. Acetest tablet c. sheet of plain white paper d. medicine dropper e. Acetest color chart f. watch with second hand			
Reads directions carefully; places one Acetest tablet on sheet of white paper; is careful not to handle tablet with fingers.			
With medicine dropper, places 1 drop of urine on Acetest tablet.			
Waits 30 seconds; compares resulting color with Acetest color chart and records results.			
Discards tablet, paper, and urine sample.			
Cleans and replaces equipment, according to facility policy.			
Washes hands.			
Reports and records completion of task.			
Urine Testing for Sugar Using Tes-Tape Strips			
Washes hands and assembles the following equipment: a. freshly voided urine sample b. Tes-Tape strips in container c. watch with second hand			
Opens Tes-Tape container and withdraws approximately 1½ inches of Tes-Tape; touches only tip closest to fingers.			
Dips approximately ¼ inch of Tes-Tape strip into urine sample; withdraws strip, holding tip downward over urine container.			
Times reaction for 60 seconds.			
Checks darkest area of wet strip against Tes-Tape color chart on back of container; reads and records the figures above color match.			
Discards tape urine sample; cleans and returns equipment to proper place.			
Washes hands.			
Reports and records completion of task.			
Urine Testing for Ketone Bodies Using Reagent Strips			
Washes hands and assembles the following equipment: a. freshly voided urine sample			

PERFORMANCE CHECKLIST			S = Satisfactory U = Unsatisfactory
Urine Testing for Ketone Bodies Using Reagent Strips (cont.)	S	U	Comments
Washes hands and assembles the following equipment (cont.): b. reagent strips c. watch with second hand			
Opens container and removes one dipstick; touches only one end; dips other end of dipstick into urine sample; removes and holds dipstick horizontally.			
Waits 15 seconds; compares color of dipstick with color code on bottle; records results.			
Disposes of urine sample, if not to be saved; cleans and returns equipment to proper place.			
Washes hands.			
Reports and records completion of task.			

PROCEDURE COMPETENCY EVALUATIONS

LESSON 26

PERFORMANCE CHECKLIST			S = Satisfactory U = Unsatisfactory
Giving Nonsterile Vaginal Douche	S	U	Comments
Washes hands and assembles the following equipment: a. disposable douche b. irrigating standard c. bed protector (e.g., Chux) d. disposable gloves e. cotton balls in Monel cup f. disinfectant solution g. toilet tissue h. bedpan and cover i. bath blanket j. plastic bag			
Identifies resident and explains what is to be done.			
Pours small amount of the specified disinfectant solution over cotton balls in Monel cup.			
Hangs douche container from irrigating standard; closes clamp on tubing; leaves protector on sterile tip.			
Measures water about 105°F in douche container; adds powder or solution, as ordered.			
Assembles remaining equipment conveniently at bedside; screens unit.			
Removes perineal pad, if present, from front to back and discards in plastic bag.			
Gives bedpan to resident and asks her to void.			
After voiding, removes, empties and rinses bedpan; measures urine if ordered; returns bedpan to bedside.			
Drapes resident with bath blanket; fanfolds top bedclothes to foot of bed.			
Assists resident into dorsal recumbent position; places bed protector beneath resident's buttocks; places bedpan under resident.			

PERFORMANCE CHECKLIST

S = Satisfactory
U = Unsatisfactory

Giving Nonsterile Vaginal Douche (cont.)	S	U	Comments
Washes hands; puts on disposable gloves.			
Cleanses perineum using proper technique; uses one cotton ball saturated with disinfectant solution for each stroke; cleanses from vulva toward anus; cleanses labia minora first; exposes labia minora with thumb and forefinger and cleanses; gives special attention to folds; discards cotton balls in plastic bag.			
Opens clamp to expel air; removes protector from sterile tip.			
Allows small amount of solution to flow over inner thigh and then over vulva; is careful not to touch vulva with nozzle.			
Allowing solution to continue to flow, inserts nozzle slowly and gently about 3 inches into vagina with upward and backward movement; rotates nozzle from side to side as solution flows.			
When all solution has been given, removes nozzle slowly and clamps tubing.			
Has resident sit up on bedpan to allow solution to return.			
Removes douche bag from standard and places on paper towels.			
Dries perineum with tissue; places used tissue in bedpan.			
Removes and covers bedpan and places on chair.			
Has resident turn on side; dries buttocks with tissue; places clean pad over perineal area from front to back.			
Removes bed protector and bath blanket; replaces top bedclothes; makes resident comfortable and observes contents of bedpan; notes character and amount of discharge, if any.			
Removes gloves and discards properly.			
Cleans and returns equipment according to facility policy.			
Washes hands; leaves unit tidy.			
Reports and records completion of procedure, including: a. date and time b. procedure: Vaginal irrigation (type, amount, and temperature of solution) c. resident's reaction d. your observations regarding douche returns			

PROCEDURE COMPETENCY EVALUATIONS

LESSON 27

PERFORMANCE CHECKLIST	S	U	Comments
Application of Postural Supports or Restraints S = Satisfactory U = Unsatisfactory			
Checks that there is written physician's order for restraint or support.			
Identifies resident and explains what is to be done and why; displays a positive, gentle attitude.			
Restrains resident only in bed or chair with wheels.			
Ties restraint under chair out of resident's reach or to the bed frame; is careful not to use slip knot to secure ties.			
Checks resident for proper positioning; pads areas under restraint to prevent friction.			
Makes sure that water and call bell are within reach.			
Checks resident frequently for signs of skin irritation and to be sure circulation is adequate.			
Removes restraints periodically.			
Exercises restrained areas regularly.			
Reports and records completion of task and any observations.			

GLOSSARY

abbreviation — shortened form of a word or phrase

abdominal — area of trunk between thorax and pelvis

abduction — movement away from midline or center

accelerated — increased motion, as in pulse or respiration

accuracy — completing assignments carefully without mistakes

acidosis — pathologic condition resulting from accumulation of acid or depletion of alkaline reserves in the blood and body tissues

activities of daily living (ADL) — the activities necessary for resident to fulfil his or her basic human needs

acute — having severe symptoms

adduction — movement toward midline or center

aiding and abetting — not reporting dishonest acts that are observed

agar — gelatinous substance sometimes used to increase intestinal bulk

aged — old; usually refers to persons over 75 years of age

ageism — discrimination against aged persons

aging — a natural, progressive process that begins at birth

akinesia — abnormal absence or poverty of movement

aldosterone — a regulating hormone of the adrenal cortex; utilization and retention of salts and water in the body

alignment — keeping a resident in proper position

alimentary canal — all the organs making up the route taken by food as it passes through the body from mouth to anus; also called the digestive tract

allergen — substance that causes sensitivity or allergic reactions

alveoli — tiny air acs that make up the bulk of the lungs

ambulation — ability to walk

amphiarthrotic — pertains to a slightly movable joint

amputation — removal of a limb or other body appendage

anatomy — study of the structure of the human body

anemia — deficiency of red blood cells in the blood

aneurysm — a sac formed by dilation of the wall of a blood vessel (usually an artery) and filled with blood

angina pectoris — acute pain in the chest caused by interference with the supply of oxygen to the heart

anterior — in anatomy, in front of the coronal or ventral plane

anus — the outlet of the rectum lying in the fold between the buttocks

antidepressant — medication effective against depressive illness

antihypertensive — medication effective against hypertension (high blood pressure)

antiseptic — anti–infectious agent used on living tissue

anuria — no urine

aorta — the great artery arising from the left ventricle

apathy — indifference; lack of emotion

aphasia — language impairment; loss of ability to comprehend normally

apical pulse — pulse rate taken by placing stethoscope over tip of heart

apnea — period of no respirations

Aquamatic K-Pad — commercial unit for applying heat or cold

arrest — sudden cessation or stoppage

arteriosclerosis — general term meaning a narrowing of the blood vessels, which can result in subsequent tissue hypoxia; degeneration and hardening of the walls of arteries and sometimes of the valves of the heart

artery — a vessel through which the blood passes away from the heart to various parts of the body

arthritis — joint inflammation

articulation — point where two bones meet

ascites — fluid accumulation in the abdomen

asepsis — without infection

aseptic technique — technique used to destroy microorganisms and prevent their transmission

Asepto syringe — glass syringe with rubber ball used to perform moist treatments

aspiration — drawing foreign material into the respiratory tract

assessment — act of evaluating

asthenia — weakness

asthma — a chronic respiratory disease characterized by bronchospasms and excessive mucous production

atherosclerosis — degenerative process involving the lining of arteries, in which the lumen eventually norrows and closes; a form of arteriosclerosis

atrium — upper heart chambers

atrophy — shrinking or wasting away of tissues

audiologist — physician specializing in hearing problems

aura — a peculiar sensation preceding the appearance of more definite symptoms in a convulsion or seizure

autoclave — a machine that sterilizes articles

autoimmune — antibodies against components of the body

axon — extension of neuron that conducts nerve impulses away from the cell body

bile — a secretion of the liver, needed to prepare fats for digestion

blood pressure — pressure of blood exerted against the vascular walls

body mechanics — using muscles correctly to move or lift heavy objects properly

bolus — soft mass of food that is ready to be swallowed

bowel — intestine

Bowman's capsule — tubule surrounding the glomerus of the nephron

bradycardia — unusually slow heartbeat

bronchi — primary divisions of the trachea

bronchitis — inflammation of the bronchi

burnout — loss of enthusiasm and interest in an activity

calculi — stones or concretions

cancer — a malignant tumor; malignancy

capillary — hairlike blood vessel; the link between arterioles and venules

carbohydrates — energy foods; used by the body to produce heat and for work

carbon dioxide — gas that is a waste product in cellular metabolism

carbon dioxide narcosis — accumulation of carbon dioxide in the bloodstream

cardiac cycle — all the (mechanical and electrical) events that occur between one contraction and the next

cardiogram — a record of cardiac pulsation produced by cardiograph

care plan — nursing plan for care of resident in long term care facility

cast — rigid covering to keep a joint or other body part immobile

cataract — opacity of the lens, resulting in loss of vision

catheter — tube for evacuating or injecting fluids

cell — basic unit in the organization of living substance

cellulose — a basic substance of all plant foods, which can supply the body with roughage

celsius — scale for measuring temperature

centimeter — one-hundredth of a meter

character (of pulse) — rhythm and volume of pulse

chart — record of information concerning resident

cheeking — storing food in one side of the mouth

Cheyne-Stokes respiration — periods of apnea alternating with periods of hyperpnea

CHF — congestive heart failure

chordotomy — surgical division of certain tracts of the spinal cord to relieve intractable pain

choroid — the vascular layer, or coat, of the eye

chronic — persisting over a long period of time

chronic bronchitis — condition in which there is excessive mucous secretion in the bronchi

chyme — semi-liquid form of food as it leaves the stomach

client — resident

climacteric — menopause; the combined phenomena accompanying cessation of the reproductive function in the female or diminution of testicular activity in the male

climax — the period of greatest intensity during sexual stimulation or intercourse

clitoris — a small, cylindrical mass of erotic tissue; part of the external female reproductive organs analogous to the penis in the male

CNS — central nervous system

coitus — sexual intercourse; copulation

cold — an acute and highly contagious virus infection of the upper respiratory tract

colon — large intestine

colostomy — an artificial opening in the abdomen for the purpose of evacuation of feces

comatose — unconscious; in a coma

comminuted fracture — fracture in which the bone is broken or crushed into small pieces

commode — a portable toilet

communicable — capable of being transferred from one person to another directly or indirectly, as infectious disease

communicate — to make known

compensation — in psychology, the act of seeking a substitute for something unacceptable or unattainable

compound fracture — fracture in which the broken bone protrudes through the skin

comprehension — the capacity of the mind for understanding

concentration — increase in strength by evaporation

concurrent cleaning — daily cleaning of equipment

confidential — keeping what is said or written to oneself; private; non-sharing

connective tissue — tissue that holds other tissues together and provides support for organs and other structures of body

constipation — difficulty in defecating

constriction — narrowing or compression

contaminated — unclean; impure; soiled with germs

continent — able to control elimination of feces and urine

contract — an agreement between two or more people, especially one that is written

contracture — permanent shortening or contraction of a muscle due to spasm or paralysis

convalescent home — long term care facility

convulsion — involuntary muscle spasm

COPD — chronic obstructive pulmonary disease; for example, pulmonary emphysema

copulation — sexual intercourse; coitus

coronary occulsion — closing off of a coronary artery

cor pulmonale — a serious cardiac condition resulting from pulmonary disease

cryosurgery — destruction of tissue by application of extreme cold

CVA — cerebrovascular accident

CVP — central venous pressure; measurement of blood pressure in the large central veins

cyanosis — bluish skin discoloration from lack of oxygen

cystocele — bladder hernia

cystoscopy — procedure using cystoscope for visualization of the urinary bladder, ureter, and kidney

day care center — a place where senior citizens may go for various services

debilitating — weakening

debridement — removal of foreign matter or devitalized tissue

decubiti — pressure sores; bedscores; decubitus ulcers

defecation — bowel movement which expels feces

defense mechanism — psychological reaction or technique for protection against a stressful environmental situation or anxiety

dehydration — excessive water loss

delirium — disordered mental condition in which speech is incoherent, fever may occur, and illusions, delusions and hallucinations may be experienced

delusion — a false belief

dementia — progressive mental deterioration due to organic brain disease

dendrite — the branch of a neuron conducting impulses toward the cell body

denial — an unconscious defense mechanism in which an occurrence or observation is refused recognition as reality, in order to avoid anxiety or pain

dental hygienist — a person licensed and specially trained to perform oral hygiene, including cleaning of teeth

dentist — a person licensed and specially trained to practice dentistry and/or dental surgery

dependability — trustworthiness; reliability

dermis — corium; true skin; the larger of skin beneath the epithelium

developmental tasks — in psychology, tasks that are normally carried out as steps in personality development

diabetes mellitus — a disorder of carbohydrate metabolsim

diabetic coma — a comatose state of acidosis due to diabetes mellitus

diaphoresis — profuse sweating

diarrhea — watery stool

diarthrotic — pertains to freely movable joints

diastole — period during which the heart muscle relaxes and the chamber fills with blood

diathermy — treatment with heat

dietetics — systematic regulation of the diet for therapeutic purposes

dietician — a person especially trained in the field of nutrition and the science of dietetics (diets)

digestion — the process of converting food into an assimilable form

digiti flexus — a condition in which toes are drawn into a tightly flexed position

dilate — to enlarge, as capillaries

directive — serving or qualified to direct; statement of direction

disability — persistent physical or mental defect or handicap

disinfectant — agent which kills germs

disinfection — the process of destroying pathogenic organisms or agents

disorientation — loss of recognition of time, place, or persons

displacement — an unconscious defense mechanism in which an emotion such as anger is directed at the wrong person

distal — farthest away from a central point, such as point of attachment of muscles

diuretics — drugs which increase urine output

diverticula — small blind pouches that form in the lining and wall of the colon

diverticulitis — inflammation of diverticula

diverticulosis — presence of many diverticula

documentation — substantiating statements

dorsal — posterior or back

draw sheet — a sheet folded under resident and extending from above the shoulder to below the hips

DRG — diagnosis-related grouping

DSD — dry sterile dressing

dyscrasia — abnormality or disorder of the body

dyspepsia — indigestion

dysphagia — difficulty in swallowing

dyspnea — difficult or labored breathing

edema — excessive accumulation of fluid in the tissues

ejaculation — forcible, sudden expulsion of semen from the male penis

EKG — electrocardiogram (see cardiogram)

electrocoagulation — the process by which unhealthy tissues are destroyed through high frequency

electrolytes — compounds which play an essential role in body function

elimination — excretion; discharge from the body of indigestible materials and of waste products of body metabolism

emesis basin — utensil for catching vomitus

empathy — intellectual understanding of something in another person which is foreign to one's self

emphysema — chronic obstructive pulmonary disease in which the alveolar walls are destroyed

endocrine gland — gland the secretes hormonal substances directly into bloodstream; ductless gland

endotracheal — within the trachea

enteric — pertaining to the alimentary canal; intestinal

environment — surroundings

enzymes — organic catalysts produced by living cells but capable of acting independently of the cells producing them

epidermis — the top layer of skin

epididymis — an elongated, cordlike structure along the posterior border of the testes in the ducts of which the sperm is stored

epilepsy — a noninfectious disorder of the brain manifested by episodes of motor and sensory dysfunction, which may or may not be accompanied by convulsions and unconsciousness

epithelium — tissues characterized by tightly packed cells with a minimum of intracellular material; forms epidermis and lines all hollow organs and passages of respiratory, digestive, and genitourinary systems

equilibrium — sense of balance

erythrocyte — red blood cell

estrogen — hormone produced by ovaries

ethical code — rules of moral, responsible conduct

exacerbation — period of increased severity of symptoms

excreta — excretions such as feces

expectorant — medication to aid in expectoration (spitting up phlegm)

expiration — exhalation

extended care facility — long term care facility

extension — movement by which the two ends of any jointed part are drawn away from each other

fallopian tube — see oviduct

fantasizing — imagination

fats — nutrient used to store energy

feces — semi-solid waste eliminated from the body

femur — thigh bone

flatulence — excessive gas in the stomach and intestines

flatus — gas or air in the stomach or intestines; air or gas expelled via any body opening

flexed — bent

flow meter — an instrument for controlling gas flow in oxygen equipment

fomite — any objects contaminated with germs, and thus able to transmit disease

forced fluids — notation meaning that resident must be encouraged to take as much fluid as possible

foreskin — prepuce; loose tissue covering the penis and clitoris

fracture — break in the continuity of bone

frequency — occurrence often repeated

gait belt — belt placed around the resident's waist to assist in ambulation

gallbladder — small, sac-like organ found on the underside of the liver, which stores bile

gangrene — the death and putrefaction of body tissue, caused by stoppage of circulation of blood to an area

gastritis — inflammation of the stomach

gastrostomy — surgical opening into the stomach

Gatch bed — bed fitted with a jointed back rest and knee rest; resident can be raised to a sitting position and kept in that position

gavage — feeding through a tube

genital — pertaining to reproduction

genitalia — the reproductive organs

geriatrics — care of the elderly

geri-chair — chair or wheelchair with table or tray affixed to it

germs — pathogenic microorganisms

gerontology — study of the aging process

glaucoma — increased intraocular pressure, which ultimately results in loss of vision

glucose — simple sugar; also called dextrose

glycosuria — sugar in the urine

golden years — name sometimes used to describe the retirement years

gonads — reproductive organs; ovaries and testes

gossip — talking about residents at lunch time or on a break

Gray Panthers — organization working for urgent reforms needed to protect the elderly

hallucination — idea or perception that is not based on reality

hallux valgus — bunions

heart — hollow, muscular organ lying slightly to the left of the midline of the chest

Heberden's nodes — nodes found on interphalangeal joints (fingers) of arthritic individuals

heloma — a corn

hematuria — blood in the urine

hemiplegia — paralysis on one side of the body

hemoptysis — expectoration of blood

hemorrhage — escape of blood from blood vessels

hemorrhoids — varicose veins in the rectum

hernia — protrusion or projection of an organ or a part of an organ through wall of cavity that normally contains it

herniorrhaphy — surgical operation for hernia

hiatal hernia — protrusion of a portion of the stomach through the esophageal hiatus of the diaphragm

home health services — help provided after an acute hospitalization

hormone — secretion of endocrine gland; substance produced by endocrine gland

hospice — special facility or arrangement to provide care of terminally ill persons

hydrochloric acid — an acid produced by the stomach

hygiene — a system of principles or rules designed for the promotion of health

hyperchlorhydria — excessive hydrochloric acid in the stomach

hyperglycemia — excessive levels of blood sugar

hyperkalimia — excessive levels of blood potassium

hypernatremia — excess of sodium ions in the bloodstream

hypertension — high blood pressure

hypertrophy — increase in size of an organ or structure, which does not involve tumor formation

hypochlorhydria — abnormally low level of hydrochloric acid in the stomach

hypochondriasis — abnormal concern about one's health

hypoglycemia — abnormally low level of sugar in the blood

hyponatremia — low blood sodium level

hypoproteinemia — abnormal decrease in the amount of protein in the blood

hypotension — low blood pressure

hypothermia — greatly reduced temperature

hypoxia — lack of adequate oxygen supply

hysterectomy — surgical removal of the uterus

I & O — intake and output

illusion — a mental impression derived from misinterpretation of an actual sensory stimulus

IM — intramuscular

impaction — condition of being tightly wedged into a part (as feces in the bowel)

impotence — inability to perform sexually

incontinent — inability to control defecation or urination

indurated — hardened

infarction — death of tissue

infection — the invasion and multiplication of any organism and the damage caused by this in the body

inferior — below another part

infusion — introduction of a solution into a vein by gravity such as an intravenous infusion (IV)

insertion — distal point of attachment of skeletal muscle

inspiration — the drawing of air into the lungs (inhalation)

insulin — the active antidiabetic hormone secreted by the islands of Langerhans, in the pancreas

insulin lipodystrophy — abnormal changes in subcutaneous fat as the result of repeated insulin injections

integumentary system — body system consisting of the skin, its various layers, and its accessory structures (hair, nails, and skin glands)

intercourse — interchange or communication between individuals

interpersonal relationships — how people interact with each other

interventricular septum — dividing portion between the ventricles of heart

interview — meeting with a prospective employer and discussion regarding a position

intravenous infusion — nourishment given through a sterile tube into the veins

involuntary muscle — type of muscle forming the walls of organs; also known as visceral or smooth muscle

IPPB — intermittent positive-pressure breathing; technique for assisting breathing

ischemia — deficient blood supply to body tissues

isolation — place where resident with easily transmitted diseases is separated from others

jaundice — yellowing of the skin

job description — the duties and responsibilities involved in a position

joint — point of articulation between bones

Kardex — a type of file in which nursing care plans are kept

keratoses — roughened, scaly, wart-like lesions

ketosis — abnormal levels of ketones in the blood; a complication of diabetes mellitus

kilogram — 1000 grams; 2.2 pounds

kyphosis — hunchback

labia majora — two large, hair-covered, lip-like structures that are part of the vulva

labia minora — two hairless lip-like structures found beneath the labia majora

laxative — medicine to relieve constipation

leisure — time free from engagement

lentigines — elevated yellow or brown spots or patches that occur on exposed skin; "liver spots"

lesion — abnormal change in tissue formation

leukemia — malignant disease of the blood-forming organs, characterized by abnormal proliferation and distortion of the leukocytes in the blood and bone marrow

leukocyte — white blood cell

libel — any oral or written defamatory statement

libido — sex drive

life care facility — apartment homes that offer health care and recreational facilities for the elderly

ligaments — bands of fibrous tissue that holds joints together

lipodystrophy — any disturbance in fat metabolism

living will — a written statement, usually by those who are terminally ill, requesting not to be kept alive on life support systems when faculties have failed

long term care facility — a facility that provides care for residents with long-standing disabilities; can be terminal care

lymph — fluid found in lymphatic vessels

malignancy — cancerous condition which, if left untreated, leads to death

malpractice — poor or improper medical treatment; for example, when assistant gives improper care or gives care in which he or she has not been instructed

masochism — self-punishment

mastication — the act of chewing food with the teeth in preparation for swallowing

masturbation — sexual gratification by self-manipulation of the genitals

maturity — state of full development, physically, mentally, and psychologically

medial — close to the midline of a body or structure

Medicaid — federal and state-funded program that pays for medical costs for those whose income falls below a certain level

Medicare — federal program that assists those over 65 years of age with hospital and medical costs

meninges — three-layered serous membrane covering the brain and spinal cord

menopause — period when ovaries stop functioning and menstruation ceases; climacteric

metabolism — the sum total of the physical and chemical processes and reactions taking place in the body

metastasis — spreading of cancer to other body parts

meter — metric distance measurement equalling 39.371 inches

metric system — a system of weights and measurements based on the meter and having all units based on some power of ten

micturition — urination

mineral — inorganic chemical compound found in nature; many are important in building body tissues and regulating body fluids

ministrokes — a series of small strokes

mitosis — division of the cyloplasm and nucleus in the cell

mobility — ability to move or to be moved easily from place to place

morbidity — state of being diseased; conditions inducing disease

moribund — dying

mortality rate — the proportion of deaths in population

motor — pertaining to any activity or behavior involving muscular movement, as motor response; pertaining to the innervation (nerve supply) of muscles, especially voluntary muscles

mottling — discoloration of skin or irregular areas

mucolytic — destroying or dissolving mucus

mucous — pertaining to or resembling mucus; also, secreting mucus

mucus — secretion of mucous membranes; thick, sticky fluid

muscle — tissue composed of contractile (contracts and relaxes) fibers or cells

myocardium — heart muscle

myth — fixed idea about a group of people

narcosis — a stuporous state produced by drugs

nasogastric tube — soft rubber or plastic tube that is inserted through a nostril and into the stomach

necrosis — tissue death

negligence — failure to give care that is reasonably expected of an assistant

neoplasm — new growth; tumor

nephron — microscopic kidney units which produce the urine

nerve — a bundle of nerve processes (axons and dendrites) that are held together by connective tissue

nerve impulse — an electrical wave which transmits a message

nervous tissue — highly specialized tissue capable of conducting a nerve impulse

networking — a line of communications between individuals with a common interest or goal

neuron — cell of the nervous system

neurotransmitter — chemical compound that transmits a nervous impulse across cells at a synapse

no code — an order not to resuscitate a resident

nocturia — excessive urination at night

nosocomial — pertaining to or originating in a hospital or infirmary

nursing assistant — nurses's aide or orderly

nutrient — food that supplies heat and energy, builds and repairs body tissue and regulates body functions

nutrition — the process by which the body uses food for growth and repair and to maintain health

obesity — overweight

O.D. — as used in text, pertains to right eye

olfactory — pertaining to the sense of smell

oliguria — scant urine

orally — through the mouth

organ — any part of the body that carries out a specific function or functions, such as the heart

orgasm — the climax of sexual stimulation

origin — proximal point of attachment to skeletal muscle

orthopnea — condition in which there is difficulty in breathing except when sitting or standing upright

O.S. — as used in text, pertains to left eye

osteoarthritis — degenerative joint disease caused by disintegration of the cartilage that covers the ends of the bones

osteoporosis — the most common metabolic disease of bone in the United States; characterized by a decrease in the mass of bony tissue; most commonly affects females past middle age

ostomy — suffix word ending meaning to create a new opening, as colostomy

output — the measured amount of fluid excreted in a given period of time

oxygen — gas essential to cellular metabolism and all life

oxygenated — carrying oxygen

ovaries — endocrine glands located in female pelvis; female gonads

oviduct; fallopian tube; — part of the female reproductive tract which carries ova from ovaries to uterus

pacemaker (pacer) — an artificial device placed in the body to regulate heartbeat

palliative — relieving symptoms but not curing disease

pallor — less color than normal, of the skin

pannus — gray, cloudy, vascular membrane which overgrows the surface of a joint; associated with rheumatoid arthritis

paralysis — loss or impairment of the ability to move parts of the body

paranoia — a state in which one has delusions of persecution and/or grandeur

paroxysmal — abrupt in onset and termination

pathogen — microorganism or other agent capable of producing a disease

pathology — disease

patient — person needing, unable to care for him/herself; resident

pelvis — the lower portion of the trunk of the body; a basin-shaped area bounded by the hip bones, the sacrum, and the coccyx

penis — male organ of copulation

pension — retirement income or fund

perceptual process — interpretation of information

pericardial — pertaining to the pericardium (the sac enclosing the heart)

perineum — in the male, the area between the anus and scrotum; in the female, the area between the anus and vagina

peristalsis — a progressive, wave-like movement that occurs involuntarily in hollow tubes of the body, especially in the alimentary canal

pes planus — flatfoot

pessary — appliance inserted into the vagina to support the uterus

petite mal seizure — a type of epilepsy attack, generally short in nature; absence attack

phalange — any bone of a finger or toe

phlebotomy — incision of a vein for the purpose of withdrawing blood

phlegm — mucus

physician — a licensed medical doctor

physiology — the science that deals with the functioning of living organisms

physiotherapist — a trained professional who provides therapy and exercise to maintain mobility

piles — hemorrhoids

pitting edema — a condition in which the tissue remains indented when pressure is applied to an edematous area

plane — imaginary line used to describe the relationship of one body part to another

plaque — irregular patch that forms on artery lining in artherosclerosis

pleura — the membranes that surround the lungs

pleural — pertaining to the pleura

PNS — peripheral nervous system

podiatrist — a physician specializing in foot problems

podigeriatrics — a medical specialty which deals with treatment and care of aging feet

polydipsia — excessive thirst

polyphagia — excessive ingestion of food

polyuria — excessive excretion of urine

posterior — back or dorsal

post mortem — after death

potassium — an element essential to the body; an electrolyte

potency — power; especially the ability of the male to perform coitus

prefix — a term placed before a word which changes or modifies the meaning of the word

presbyopia — impaired vision as a result of the aging process

procedure — a series of steps outlining how to do something and in what order and manner

procedure book — a reference for procedures

procidentia — prolapse of the uterus

progesterone — hormone produced by female ovaries

prognosis — probability outcome of a disease or injury

projection — an unconscious defense mechanism in which an individual sees own defects as belonging to another

prolapse — the falling down or downward displacement of a body part or organ

proprioception — information received from internal stimuli

prostatectomy — removal of all or part of the prostate gland

prostate gland — gland of male reproductive system which surrounds the neck of the urinary bladder and the beginning of the urethra

prosthesis — artificial substitute for a missing body part, such as denture, hand, leg

protein — the basic material of every body cell; an essential nutrient

proximal — closest to the point of attachment

pruritus — itching

psychosocial — relating social conditions to mental health

psychotic — completely out of touch with reality

puberty — the condition or period of becoming capable of sexual reproduction

pulmonary artery — blood vessel that carries deoxygenated blood from the right ventricle to the lung

pulmonary emphysema — a chronic lung disorder in which the terminal bronchioles become plugged with mucus and lung elasticity is lost

pulse — wave of pressure exerted against the walls of the arteries in response to ventricular contraction

pulse deficit — difference between contractions of the heart and pulse expansions of the radial artery

pulse pressure — the difference between the systolic and diastolic pressure

PVD — peripheral vascular disease

pylorus — the narrow, tapered end of the stomach opening into the duodenum

pyorrhea — peridontitis; loosening of the teeth due to gum disease

quadrant — one of the four imaginary sections of the surface of the abdomen

rales — abnormal respiratory sound heard in auscultation of the chest

range-of-motion (ROM) exercises — series of exercises specifically designed to move each joint through its range

rationalization — an unconscious defense mechanism in which one devises a logical, self-satisfying but incorrect explanation for one's behavior or feelings

reaction — a response to a stimulus; opposite action or counteraction

receptor — peripheral nerve ending responsive to stimuli

rectocele — protrusion of part of the rectum into the vagina

rectum — the lower part of large intestine, about 5 inches long, between the sigmoid flexure and the anal canal

references — in a résumé, statements about abilities and characteristics; persons who give such statements

regurgitating — "throwing up" undigested food from the stomach

relax — rest; loosen tension

remission — period of decreased severity of symptoms in chronic disease

renal calculi — kidney stones

resident — patient in long term care facility

resident unit — room occupied by resident and his or her personal possessions; may be shared by other residents

respiration — process of taking oxygen into the body and expelling carbon dioxide

rest home — long term care facility

résumé — a short account of one's career and qualifications which is prepared by an applicant for a position

retention — the inability to excrete urine that has been produced

retina — innermost or third layer of the eye, which receives images

retinopathy — non-inflammatory disease of the retina

retirement — period of time after leaving employment

retroperitoneal space — area of the anterior cavity behind the peritoneum; in it are the kidneys, aorta, inferior vena cava

ribs — the 24 long, flat bones forming the wall of the thorax

rotation — the act of turning about the axis of the center of a body, as rotation of a joint

rubra — unusual redness or flushing of skin

rupture — the bursting of a part

sacrament of the sick — last rites given by a clergyman to a person who is terminally ill (dying)

saliva — digestive secretion produced by the salivary glands and found in the mouth

sclera — white of the eye

scrotum — sac-like pouch that holds the male gonads

sedative — medication that has calming effect; used to control nervousness, irritability, and excitement

seizure — sudden attack of a disease; an epileptic fit

seminal vesicles — pouch-like sacs found on the posterior wall of the bladder that produces the bulk of the seminal fluid

senescent — growing old

senile — affected with the infirmities of age

senile keratosis — roughened, scaly, slightly elevated wart-like lesions, believed to be related to sun damage in fair-skinned individuals

senior — person over the age of 65

senior citizen center — place where seniors can meet for social and other activities

sensitivity — the state of acute or abnormal responsiveness to stimuli

sensual — pertaining to the senses or sensation

sensuality — quality or state of being sensual

septum — wall or partition dividing a body cavity or space

sexuality — the attitude of a person in relation to sexual attitude and behavior

signing — using hands and facial expression to communicate without speaking words

simple fracture — fracture which does not produce an open wound in the skin

sitz bath — bath providing moist heat to the genitals or anal area

skilled care facility — long term care facility

slander — a false statement, oral or written, that injures the reputation of another person

society — a group of people who have common interests

speech therapist — a person specially trained to teach speech and correct speech disorders

sperm — the male germ or reproductive cell

sphincter muscle — a circular muscle that constricts a passage or closes a natural orifice; when relaxed, it allows passage of materials

sphygmomanometer — instrument for determining arterial pressure; blood pressure gauge

spinal column — backbone or vertebral column

spirituality — the state of being spiritual-minded or religious

spouse — a marriage partner; husband or wife

status — condition or state of health

stereotype — characteristic assigned to entire groups of people

sterile — free from bacteria or other microorganisms; incapable of producing sexually

sterilization — process that renders an individual incapable of reproduction

steroids — a group name for certain compounds that include progesterone, the adrenocortical and gonadal hormones, bile acids, and sterols such as cholesterol

stethoscope — instrument used in ausculation to make audible the sounds produced in the body

stimulant — agent that produces stimulation

stoma — an artificial, mouth-like opening

stroke — cerebrovascular accident; damage to the blood vessels of the brain

stump — the distal end of a limb remaining after amputation

subcutaneous — beneath the layers of the skin

suffix — a term added to the end of a word that changes or modifies the meaning of the word

superior — toward the head; upward

superior vena cava — large blood vessel that drains the blood from the upper part of the body into the right atrium of the heart

suppository — medication used to help the bowels eliminate feces

synapse — space between the axon of one cell and the dendrites of others

synarthrotic — pertains to an immovable joint

synovium — joint lining

system — group of organs organized to carry out a specific body function or functions, as respiratory system

systole — contraction, or period of contraction, of cardiac muscle

tachycardia — an unusually rapid heartbeat

tachypnea — respiratory pattern of rapid, shallow respirations

tact — sensitive mental perception

tactile — pertaining to touch

TED hose — support hose

tendon — fibrous band of connective tissue that attaches skeletal muscle to bone

terminal — final; life-ending stage

terminal cleaning — cleaning and sterilization of a room after resident's death or departure

testes — male gonads; reproductive glands located in the scrotal sac

testicles — testes

testosterone — hormone produced by the testes

therapeutic — pertaining to results obtained from treatment; a healing agent

therapy — treatment designated to eliminate disease or other bodily disorder

thermometer — instrument used to determine temperature

thoracic — pertaining to the chest

thrombocyte — blood platelet that is formed in the bone marrow and is important in blood clotting

thrombus — blood clot

thyroxine — hormone of the thyroid gland that contains iodine

TIA — transient ischemic attack (temporary decrease in blood flow to brain)

tipping — giving a sum of money for service rendered; not salary-connected

tissue — collection of specialized cells that perform a particular function; piece of paper used for cleansing (e.g., toilet tissue, facial tissue, Kleenex)

torso — the body, exclusive of the head and limbs

tranquilizer — agent used to calm or quiet anxious person without causing drowsiness

transurethral — through the urethra

trapeze — a horizontal bar suspended overhead down the length of the bed

tubal ligation — tying off of a fallopian tube

tubercle — small, rounded nodule formed by infection with *Mycobacterium tuberculosis*

tumor — neoplasm

tunica intima — the inner coat of the blood vessels

tyloma — a callus

ulcer — open sore caused by inadequate blood supply and broken skin

ulceration — development of an ulcer

uremia — the presence of excessive amounts of urea, a waste product, in the blood

ureter — narrow tube that conducts urine from the kidney to the urinary bladder

urethra — mucus-lined tube conveying urine from the urinary bladder to the exterior of the body; in the male, the urethra also conveys the semen

urgency — the need to urinate

urinalysis — laboratory analysis of the urine

vagina — the tube that extends from the vulva to the uterine cervix; the female organ of copulation that receives the penis during sexual intercourse

vas deferens — the tube that carries sperm from the epididymis to the junction of the seminal vesicle; ductus deferens

vasectomy — excision of part or all of the vas deferens; bilateral vasectomy results in sterility

vasoconstriction — decrease in the caliber of the blood vessels

vasodilation — dilation of the blood vessels

vasodilator — a neuron or medication that causes dilation of the blood vessels

vein — a vessel through which blood passes on its way back to the heart

ventilation — process of admitting fresh air and expelling stale air; the movement of gases into and out of the lungs

ventral — front; anterior

ventricle — a small cavity or chamber, as in the brain or heart

venule — small vein

vital capacity — the volume of air a person can forcibly expire from the lungs after a maximal inspiration

vital signs — measurements of temperature, pulse, respiration, and blood pressure

vitamin — a general term for various, unrelated organic substances found in many foods in minute amounts that are necessary for normal metabolic functioning of the body

voiding — the release of urine from the bladder

volume — the capacity or size of an object or of an area; the measure of the quantity of a substance

voluntary muscle — any part of the skeletal muscle that is under direct control

volunteerism — the contribution of ones time and energy to helping others

vomitus — the material vomited or brought up from the stomach

vulva — the external female genitalia

withdrawal — the retreat from reality or from social contact that is associated with severe depression and other psychiatric disorders

withhold — order to refrain from serving a resident certain foods or all food

INDEX